PATTERNS OF LEARNING DISORDERS

The Guilford School Practitioner Series

EDITORS

STEPHEN N. ELLIOTT, PhD
Vanderbilt University

JOSEPH C. WITT, PhD
Louisiana State University, Baton Rouge

Patterns of
Learning Disorders

WORKING SYSTEMATICALLY
FROM ASSESSMENT TO INTERVENTION

◆ ◆ ◆

David L. Wodrich
Ara J. Schmitt

◆

THE GUILFORD PRESS
New York   London

© 2006 The Guilford Press
A Division of Guilford Publications, Inc.
72 Spring Street, New York, NY 10012
www.guilford.com

Printed in the United States of America

This book is printed on acid-free paper.

Last digit is print number: 9 8 7 6 5 4 3 2 1

Library of Congress Cataloging-in-Publication Data

Wodrich, David L., 1948–
   Patterns of learning disorders : working systematically from assessment to
intervention / David L. Wodrich, Ara J. Schmitt.
       p. ; cm. — (The Guilford school practitioner series)
   Includes bibliographical references and index.
   ISBN-13: 978-1-59385-201-6 (alk. paper)
   ISBN-10: 1-59385-201-0 (alk. paper)
   1. Learning disabilities—Diagnosis. I. Schmitt, Ara J. II. Title. III. Series.
   [DNLM: 1. Learning Disorders—diagnosis. 2. Child. 3. Educational
Measurement—methods. 4. Learning Disorders—therapy. 5. Needs Assessment. 6.
Psychological Tests. 7. School Health Services. WS 110 W839p 2006]
   RJ496.L4P38 2006
   618.92'85889—dc22

                                                        2006009770

To the girl from Arcadia and Germany,
with love still
—D. L. W.

To those who have loved and supported me
—A. J. S.

About the Authors

♦

David L. Wodrich, PhD, is Associate Professor of Psychology in Education at Arizona State University, where he teaches graduate students in school psychology. Before his university appointment, his practice in public schools and at Phoenix Children's Hospital for more than 20 years involved evaluation of, and planning for, children with learning and developmental problems. Dr. Wodrich is past president of the American Board of School Psychology and the Arizona Psychological Association and a diplomate in school psychology of the American Board of Professional Psychology. Dr. Wodrich's research interests include the effect of chronic illness on school success and attention-deficit/hyperactivity disorder. He is the author of several books and numerous peer-reviewed articles.

Ara J. Schmitt, PhD, is a practicing school psychologist within the Tempe Union High School District, where he provides a full range of services, including psychoeducational evaluation, consultation, intervention, staff development, and trainee supervision. He serves as a faculty associate for Arizona State University's doctoral program in school psychology and teaches a course on academic intervention and progress monitoring. The author of several publications, Dr. Schmitt's research interests include psychoeducational assessment, intervention, and pediatric school psychology.

Preface

◆

Helping struggling students has long been a primary role for school psychologists. Precisely how best to execute this role, however, remains unresolved. One historically popular approach has been to formulate educational intervention plans based on psychometric and case data. This book provides a comprehensive, coherent, user-friendly system for this practice by tapping the existing literature on assessment and intervention practices for children with learning and developmental problems. We believe that all school psychologists, as well as many child clinical and pediatric psychologists, should master the essential skills detailed here.

Although the judicious use of psychometric testing to help students is important, school-based psychologists should possess other skills too. Recently, some school psychology leaders have advocated consultation with teachers and classroom-based interventions as a key role. Proponents of this approach may substitute curriculum-based assessment (CBA) for formal psychometrics. A spate of practitioner-directed books compatible with the concept of consultation ensued (e.g., Shapiro, 2004; Shapiro & Kratochwill, 1988; Rathvon, 1999; Shinn, 1998; Brown, Pryzwansky, & Schulte, 2001). Given these changes, most contemporary school psychologists embrace at least some aspects of direct classroom consultation when problems with learning are the issue. Furthermore, the recent reauthorization of the Individuals with Disabilities Education Act (IDEA; Public Law 108-446) and the prospect of identifying students with specific learning disabilities (SLD) by their lack of response to intervention (RTI) may prompt reconsideration of the use of psychometrics. As important as consultation skills are, we propose in this book that they are complements rather than alternatives to comprehensive evaluations.

In fact, no matter which regulations for identifying students with SLD are ultimately adopted, including an option dominated by RTI, the wisdom of comprehensive evaluations (including psychometrics) for students under consideration for special education designation is widely endorsed (National Association of School Psychologists, 2003). It is likely that a great many students will continue to undergo psychometric evaluation for the foreseeable future. Indeed, standardized psychometric testing has long consumed much of school psychology practitioners' time (Bramlett, Murphy, Johnson, Wallingsford, & Hall, 2002; Wilson & Reschly, 1996), and its wholesale abandonment is quite unlikely.

Crucially, comprehensive evaluations afford the greatest value when they contribute to planning and promote understanding, not just document program eligibility. In this book, we argue that both planning and under-standing are enhanced by evaluations that help detect *"specific* [emphasis added] disabilities and disorders that affect learning" (American Psycho-logical Association, Division 16, 1998). Unfortunately, current texts addressing standardized mental tests are long on instruments' psychometric properties and short on specific patterns that interfere with learning. For example, Sattler's (2001) popular and valuable text addresses general pro-cedures for assessing children, the data sources required for inference mak-ing, psychometric principles, and methods of organizing scores and writing reports, and includes a compendium of contemporary IQ, special ability, and achievement tests. However, it is largely silent on the particular profile configurations likely to be encountered in applied practice, and it does not cover in-depth remedial procedures. Other assessment books contain descriptions of single tests and implicit arguments to adopt one test or bat-tery over another (Naglieri, 1999; Schrank, Flanagan, Woodcock, & Mascolo, 2002). Still others present a system for organizing and interpret-ing scores, such as by using the Cattell–Horn–Carroll scheme, but confine their coverage to assessment rather than intervention (Flanagan, McGrew, & Ortiz, 2000). Given this situation, practitioners and psychologists-in-training may have relatively little information on how psychometrically based evaluations can actually help those students for whom classroom mastery remains elusive. Particularly lacking is guidance on "assessment *for* intervention" (D'Amato, 2003, p. ix). This limitation is all the more regrettable given school psychology's intensifying search for empirically supported interventions suitable for school problems, including academic failure (Stoiber & Kratochwill, 2000; Kratochwill & Stoiber, 2002). A method of linking comprehensive assessments, including psychometric, with peer-reviewed reports of academic interventions, including some that enjoy empirical support, would offer practitioners an alternative and a complement to behavioral consultation and CBA techniques. Precisely for these reasons, we present a method for use when behavioral consultation and direct instructional techniques alone fall short.

PURPOSES OF THE BOOK

This book was prepared for several purposes:

- To familiarize psychologists, especially school-based psychologists, with common patterns reported in the published literature (often expressed in standardized test scores) known to be associated with academic problems.
- To present a rationale for the use of comprehensive psychometric evaluations and related interventions (available in this book) that are complementary to classroom-based consultation (available in other sources).
- To describe the most effective and efficient test batteries to be used during in-depth evaluations.
- To reveal how and why certain psychometric patterns predict specific classroom skills or performance problems.
- To outline the defining criteria for common patterns of learning dysfunction.
- To provide helpful diagnostic information about the various conditions, including typical concerns of teachers, grade of typical referral, gender ratio, and prevalence in clinic samples of each condition.
- To supply information about assessment pitfalls and effective strategies for evaluating students.
- To outline interventions for each disorder, including those that are evidence based.
- To provide psychologists with case examples, including psychometric profiles and case-specific intervention suggestions, for each of the patterns included in this book.

UNIQUE FEATURES OF THE BOOK

Unlike other books currently available, this one:

- Describes an assessment system not primarily concerned with gate-keeping.

♦ Is not wed to any one approach to assessment.
♦ Is not bound to any one theory of learning dysfunction or psycho-metric approach, and recognizes that some problems are attribut-able to general cognitive factors, some to narrow information-processing problems, and some to performance deficits.
♦ Links intervention and assessment.
♦ Incorporates extant literature on assessment (via commonly re-ported patterns) and treatment (via interventions reported in the literature).
♦ Provides both an advanced assessment guide and a source of inter-vention material in down-to-earth, "how-to" form.
♦ Is well suited for course adoption and as a resource for current prac-titioners.

THE BOOK'S ORGANIZATION

The book is divided into six chapters. Readers are encouraged to proceed from beginning to end. Relatively experienced practitioners may simply read Chapters 1–4, choosing to forgo case examples and practice-related suggestions. All readers should find the volume useful as a handbook to assist in assessment and planning. Thus, Chapters 2, 3, and 4 should be revisited when evaluations are conducted. The flowchart in Figure 1.1 can be photocopied and used repeatedly to provide a guide on assessment-related decision making. Even though general intervention strategies are provided as each condition is reviewed in Chapters 2, 3, and 4, psycholo-gists may find additional useful intervention information in the case exam-ples of Chapter 5. The conditions and related case examples are cross-referenced in the text to aid usage (there is a case example for every condition).

Chapter 1, "Overview of the System and Reasons for Assessing," is a foundation for psychological assessment in general and for detailed, com-prehensive evaluations that include psychometric testing in particular. Evaluation for special education eligibility is distinguished from assessment to provide the in-depth understanding necessary to plan interventions. Likewise, a rationale favoring homogeneous groupings of students who fail is presented to promote better understanding, planning, and intervening for students. Reasoning is provided for a hierarchy beginning with three broad types of classroom learning failure: (1) IQ-related conditions and their rela-tionship to classroom expectations, (2) narrow information-processing fail-ures, and (3) problems characterized by poor classroom performance in the face of intact ability and academic skill development.

Chapter 2, "IQ-Related Conditions," describes three types of problems that are defined by students' general cognitive levels (and classroom expectations): mild mental retardation, slow learner, and students with ability–expectation mismatch. Each condition in this chapter (and in Chapters 3 and 4) is given a definition, a description of classroom manifestation, measurement considerations, conditions to rule out and possible co-occurring conditions, a brief discussion of its relationship to special education eligibility, and potential interventions. Although considerations of special education eligibility are not prime in this book, eligibility decisions are indirectly facilitated because recognition of some of these conditions (especially those in Chapter 3) promotes early identification for special education services and early, targeted intervention.

Chapter 3, "Information-Processing-Related Conditions," in contrast to Chapter 2, reviews disorders characterized by intact general cognitive functioning but narrow information-processing skill deficits. There are five conditions presented here: specific language impairment, phonological reading disorder, nonverbal learning disability, graphomotor underproduction, and inconsistent success with splinter skills. These conditions were selected from conditions frequently reported in the learning disorders literature.

Chapter 4, "Performance-Related Conditions," presents conditions distinguished by failure to perform well in class in the absence of detectable cognitive, information-processing, or academic skill problems. Based on the existing literature and noting those conditions most commonly seen in clinic settings, three conditions were selected for inclusion: attention-deficit/hyperactivity disorder, combined type; attention-deficit/hyperactivity disorder, predominantly inattentive type; and compulsive underproduction (the classroom manifestation sometimes seen among students with obsessive–compulsive disorder characteristics). Because our classification system concerns students with classroom problems, this chapter's conditions are presented in an educational context, and the interventions offered were selected to speak to educational matters.

Chapter 5, "How to Use the System through Case Examples," provides 12 case studies. Each case includes the procedures used to identify a student's problem, an analysis of assessment data using a flowchart to support decision making, and a list of interventions. By working systematically through these case examples, the reader will be better prepared to implement the book's procedures in his or her own practice. Although based on patterns seen in school and clinic settings, none of these cases represent actual children. They are composites provided only for educational purposes and to demonstrate how to use this system.

Chapter 6, "Suggestions for Implementing the Classification and Intervention Planning System," contains information designed to help the reader implement this system. Among the topics addressed are ways to share information with teachers and parents, approaches to managing diagnostic information submitted from outside the school, and practices that contribute to efficient data collection. The chapter also helps narrow the distance between the book's information and its application.

Contents

◆

CHAPTER 1

♦ ♦ ♦

Overview of the System and Reasons for Assessing

♦

Jason is a 9-year-old third grader whose teacher is concerned about his writing. The concern is not new. School records indicate that he was less successful than most of his kindergarten classmates in learning to form legible letters. Likewise, he struggled in attempts to write the letters associated with sounds during first grade. His teacher and parents now concur that the amount, legibility, and sophistication of his daily journal entries are far below third-grade standards.

Jason's teacher told members of his school's academic problem-solving (prereferral) team that his best subject is computational arithmetic. He displays good memory on flashcards and oral recitation of math facts with his mother, but he forms numerals poorly on worksheets. He apparently possesses a reasonably developed sight vocabulary, and this enables him to read fluently. Nonetheless, his teacher said that he is reluctant to sound out unknown words, and he frequently fails to answer reading comprehension questions that depend on judgment or require him to draw inferences. Seatwork, especially tasks that require sustained writing, is often left incomplete. Favorably, Jason has positive qualities. He is a large, handsome boy who plays well during recess, although often with younger children. He is described as generous and kindhearted. Unfortunately, he is sometimes inattentive and slow to begin assignments.

Hoping to help Jason, his teacher and members of the school-based intervention team devised several straightforward classroom modifications.

- ◆ Pair him with a better writer to help him generate ideas before writing begins.
- ◆ Assure him that he will not be marked down for poorly shaped letters or misspelled words, so long as he attempts to use phonics.
- ◆ Institute an in-class reward program to encourage written work completion.
- ◆ Encourage practice writing with parents during evenings via joint composition activities (i.e., those in which both he and his parents participate).

These interventions were implemented, one at a time, over the course of an entire semester. During this time, his progress was monitored closely. Unfortunately, none produced noticeable improvement in his writing.

The psychologist at Jason's elementary school then became directly involved in the hope that she might shed light on his lack of success. Listening to the facts, reviewing records, and observing him in class, she quickly generated several pivotal questions:

1. Does Jason possess basic reasoning and problem-solving skills commensurate with his classmates?
2. Does he have the general language concepts, vocabulary, and verbal maturity necessary to produce acceptable writing?
3. Has he mastered the requisite phonics skills (including underlying phonological processing) to write?
4. Is there a fine-motor or hand–eye coordination problem that limits effective writing?

Jason's school psychologist reasoned that now was the best time to answer these questions. He had so far failed to respond to interventions. Pre-evaluation attempts at intervention make intuitive sense and are advocated explicitly in the response to intervention (RTI) model discussed later. The school psychologist's position was that if one or more of these possible causes could be confirmed, a logical, highly focused intervention plan could be devised to meet Jason's particular needs. Her thinking revealed a core tenet used throughout this book: every academic deficit can arise for several distinct reasons. This is true in part because academic skills develop from complex interactions of many factors, including school instructional variables and the immediate array of abilities, such as cognition, language, visual and auditory perception, and attention (Lyon & Flynn, 1991). The individual integrity of each of these abilities is necessary but not sufficient for academic success (Berninger & Richards, 2002). Determining the underlying reasons for academic failure helps psychologists and educators create an effective plan. In this instance, Jason's school psychologist first wanted to rule out low IQ. If global cognitive problems were eliminated, then a language, phonological processing (and associated spelling problems), or fine-motor (e.g., pencil control) problem might explain his poor writing. If any of these problems were confirmed, a precise plan for Jason could be created. This book provides a system to help students like Jason. It illustrates how to perform comprehensive evaluations, which include psychological and educational tests, to detect the nature of underlying learning problems. In turn, this information allows the school psychologist (or other diagnosticians) to suggest narrowly focused interventions that have been reported in the peer-reviewed literature. The book is not primarily concerned with special education eligibility. However, it does concern the role of basic psychological processes in learning, advocates the use of pre-evaluation intervention, and encourages application of research-based interventions reported in the peer-reviewed literature. In that regard, it matches individual elements and the general spirit of the recent changes in the Individuals with Disabilities Education Act (IDEA; Public Law 108-446).

OVERVIEW OF THE BOOK

This is a "how-to" book. It is for professionals (or professionals-in-training) already familiar with administering and scoring IQ and achievement tests, collecting educational information about students, and offering plans to alleviate academic problems. Users will also need to know (or learn) how to administer, score, and interpret special ability tests, such as those that tap language and visual perception. In most instances, knowledge of special education rules and regulation is also necessary. Prior experience or coursework in educational planning for students with handicaps is also helpful. Thus, most users of this book will have a background in the diagnosis of children's learning and developmental problems and will be acquainted with special education classification and with formulating school-based interventions. School psychologists, child clinical or pediatric psychologists, or graduate students in such programs are typically well prepared to use this system. Educational diagnosticians and learning disability specialists may also find valuable information in this book.

Crucially, this book includes a detailed presentation of several common patterns that underlie school failure. These patterns are recognizable by their psychometric configuration, school and developmental history, and, in some cases, response to intervention. A simple classification structure is used to help assure that information is provided in an understandable form. Thus, the book enables the use of psychometric (and supporting background information) data in the identification of problems that often result in school failure. It also presents information about the characteristics, classroom manifestations, prevalence, and natural history of each disorder. The book, however, is *not* a mere diagnostic guidebook. It is an organized system for linking assessment and intervention in the everyday practice of assessing students with suspected learning problems. As such, it provides professionals with disorder-specific treatment information that they can use to make suggestions to team members and parents. It can also be a springboard for ongoing consultation with teachers and parents.

This chapter provides an overview of the evaluation process, presents a rationale for assessment, discusses the role of classification in supporting intervention, and outlines several practical points about this system's use. Chapter 2 addresses a group of problems attributable to IQ or general cognitive functioning (see Table 1.1). Three conditions are included here: children with mild mental retardation (MiMR), children with ability in the slow learner (SL) range, and children who experience ability–expectation mismatches (AEM). In our experience, these conditions are often given short shrift by contemporary diagnosticians, who sometimes narrow their search to information-processing problems only.

Chapter 3 addresses narrow information-processing deficits. The five conditions included were selected from a much more extensive list of possibilities. The method of deciding which conditions to include involved review of the recently published literature for references to syndromes underlying reading, writing, or arithmetic problems. We looked at hundreds of references related to learning and developmental disabilities in the American Psychological Association abstracting system, PsyScan. The most

---

TABLE 1.1. General Categories and Specific Conditions

IQ-related conditions

- Mild mental retardation (MiMR)
- Slow learner (SL)
- Ability–expectation mismatch (AEM)

Information-processing-related conditions

- Specific language impairment (SLI)
- Phonological reading disorder (PRD)
- Nonverbal learning disability (NLD)
- Graphomotor underproduction (GU)
- Inconsistent success with splinter skills (ISSS)

Performance-related conditions

- ADHD, predominately hyperactive–impulsive or combined type (ADHD-C)
- ADHD, predominately inattentive type (ADHD-I)
- Compulsive underproduction (CU)

---

commonly cited conditions (e.g., phonological processing deficit, nonverbal learning disability) were included in this book. Thus, the book attempts to rely on the scientific and research base provided in the school, educational, and clinical child psychology literature. A shortlist of information-processing deficits, in our experience, helps evaluators keep their focus narrowed to legitimate deficits that can be detected and used as a basis for planning. Not unexpectedly, we sometimes encountered conditions with overlapping characteristics and indistinct boundaries. Conditions described in the literature with similar features but different terms were included, but a single, parsimonious label was adopted for each for use in this book. For example, the literature contained references to fine-motor problems, dysgraphia, and hand–eye coordination problems. We chose to focus on the fine-motor and pencil-control core of these problems (i.e., the graphomotor deficit). However, because in our experience many of these children are referred for evaluation because of failure to compete schoolwork, not just graphomotor quality, we refer to such children as having problems with graphomotor underproduction (GU). Overlap was also found regarding general language disorders (sometimes called expressive and receptive language disorders, general language delays, specific language impairment, or selective language impairment) and problems with phonological processing that affect reading (sometimes called phonemic awareness deficits or phonological dyslexia). In each instance, a single descriptor was adopted for our use.

Chapter 4 addresses performance deficits. Included here are three conditions: attention-deficit/hyperactivity disorder (ADHD), combined type, or ADHD, predominately hyperactive–impulsive type (both referred to as ADHD-C in this system); ADHD, predominately inattentive type (ADHD-I); and a condition referred to as children with compulsive underproduction (CU). As seen in Chapter 4, we encourage school psychologists and other school-based professionals to take active roles in documenting these latter three conditions, even though there are potential boundary issues with psychiatry and medicine.

WHEN SHOULD CLASSIFICATIONS (AND MATERIAL FROM THIS BOOK) BE USED?

This book is predicated on the use of comprehensive psychoeducational evaluations. Such evaluations typically comprise IQ, special ability (e.g., memory, visual perception), and achievement testing, plus background facts and observations. As helpful as such intensive evaluations can be, they should be reserved for certain circumstances. It makes sense for school psychologists to prioritize and spend time wisely. Accordingly, full-length evaluations should be assigned low priority until simpler, less

time-consuming approaches have been tried. Furthermore, straightforward and potentially less stigmatizing ways to assess and intervene often
work. For example, prereferral teams, which do not depend on detailed
psychoeducational evaluations, often produce significant improvement on
student-related and system-related variables (see Burns & Symington,
2002, for meta-analysis).

Psychologists are trained to consult with teachers and apply behavioral
techniques to improve conduct, expand time on task, and promote effective
work habits, not just perform psychometric evaluations (APA, Division 16,
1998; National Association of School Psychologists, 2000). Equally important, general education teachers, without psychological involvement, have
become proficient in collaborating with each other to solve many of their
students' common academic problems (Rathvon, 1999). Assigning routine
problems to prereferral teams acknowledges that many academic problems
are caused by modifiable instructional, classroom environmental, and curriculum factors. Full psychometric evaluations are unnecessary in these
instances. Many times, behavioral-based consultative approaches, including use of curriculum-based measurement, are successful in addressing and
correcting students' problems. These skills are now widely taught (Shapiro,
Angello, & Eckert, 2004). A tiered approach, in which a comprehensive
evaluation is the last to be implemented tier, is conceptually compatible
with what we are proposing. Such an approach is endorsed by the National
Association of School Psychologists (NASP; 2003).

To illustrate the value of nonpsychometric procedures, consider a second grader who is failing reading. Speculation about cognitive or information-processing problems may not be required until immediate classroom
and direct instructional causes are considered. Research documents that
many students struggle because they spend insufficient time actively engaged in academic tasks; therefore, they often benefit from increased direct
instruction, teacher monitoring, and feedback in simple and straightforward ways (see Shapiro, 2004, for detailed discussion). Academic engaged
time (the amount of time in which students are actually involved in active
responding) is a key predictor of academic skill gains (Greenwood, Terry,
Marquis, & Walker, 1994; Greenwood, Horton, & Utley, 2002). The
explanation for our struggling second grader may be as simple as spending
too little time practicing (e.g., she is not actively taught the subject matter).
Alternatively, she may be floundering because she is misplaced in the reading curriculum, and her reading assignments are either too easy or too difficult for her. Then again, she may suffer because of disruptive classmates or
poorly explained assignments. If any of these possibilities is true, then less
intrusive approaches using teachers, rather than detailed psychometric
evaluations conducted by psychologists, can be viable first intervention
steps. In other words, some such children may respond to teacher-devised

interventions (see RTI, below), precluding the need for detailed psychometric testing. Formal school psychology consultation using structured observations, interviews, and monitoring of students' progress may also be needed (Brown et al., 2001; Kratochwill & Bergan, 1990), but this would generally follow less formal attempts by teachers. School psychologists and other school-based professionals should learn all the ways in which they can help students and avoid adopting practice styles that depend on only one skill set (e.g., behavioral consultation or psychoeducational evaluation) to address all situations.

CHILDREN FOR WHOM THIS SYSTEM MIGHT APPLY

We devised a hierarchical system for classifying children with learning problems based on comprehensive evaluations, including extensive use of psychological tests. Most of the system's individual categories are drawn from the extant literature, although some existed previously as disorders listed in text revision of the fourth edition of the *Diagnostic and Statistical Manual of Mental Disorders* (DSM-IV-TR; American Psychiatric Association, 2000), and one is also included in the various special education categories in the IDEA. We have used this system (or its precursor) in clinic settings at Phoenix Children's Hospital, in the Psychological Services Center at Illinois State University, and in public school settings where each of us worked (in Arizona and Illinois). Several school-based colleagues also have tried out the scheme and confirmed that it helped them to conceptualize cases and to recommend interventions, as have school psychology graduate students at Arizona State University. We also pilot tested, at workshops held for practicing psychologists, use of a flowchart (see Figure 1.1) designed to guide the decision-making process. Participants' feedback helped us revise the flowchart and clarify our original description of the various patterns. That flowchart (also reproduced in Chapter 5, where its application is addressed in detail) guides the analysis of information in determining if one of the patterns discussed in this book is present.

The system has wide applicability. It is suitable for the following:

- Students who have received a full evaluation, including developmental/educational history and psychometric scores sufficient to address all components (see discussion of evaluation components below).
- Those between ages 6 and 18.
- Those who speak English as their primary or exclusive language.
- Those who are presumed to be free of diagnosable neurological conditions or genetic syndromes.

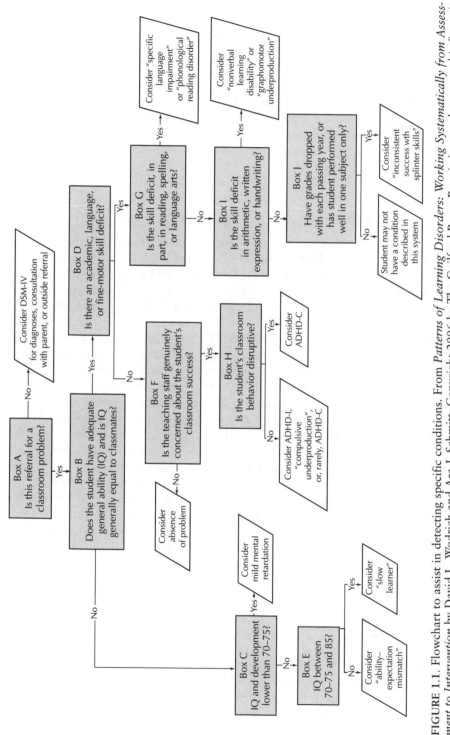

FIGURE 1.1. Flowchart to assist in detecting specific conditions. From *Patterns of Learning Disorders: Working Systematically from Assessment to Intervention* by David L. Wodrich and Ara J. Schmitt. Copyright 2006 by The Guilford Press. Permission to photocopy this figure is granted to purchasers of this book for personal use only (see copyright page for details).

Because this book addresses developmental problems associated with school learning only, no information is included about the patterns of acquired disorders such as traumatic brain injury. Valuable sources of information for these conditions are Bigler, Clark, and Farmer (1997) and Semrud-Clikeman (2001). Nor is information included about children with health problems that can affect school learning. Excellent sources of this information are Phelps (1998) and Brown (2004). Likewise, this book makes no attempt to describe neurological diseases or physiological/genetic syndromes. Excellent sources for this information are the classic text by Jones (1997), a user-friendly volume by Batshaw (2002), and more educationally oriented volumes by Goldstein and Reynolds (1999) and Phelps (in press). Finally, this book does not concern the vast array of psychiatric, behavioral, or emotional conditions that school psychologists will certainly encounter. Nonetheless, ADHD and OCD-spectrum problems (CU) are included (see Chapter 4) because they often impact classroom learning and productivity, not because our focus is on psychiatric disorders. Readers should use the DSM-IV-TR as the primary source for psychiatric disorders and consider supplements, such as House (2002), regarding school-based application of psychiatric diagnoses.

Purposes of Assessment

Psychological testing has been among school psychologists' prime activities for at least the past 30 years. When school psychologists conduct evaluations, parents and teachers expect to learn why the involved student is struggling and what can be done about it. To assure that findings are organized and interpreted to help students, a comprehensive system is needed. Such a system ideally would show how to arrange facts about the student's characteristics, talents, and limitations as derived from psychometric tests and integrate this information with nonpsychometric information, such as background facts, observations, and classroom data. This is the assessment system that we demonstrate throughout the book.

Why expend the time and effort for such an in-depth evaluation? We argue that it is unacceptable for psychoeducational evaluations simply to assign special education-related administrative labels (referred to as part of the "entitlement decisions" process by Salvia & Ysseldyke, 1998). Evaluations are too time consuming (and therefore costly) and the potential to do good is too great to settle for such humble goals. Indeed, criticism of psychological tests as the cornerstone of eligibility determination for specific learning disabilities (SLD) is one of the reasons for changes in the law regarding SLD (National Association of School Psychologists, 2004). This section briefly addresses the rationale for comprehensive assessments.

Beginning diagnosticians are often uncertain about the core reason for conducting psychological assessment. Although they may be comforted by performing familiar tasks (e.g., test and then prepare a report), many novice psychologists feel anxious about which tests to use and what to report in written documents. Nonetheless, many have mastered the testing and report writing steps necessary to assure a legally defensible placement (e.g., satisfies legal requirements for SLD designation). This was especially true when the regulations for special education services required that students with an SLD had to evidence a discrepancy between their scores on ability (IQ) and achievement tests (i.e., before the December 2004 reauthorization of IDEA). Even when able to conduct an administratively correct evaluation, some school psychologists remain unable to develop the in-depth insights necessary genuinely to help students. Psychologists commonly are troubled by how to organize and interpret evaluation-based information and how much confidence to place in their conclusions.

Some experienced diagnosticians harbor similar doubts, and they may experience a lot of aversion to testing. Many psychologists became bored with the psychodiagnostic process long ago. Some school psychologists and special educator-diagnosticians feel trapped in an unfulfilling test-and-place cycle; institution-based evaluators, such as those who work in clinics or hospitals, may likewise feel trapped by bureaucratic mandates to assign labels. We argue that reviewing the underlying justification for evaluations is a first step for improving the utility of the process and making it more interesting for beginning and experienced practitioners. Accordingly, a digression into the rationale for evaluation is in order.

The purposes of psychoeducational assessment are inseparable from the broader objectives of scientific psychology. Psychology is a science of behavior. Its classic purpose has been described as understanding, predicting, and controlling behavior (Allport, 1940). As psychoeducational assessment is a science-related cousin of child and educational psychology, the contemporary purposes of assessment should match psychology's longstanding broader goals (of understanding, predicting, and controlling or influencing). Accordingly, assessment should permit the educational and developmental status of the child to be understood, predicted, and influenced. Evaluations that concern only special education entitlement fail to address these goals and thus are generally incomplete. If understanding, predicting, and influencing, rather than simple eligibility questions, are the focus of evaluation, then school psychologists can enjoy expanded roles. Rather than special education gatekeeping (i.e., special education entitlement), we propose that psychologists adopt tasks analogous to a sophisticated classification evaluation or the "focused, or problem solving assessment" described by Sattler (2001). The timing for such an approach is ideal as the reauthorization of IDEA in 2004 encouraged identifying students with special needs before their problems prove intractable (i.e., professionals are no longer obliged to wait for students to evidence longstanding and extreme academic failure before initiating services). In support of the emphasis on recognizing problems early, Chapter 3 in this book presents various patterns that indicate the likelihood of an underlying information-processing problem that may require special education instructional procedures (e.g., an SLD); using the patterns presented here can help facilitate accurate and early diagnosis and intervention planning.

Assessment to Understand

Some prominent trainers of school psychologists have grown increasingly disenchanted with standardized psychological testing for children with learning problems. The logic supporting this position is that testing is devoid of a link to proven treatments. For example, Reschly (1997, p. 438) stated, "Assessment that does not result in effective interventions is useless for the individual." In part because inconsistent and modest academic gains are a likely outcome of placement in special education programs (e.g., for students with mental retardation or SLD, see Schulte, Osborne, & Erchul, 1998) and because testing may result in this outcome, the process of testing is questioned. Although highlighting the primacy of intervention and offering a wonderful goal, Reschly's position may be far too narrow to be taken literally. Consider how psychoeducational evaluations can promote understanding for key stakeholders, like a student's parents. For parents, the assessment process is the final step in a long journey. By the time a formal psychometric evaluation is conducted, most failing students have been the subject of numerous (and often unsolicited) opinions, as well as unsuccessful efforts to fix the problem. Everyone from grandparents to neighbors to clergy may have offered opinions and suggestions. Although well intended, these individuals seldom provide clarification. Understandably, parents hold high hopes when they hear that their son or daughter is finally to be evaluated by a competent professional. When results are presented, psychologists (or the evaluating team) must provide an explanation of the child's problem. Failure to explicate each student's particular problem, in our experience, is a direct path to a disappointed parent (and teacher). Sadly, sometimes assessments fail to provide the enlightenment that parents rightfully expect from skilled and compassionate evaluating professionals.

Parents' and teachers' desire to understand reflects a basic human need. That need was well described in the early work of attribution theorists as a "constant pursuit of 'why?' " (Weiner, 1985, p. 548). It is argued that the pursuit is a "pan-cultural" and "timeless" aspect of human cognition that possesses adaptive value. According to attribution theory, regardless of the issue at hand, human cognition presupposes that "once a cause, or causes, are assigned, effective management may be possible and a prescription or guide for future action can be suggested" (Weiner, 1985, p. 548). Consistent with the urge to understand, parents often ask revealing questions: "Is there a name for this problem?" "So, could this be a form of dyslexia?" "I had a reading problem; could this be inherited?" "Is my child's problem due to spending too much time on videogames when he was younger?" When school-based teams convene to consider special education eligibility, the ensuing discussion risks overconcern with administrative rules and legal definitions and concomitant underconcern with the "why question." Consequently, parents may feel left out and disappointed (Wodrich, 2004). If special education is at issue, the assessment process understandably must speak to the question of rule-determined eligibility. This goes without saying. At a minimum, however, the process should endeavor to get to the bottom of the problem. Providing a name alone can be helpful, such as informing a parent, "Your child has a deficit in phonological processing. His problems in reading are commonly seen when such a deficit exists. We know that his reading failure is not due to low ability or laziness." A method to classify problems that is logical, meaningful, and research-related can support searches for answers to the "why question." Unfortunately, straightforward approaches that emphasize only intensifying instruction or explain problems as arising only from environmental contingencies are likely silent on this critical point.

Assessment to Predict

Understanding's value multiplies when it is combined with prediction. Besides providing compassionate information for parents, prediction can afford utility to the professionals planning the child's future. A system for classifying problems can help forecast educational, social, and psychological outcomes and better allow children to be helped. Consider several examples.

Children with Down syndrome (viz., those with classic trisomy 21) as a group express disorder-specific patterns. For example, most have slow, steady cognitive growth from birth to 5 years of age. Because the rate of development during these preschool years may be only modestly delayed, parents sometimes assume that their child will later confront only mild problems; that is, the child will be spared long-term severe delays. Beyond age 5, however, children with Down syndrome encounter a diminished rate of cognitive development (see Hodapp, Evans, & Gray, 1999, for review). As a result, few achieve sufficient self-care and academic skills to permit the kind of adult independence that might have been anticipated by their early cognitive scores. On the other hand, longitudinal research indicates that continued stimulation throughout the high school years results in continuing adaptive gains for individuals with Down syndrome (Dykens, Hodapp,

& Finucane, 2000); some of these gains may not be expected if cognitive scores alone, rather than the etiology of the impairment, were considered. Syndrome designations (e.g., the recognition of Down syndrome, not just undifferentiated mental retardation) enable prediction. Crucially, this information can be worthwhile even if nothing can be done specifically to alter long-term outcomes. In this case, the rate or degree of development or its ultimate level may not be changed, but those caring for a child with Down syndrome know what to expect, and as a result they also know how to plan.

Still regarding the value of recognizing specific conditions, consider the insights available to those working with Shawn, an 8-year-old with ADHD-C. After diagnosis and implementation of a successful behavioral and medication (Ritalin) treatment plan midway through his third-grade year, Shawn's parents came to doubt that he actually suffered from ADHD-C. Their skepticism sprang from a relatively trouble-free summer before his fourth-grade year, which he spent mostly at home. This summer was remarkable for surprisingly few complaints that Shawn was out of control or overly impulsive. His parents, however, overlooked the fact that no schoolwork was required during this time and that their home imposes few of the stringent rules that characterize school. Because ADHD is known to be largely unremitting and because current behavior is recognized to be highly influenced by situation-specific demands (Barkley, 2006), Shawn's parents were cautioned against a premature assumption that their son no longer had ADHD. They were also warned that Shawn may as a teen continue to encounter problems with planning, foresight, and judgment (e.g., problems with responsible driving, homework completion, etc.), even though conspicuous symptoms of hyperactivity may disappear. Facts about the syndrome (ADHD-C) permit parents to be counseled against counterproductive abandonment of a good intervention plan.

Parallel logic applies to planning for developmental problems, such as in speech and language development. A system for classifying speech problems is widely known; once classification is made, it becomes possible to address the crucial question of the problem's natural history (Wolraich, Felice, & Drotar, 1996). Articulation impairments seen in 3-year-olds typically normalize without treatment. Speech therapy is generally not indicated, and telling parents to relax is the treatment of choice. However, speech articulation problems that persist to age 8 years warrant evaluation, and such children probably will be recommended for treatment. Early language delays, as opposed to speech delays, portend significant enduring problems. When 5-year-olds with language impairments were followed to age 19 years, they lagged behind unaffected peers in all academic areas, suffered more learning disabilities (Young et al., 2002), and had greater risk for psychiatric impairments, such as anxiety (Beitchman et al., 2001). Practitioners can use longitudinal information like this to conclude that many early articulation problems are benign, whereas later articulation problems are precursors to lasting deficits that require professional attention. Early general language deficits, in contrast, represent the prospect of various undesirable outcomes and warrant professional attention. Recognition of children's membership in precise, homogeneous groups yields enhanced understanding and planning. In this example, children with early language deficits have a "risk ratio" of 11.7 for suffering learning disabilities in all academic areas at age 19 years (Young et al., 2002). The risk ratio indicates, relative to controls, how many times more likely a clinical group child is to have a particular (negative) outcome. It is easy to see how this type of information can be helpful as mid- and long-term plans are prepared. Knowing which children are likely to need help, and which type of help might be best, is a cornerstone to early intervention and prevention of long-standing, intractable problems. Again, school-based evaluations frequently emphasize program eligibility at the expense of addressing prognosis and programming. We argue that the most helpful evaluations produce conclusions about the patterns that underlie failure (i.e., syndromes), not just administrative labels.

Assessment to Influence

The final purpose of psychology (and associated reason for psychoeducational assessment) is to control or influence behavior to promote positive outcomes. This is the prime purpose of assessment. In other words, psychoeducational assessment's greatest potential benefit is the facilitation of targeted plans to foster development and enhance learning. There are two ways that this may occur. The first is to locate a deficit that can be corrected via practice, special training, or instruction. For example, developmental articulation disorder, as well as a few information-processing problems (e.g., those related to phonological processing or general linguistic development) and many academic skills (e.g., in math or reading), appear to respond to direct treatment (e.g., see Camarata & Yoder, 2002; Fitzgerald, 2001; Nunes, Bryant, & Olsson, 2003; Wise, Ring, & Olson, 1999). Importantly, however, most processing deficits do not appear amenable to direct treatment. Consequently, attempts to remedy processes can misuse instructional time. For example, visual–perceptual deficits occasionally hamper classroom learning, but direct drills to correct the underlying perceptual deficit are largely ineffective (Forness, 2001). Arter and Jenkins (1979), writing more than 25 years ago, provided a still-applicable discussion of the problems associated with attempting to correct information-processing problems. Contemporary researchers using sophisticated models of human cognition and instruments, however, sometimes find that training special abilities, such as the ability to plan, does produce significant results (e.g., Haddad et al., 2003). Accordingly, some have argued that matching instruction with cognitive profiles has been prematurely dismissed (see Andrews & Naglieri, 1994). Still, accommodations that circumvent underlying problems, rather than remedy them, are often required (see below).

Regarding treating problems directly, a sound treatment design depends on distinguishing deficits that respond to direct intervention from those that do not. Homogeneous, narrowly grouped problems can allow facts about interventions and their effectiveness to be organized. We have included an intervention section accompanying each condition (Chapters 2, 3, and 4) that provides findings from the published literature, although locating interventions matching specific disorders proved daunting. Nonetheless, in including this information, we attempted to follow the lead of Division 16 (School Psychology) of the APA. The interested reader is encouraged to examine Volume 16, Number 4 (2002), of *School Psychology Quarterly* for a discussion of the crucial topic of employing "evidence-based interventions." Additional general findings about documented treatments are also available from Swanson, Hoskyn, and Lee (1999).

The second way in which psychoeducational information can be used to promote effective treatment is by circumvention. Circumvention involves finding ways to deliver instruction that minimizes or alleviates the negative impact of a cognitive or information-processing deficit. That is, it is not necessary for diagnostic information to lead to bona fide remedial activities to be valuable. Sometimes it is enough just to recognize a deficit's role in school failure so that accommodations can be made. If a student with a specific language impairment (SLI) is required to comprehend instructions in junior high classes (e.g., science, geography), then simplifying directions, demonstrating in lieu of telling, or providing peer assistance to clarify can improve academic performance. This is true even if the underlying language problem is neither treated nor improves. Effective supports and accommodations, however, presuppose a complete understanding of the student's deficits and how they contribute to classroom failure. Here, too, the clinical labels associated with homogeneous underlying problems are often helpful. This fact appears to be increasingly recognized by school psychology leaders as a search for evidence-based interventions intensifies (Stoiber & Kratochwill, 2000). For example, Kratochwill and McGivern (1996) argued that "as syndromes/disorders become more discretely defined, there may be a greater correspondence between diagnoses and treatment" (p. 351). Not all treatments fit all problems. Obviously, having a system for categorizing problems might help link assessment with treatment. In the words of Kamphaus, Reynolds, and Imperato-McCammon (1999, p. 304), "classification schemes, whether psychiatric, educational, or behavioral in origin, give psychologists ready access to a burgeoning research literature."

In summary, if psychologists are to understand, predict, and influence student behavior, then they need access to a system that provides homogeneous and clinically meaningful categories.

ADMINISTRATIVE VERSUS CLINICAL LABELS

The previous discussion implies a distinction between administrative and clinical (or syndrome-related) labels. Practitioners, especially as they begin their careers, benefit from keeping the two types of labels distinct in their own thinking. SLD is an example of an administrative category; its diagnostic criteria are established by a consensus of practicing professionals, researchers, and appointed officials. The exact demarcation line between a child with SLD and one without is arbitrary. The line, at least in part, is drawn to indicate those students needing services and to group them together for administrative purposes.

SLD is a crude categorization and not terribly helpful for most of the important scientific reasons for which assessment usually occurs (i.e., understanding, predicting, and influencing). This is so because SLD lacks a single or even finite number of causes, its natural history and course is variable, and it is unlikely that a single treatment will be found to be effective for the multitude of students placed in this category. Accordingly, debates as to whether any individual "really" has SLD should be thought of more as administrative disputes than clinical diagnostic conflicts. To consider these to be disagreements of clinical judgment is to miss the important point that nature did not create SLD. It is a human construct used conveniently to denote those students with inherent information-processing problems who are struggling academically despite adequate general cognitive functioning (i.e., does not have mental retardation), adequate emotional adjustment, and sufficient educational opportunities (note that the statutory definition of SLD remains unchanged despite revisions in the procedures that may be used to identify students with the 2004 reauthorization of IDEA).

The term "learning disability" did not even exist until 1962, and it did not attain popularity until the passage of public laws mandating special education services in the mid-1970s. In the 1970s, SLD identification procedures typically relied upon evidence of low grade-equivalent scores on achievement tests in the presence of average IQ. For example, average IQ coupled with achievement test scores 2 years below grade level suggested the presence of SLD (other requirements also existed, however). In the early 1980s, simple differences between IQ and achievement test standard scores (the use of grade-equivalent scores was abandoned) were used to define underachievement sufficient for SLD designation. Thus, a student with an achievement test score 15 standard score points lower than his or her IQ, for example, might be deemed sufficiently underachieving for SLD designation. By the late 1980s, sophisticated regression formulas that consider factors related to the reliability of IQ and achievement tests and regression to the mean were devised to select the students most underachieving compared to statistically determined, predicted achievement levels as indexed by standard scores. At the current time, SLD identification can be accomplished by either the ability–achievement approach or students' poor response to intervention; with either method, a team must make a judgment based on the statutory definition of SLD (Public Law 108-466). Although each of these approaches may be able to classify children with SLD reliably, each distinct procedure's use might result in fewer or more students, and different individuals, being identified. The standard for correct identification can change over time because the label was invented to select service recipients.

It should be clear the SLD label comprises children with quite heterogeneous core problems. Accordingly, the administrative label offers little help in understanding individual children. For example, should we expect that children with SLD suffer from poor memory? Some do; some do not. It depends on the specific nature of their learning disability. Alternatively, should we expect an inability to think abstractly? To manipulate numbers? To pay attention? Again, the answer depends on the nature of each child's underlying problem(s). The category is too large and its members too heterogeneous to promote much scientific advancement if SLD is used as a research variable. Thus, it makes little scientific sense to conduct research to locate the common basis of learning disabilities (and, by parallel logic, it is impossible to find a single key for teaching those with SLD).

The alternative (or complement) to broad administrative labels proposed here is to seek narrower, more homogeneous groups of children who are recognizable by their psychometric patterns, educational and developmental histories, and presenting problems. For many of the applied tasks that confront school psychologists, it is helpful to define subcategories or syndromes. Extensive work beginning in the 1970s by Rourke (e.g., Rourke & Findlayson, 1978; Rourke & Strang, 1978) and later by Lyon (e.g., Lyon, Watson, Reitta, Porch, & Rhodes, 1981; Lyon, Steward, & Freedman, 1982) sought recurring clusters of problems. These clusters constituted relatively homogeneous subgroups of students with learning disabilities. Each subgroup had several important characteristics (typically specific cognitive or information-processing deficits) in common, and these were related to specific academic, social, or learning problems. The patterns discovered during this phase of research parallel some of those pre-

Box 1.1. The Issue of Comorbidity

Comorbidity, or the appearance of a *coexisting* or *additional* disorder, is widely reported in the psychiatric literature. For example, 50% or more of children with ADHD seen in clinic settings have a comorbid diagnosis of oppositional defiant disorder (ODD; Waschbusch, et al., 2002). Recognizing coexisting ODD's presence in children with ADHD helps children to be understood and encourages development of a treatment plan that addresses the entire array of existing problems. Similar advantages accompany the recognition of coexisting problems in most diagnostic systems, including ours. Our system provides descriptions of various patterns associated with school failure, and we emphasize seeking the pattern that best fits each child's facts. Emphasizing a single best pattern is, in part, a pedagogical strategy designed to help those unfamiliar with our system. In reality, individual children may match criteria for one, several, or none of these patterns. When two or more conditions are present, it is helpful to recognize both and to consider their combined features so that comprehensive intervention strategies are developed. In other words, if both SLI and PRD are present, then diagnosticians can be helped by recognizing the existence of both problems. Such children may struggle to develop word recognition skills (attributable to PRD) and encounter limitations in the use of context clues when reading or weak reading comprehension (attributable to SLI). Advantages of noting more than one disorder notwithstanding, psychologists should remember that patterns or syndromes are hypothetical constructs designed to explain recurrent patterns observed in human behavior. They are not tangible or real in the sense of a physical condition. For example, GU is a description of a pattern of behavior. It lacks the reality of medical conditions, such as a specific genetic syndrome (e.g., fragile X syndrome) or a brain tumor (e.g., medulloblastoma), which can be reliably established by medical diagnostic procedures and where threshold level for disease presence can be cleanly drawn. Accordingly, psychologists are encouraged to avoid excessive debate about whether any of the patterns is precisely present or absent (exceptions may be MiMR, ADHD-C, and ADHD-I; see above discussion). The patterns can exist to various degrees; there is little black and white in this business. The value of the patterns we present, whether encountered in isolation or in comorbid combinations, is heuristic. In other words, the patterns are worthwhile because they promote understanding, prediction, and influence.

sented later in this book (e.g., those related to linguistic or visual–spatial problems). Some of the labels from DSM-IV-TR are clinical in nature, and we have included some of them here for that reason. The clinical labels in this book can be used as complements to the administrative labels required for special education gatekeeping. Thus, for each of the clinical conditions discussed in this text, we include a review of special services program eligibility to help the practitioner integrate clinical and administrative labels. With changes accompanying the reauthorization of IDEA, the clinical–administrative label relationship may be crucial. In other words, a clinical label on the one hand might promote understanding and facilitate planning and on the other hand establish whether an SLD administrative label is appropriate. Specifically, we present five disorders in Chapter 3 whose presence is extremely suggestive of eligibility for SLD services. In contrast, of the three conditions presented in Chapter 2, two (MiMR and AEM) are not associated with SLD service eligibility and one (SL) is equivocal. The three conditions in Chapter 4 (as we have defined them as performance problems) are usually, but not universally, ineligible for SLD services.

TOOLS AND PERSPECTIVES THAT ENHANCE ASSESSMENT

Besides embracing clinical labels, school psychologists are encouraged to consider two other interconnected ideas. Both ideas are typically more familiar to neuropsychologists than to school psychologists. The first is the notion that each child needs scores from diverse psychometric instruments to be fully understood. This necessarily includes test scores from many psychological domains. The second idea involves a willingness to recognize faulty or problematic aspects of development (which are sometimes subtle) when they exist so that students truly can be understood and helped. In common parlance, it is necessary to call a spade a spade.

Regarding the first point, many of the techniques discussed in this book come from clinical settings and are related to neuropsychology. Neuropsychologists generally collect more extensive and varied psychometric data than is typical in a school-based evaluation. Rather than IQ tests (e.g., Wechsler Intelligence Scale for Children–IV; WISC-IV; Wechsler, 2003, which typically involves administration of 10 or 12 closely related subtests), neuropsychologists may administer two or three times as many tasks (subtests). This extensive battery is designed to appraise skills from domains such as general ability, motor speed and dexterity, automaticity of speech, or declarative memory. Clinic-based neuropsychologists often see a larger volume of children (one or two evaluations per day are possible if one is not encumbered with extensive school-based paperwork). In some settings, these children present with more severe problems than a typical student referred for academic failure; the diversity of these problems may also be greater. Because children seen in clinical settings may have suffered (or are suspected to have suffered) brain impairments that affect narrow skill areas, these children must be especially carefully studied for intra-individual differences.

Consistent with the traditional methods of neurology (and indeed all of medicine), child neuropsychologists seek syndromes that are associated with various types of injuries or lesions at specific sites. By turning their attention to school failure, neuropsychologists use the same batteries to search for syndromes associated with school failure (Rourke, 1994). Furthermore, neuropsychologists often rely on analysis of children with problems rather than unimpaired learners. A typical research strategy arising from clinical neuropsychology is to locate a clinical group with a common academic deficit (e.g., reading) and carefully analyze that group to determine the psychometric patterns that distinguish its members from normal peers. For example, using such an approach, Rourke found striking differences in psycholinguistic skills (e.g., sentence memory and auditory analysis of words) among poor readers; a dissimilar pattern of neuropsychological weaknesses (e.g., visual–spatial) characterized those with arithmetic problems (Rourke, 1989).

Regarding the second point, the willingness to recognize problems, school psychology and clinical neuropsychology may have more in common than is apparent on the surface. After all, school-based psychologists must understand and plan (with other professionals) for children with potential, if not actual, problems. Furthermore, comprehensive school-based evaluations are actually quite clinical because they mostly concern children with genuine and often distinctive problems. Such evaluations are clinical because problem-free students, or those suffering only minor deficits, are handled earlier by less formal, prereferral school services. Such children may never see the school psychologist. Though not necessarily trained in neuropsychology or experienced in clinical settings, school psychologists can benefit by detecting syndromes or recognizable patterns of learning problems. Although premature or excessive emphasis on pathology is a mistake, when puzzles remain after preliminary attempts to understand and help, psychologists might consider a detailed, psychometrically based approach. When that evaluation is completed, they should not balk at identifying genuine problems.

When psychometric research is conducted without including children with pathology (e.g., learning, academic, or behavioral disorders), findings may have limited real-world implications. For example, a common strategy in LD research is to factor analyze test scores of normal children. It is common for such researchers to start with a large data set of randomly selected children that contains no group of children with documented learning problems. Although this approach often produces interesting findings, the analysis of children without disabilities provides only limited information about the configurations that occur among children with disabilities. Consider a factor analysis of Wechsler IQ and achievement scores, which produced several identifiable clusters (Pritchard, Livingston, Reynolds, & Moses, 2000). One cluster was characterized by diminished processing speed (i.e., mean processing speed factor score = $-1.7z$), this occurred in 12% of participants, most of whom were boys with higher than average Full Scale IQ and with achievement generally commensurate with IQ scores. Unfortunately, this information is not yet directly applicable to frontline diagnosticians because it denotes patterns that arise among children never referred for evaluation. Whether patterns characterized by slow processing speed, for example, occur among referred children and whether those patterns predict specific academic or developmental problems cannot be ascertained from this type of study (a point made clearly by Pritchard and colleagues, 2000).

A somewhat related approach that also involves unimpaired children uses sophisticated batteries constructed to match cognitive/information-processing theories (Flanagan & Ortiz, 2001). Although these theory-related approaches hold tremendous long-term potential to understand the bases of students' success and failure, they presently suffer some of the same limitations mentioned above. For example, the so-called "cross-battery" approach, tied to the Cattell–Horn–Carroll (CHC) model, is helpful in describing patterns of strengths and weaknesses, but it has been largely silent on the patterns that recur among children seen in clinical settings (much of the research involves correlations among students without disabilities; e.g., see Evans, Floyd, McGrew, & LeForgee, 2002; Flanagan, 2000; Taub & McGrew, 2004). Until samples of children with disabilities are scrutinized (see recent article by Proctor, Floyd, & Shaver, 2005, as an example of movement toward that end), the cross-battery approach represents primarily a method for constructing an extensive battery that may produce useful data. The approach does not yet seem to help the evaluating psychologist by providing research evidence of exactly those pathological patterns for which to watch.

One more approach to looking at psychometric results requires mentioning because it is so frequently used. The ipsative test score interpretation approach involves administering tests (often only one, such as the WISC-IV) followed by describing the child's intraindividual, test-based strengths and weaknesses (e.g., by subtracting the average value of subtests and looking for scores that are above or below average). This method of analyzing results is not devised to distinguish those with impairments from those without them or to create reliable, recurrent patterns among those who suffer impairments. Nor does it produce theory-based factor analysis–related dimensions derived from multiple batteries (i.e., the cross-battery approach). The simplest idea of profile analysis is to look at each child's pattern for unique manifestations of strength and weakness. This approach is often used in beginning courses on psychoeducational assessment because it provides a method of allowing students to practice describing test results. Of course, many of the practice test administrations involve volunteer participants for whom no real referral concern exists and for whom no pertinent background information is available to add context to the evaluation. Ipsative interpretation makes sense under these limited training circumstances because there are few other pedagogical solutions to what to do with practice test results.

Beyond its use in training graduate students, we contend that simple ipsative interpretation (i.e., a profile analysis of one test) is an incomplete and potentially faulty way to analyze assessment results. Among the limitations of the simple ipsative approach is that diagnosticians often attend to and explain all scores. The number of individual test and subtest scores requiring attention in a scheme such as this are simply too numerous to make it workable. In our experience, even extremely experienced diagnosticians (e.g., with hundreds of WISCs under their belts) may be left seeking, but not finding, a meaningful configuration. Further, when school psychologists attempt to describe their findings for parents or teachers what is said is often unclear, confusing, and suffused with psychobabble. The minutiae of test scores often predominate to the extent that background information, the children's presenting problem, what has succeeded or failed in the past, and the big picture are obscured.

The following exemplify potentially confusing statements that appeared in psychological reports that used ipsative interpretation: "Dylan performed better on constructional tasks involving spatial and manipulative elements" than on "recognizing nonverbal relationships and reasoning with patterns." The author was indicating the student scored better on the WISC-IV Block Design subtest than on the Matrix Reasoning subtest. Another example is that Sarah's "scores on subtests requiring the description of how two words are alike represent a strength compared to self, but the absolute level of ability reflected in her score on this subtest indicates below-average development of this skill area." Such statements are designed to describe the underlying construct associated with the Similarities subtest and to indicate this girl's status on that dimension. Reports like this abound, especially among beginning diagnosticians, perhaps as a remnant of the extremely descriptive reports that are written during training for professors or supervisors to demonstrate mastery of test interpretation. At best, most ipsative interpretation provides only a limited road map to intervention (however, see Carroll, 2000, for an alternative and expanded definition of ipsative and Naglieri, 2000, for suggestions about extending ipsative interpretation and attaching evaluation findings to a cognitive theory). Instead of either ipsative or theory-based approaches, we rely on patterns derived from work with children referred because of learning problems (e.g., the various patterns listed in this book).

OUR SUGGESTED BATTERY

Each of the elements listed below can sometimes help determine if one (or more) of the patterns outlined in this book is present or, alternatively, support the conclusion that the child is free of identifiable problems. Additional information on the nature of the various components and how to assess them is provided in Chapters 2, 3, and 4 as each condition is presented and in the case examples of Chapter 5. As most experienced practitioners recognize, flexibility is required in selecting tests that help answer specific questions. Nonetheless, in most settings where students are trained (or when psychologists are initially learning the system), a battery commonly involves each of the following:

- History and interview (including information about health, development, school history, and family).
- Information about the student's home, school, and his or her classroom.
- Teachers' classroom observations.
- School records/work samples and permanent products.
- Response to previous intervention efforts.
- Psychometric measure of IQ or *g* (i.e., the common factor that is common to all problem-solving abilities), usually the WISC-IV, although shorter screening instruments can be used at times.
- Psychometric measures of language and phonological processing.
- Psychometric measures of visual–spatial functioning.
- Psychometric measures of fine-motor and graphomotor functioning.
- Ratings or psychometric measures of attention/executive functioning.
- Standardized tests of school achievement.
- Behavior rating scales from classroom teachers and parents.
- Observations made by the evaluator during testing.

Table 1.2 lists the instruments that we have found helpful. There are many other instruments that can adequately assess these domains, and individual practitioners are encouraged to use their own judgment in selecting batteries. As can be seen, this approach makes use of standardized test instruments, many with close links to neuropsychology, *but it is not exclu-*

TABLE 1.2. Examples of Psychological Tests Used to Assess Various Domains

General cognitive ability (g)

- Wechsler Intelligence Scale for Children–IV (WISC-IV; Wechsler, 2003)—Full Scale IQ
- Woodcock–Johnson Tests of Cognitive Ability III (WJ III; Woodcock, McGrew, & Mather, 2001)—Composite score
- Reynolds Intellectual Assessment Scales (RIAS; Reynolds, & Kamphaus, 2003)— Used for screening under some circumstances

Language

- Peabody Picture Vocabulary Test—Third Edition (PPVT-III; Dunn & Dunn, 1997) Expressive Vocabulary Test (Williams, 1997)
- WISC-IV Verbal Comprehension Index (Wechsler, 2003)

Phonological processing/phonemic awareness

- A Developmental Neuropsychological Assessment (NEPSY Phonological Processing and Repetition of Nonsense Words subtests; Korkman, Kirk, & Kemp, 1998)— NEPSY subtest scores
- WJ III Sound Blending and Incomplete Words subtests (Woodcock, McGrew, & Mather, 2001)—WJ III Phonemic Awareness standard scores (see Table 3.2 for more instruments)

Visual–spatial

- Wide Range Assessment of Visual–Motor Abilities (WRAVMA) Design Copying and Pattern Recognition subtests (Adams & Sheslow, 1995)
- NEPSY Design Copy subtest (Korkman et al., 1998)
- Developmental Test of Visual–Motor Integration (Beery, Buktenica, & Beery, 2004)

Memory/new learning

- Wide Range Assessment of Memory and Learning—Second Edition (Adams & Sheslow, 2003)
- Wechsler Memory Scale—Third Edition (WMS-III; Wechsler, 1997)
- California Verbal Learning Test (Delis, Kramer, Kaplan, & Ober, 1994)

Fine-motor/graphomotor

- NEPSY Visuomotor Precision subtest (Korkman et al., 1998)
- WRAVMA Pegs subtest (Adams, & Sheslow, 1995)
- Grooved Pegboard Test (Lafayette Instrument Company, n.d.)

Attention/executive functions

- NEPSY Tower, Auditory Attention, and Visual Attention subtests (Korkman et al., 1998)
- Gordon Diagnostic System (Gordon, 1991)
- Wisconsin Card Sorting Test (Heaton, Chelune, Talley, Kay, & Curtiss, 1993)
- Children's Category Test (Boll, 1993)
- Trailmaking Test B (Reitan & Wolfson, 1992)

(continued)

TABLE 1.2. (*continued*)

Attention/executive functions *(continued)*
◆ Test of Variables of Attention (TOVA; Greenberg, Corman, & Kindschi, 1997)
◆ Conners Continuous Performance Test (Conners, 2000)
◆ Delis–Kaplan Executive Function System (Delis, Kaplan, & Kramer, 2001)

Academic

◆ Wechsler Individual Achievement Test: II (Psychological Corporation, 2002)
◆ Woodcock–Johnson Tests of Achievement III (Woodcock et al., 2001)

Social–emotional

◆ Behavior Assessment System for Children: II (Reynolds & Kamphaus, 2004)
◆ Child Behavior Checklist (Achenbach & Rescorla, 2001)

sively a psychometric approach. Rather, we endorse assessment that relies on at least several sources of information, such as Sattler's (2001) four pillars of assessment (norm-referenced tests, interviews, observation, and informal assessment procedures). This means that besides psychometric information, each child is typically observed, interviews are conducted with the child and his or her parent, and records are reviewed. Similarly, we concur with Kamphaus (1993) that substantiation of evaluation inferences by two independent sources is generally needed. Practically, this means that all sources of information are germane and that psychometric components may shrink or grow as needed. For example, if a child presents with a history of well-developed drawing skills, good handwriting, and adequate scores on WISC-IV Block Design and Coding, then his or her graphomotor skills require little or no supplemental testing with specific measures of graphomotor functioning. For such a child, a graphomotor disability is unlikely, and the time allocated to special ability tests that tap graphomotor skills should reflect this reality.

As important as tests are, their use should not disguise that the psychologists' task is one of assessment, not mere testing. Assessment, as contrasted with testing, consists of collecting data and applying professional insights to understand the nature of the child's characteristics, developmental levels, and skills. Information that converges from all sources permits inferences to be drawn. Simply interpreting test scores fails to reach the standard of assessment. Research suggests that multimethod assessment batteries used by skilled diagnosticians maximize assessment validity and minimize the risk that contradictory (wrong) conclusions are reached when these complex procedures are compared to a single-method approach (Meyer et al., 2001). That is, individual students (clients, patients) are apt to be misunderstood and mistreated if speed (efficiency) is stressed over comprehensiveness in the evaluation process.

Consistent with this notion, comprehensive evaluations are held to be important by skilled practitioners. For example, the select group of school psychologists who hold advanced, practice-based certification (from the American Board of School Psychology) almost universally support the need for comprehensive evaluations if decisions are to be made about important issues like special services eligibility (American Academy of School Psychology, 2004).

USE OF THE BOOK IN APPLIED SETTINGS

For each of the conditions in Chapters 2, 3, and 4, we list either criteria for diagnosis or characteristics associated with conditions. Criteria are listed for MiMR, ADHD-C, and ADHD-I only because each of these three disorders is well recognized, has previously established criteria for its diagnosis, and is associated either with entitlement for services (MiMR) or specific, recognized treatment (ADHD-C and ADHD-I). When considering these three disorders, school psychologists should attempt to establish definitively their presence and share their diagnostic conclusions with parents in a clear manner (see Chapter 6). In contrast, conditions like NLD and SLI are much more nebulously defined in the literature and much less associated with either service entitlement or specific interventions. Moreover, recognizing these patterns is mostly helpful to psychologists by promoting understanding and planning in a general way. Thus, the obligation to rule in or rule out NLD or SLI is far less critical than with MiMR or ADHD-C. We have, therefore, listed only characteristics of each of these conditions. Evaluating school psychologists must decide whether a student's facts match characteristics of conditions like NLD and SLI well enough to help explain and plan for each student.

Besides characteristics or criteria for each condition, we have also listed general trends from our experiences with school-age children seen in settings where we have worked. This includes (1) how commonly each pattern might be seen (based, in part, on local prevalence rates in a hospital clinic and university-based psychoeducational center, as discussed below), (2) age ranges at which children with each pattern might have been referred, (3) boy/girl ratios, and (4) common presenting complaints of teachers or parents for each pattern. As mentioned above, we have also included a discussion of assessment tools (by name) that we found helpful and some of the special challenges associated with recognizing the various conditions. This information is designed to help you apply in your setting what we have learned in ours. Figure 1.1 provides a flowchart to help guide decision making; the chart is repeated in Chapter 5 with a series of cases that demonstrate how it is used.

Local Prevalence Rates

We established local prevalence rates when we used the system at Phoenix Children's Hospital outpatient clinic, and we have a less formal sense about the prevalence in the Psychological Services Center at Illinois State University. We encourage school psychologists to collect local prevalence tallies for themselves where they work. Diagnosticians benefit from knowing two types of prevalence facts at the outset of assessment: first, how often the particular condition occurs, and second, how often they might see the condition. The first fact concerns occurrence among children in general. It is the prevalence rate that everyone hears about, such as "the prevalence of depression appears to be growing as 20% of teenagers now have experienced at least one major depressive episode." The second concerns setting-specific occurrences, and it is rarely addressed. In fact, unless practitioners at a particular site collect descriptive data about diagnoses, this information remains unknown.

The settings in which we have practiced may be different from those of most readers of this book. Generalizations from any one setting to another can be hard to make. Thus, we provide only general descriptions of how commonly we encountered the various patterns. For example, in our hospital-associated clinic setting, many children were referred by primary care physicians (e.g., pediatricians and family physicians). Parent-initiated referrals also made up a large portion of the youngsters seen in the clinic. Students referred to this setting, thus, may have experienced various problems at rates and levels of intensity greater or lesser than youngsters evaluated at other sites. For example, pediatricians are quite cognizant of ADHD, and concern about ADHD is one reason that parents take their children to see a pediatrician. Accordingly, among subsequent referrals from pediatricians to us, ADHD may be highly represented. In contrast, school-based diagnosticians may encounter relatively low rates of ADHD but higher rates of children with cognitive delay (e.g., MiMR or children with SL status). Likewise, in a clinic setting more parent- than teacher-initiated referrals might exist and relatively more children with AEM, a phenomenon attributable in part to parental expectations. In contrast, when one of us was working in a middle school setting where many children with SLD were already identified and placed in special programs, referrals were predominated by children with SL and by those with productivity problems (e.g., ADHD). For more information about the use of "local prevalence rates" and "prior probabilities" in the assessment process, see Elwood (1993) and Upshur (2000).

Problem Onset

Age at first diagnosis is information often used to help physicians, and the same type of information can help psychologists. Neurologists working with adults, for example, recognize that complaints of forgetfulness might presage a diagnosis of dementia. Besides the presenting symptoms, the patient's age is important. Memory complaints are unlikely to harbinger dementia in a 50-year-old patient but may in an 85-year-old. This is so because the probability of dementia differs so drastically between the two groups. The same is true for detecting developmental and learning problems. Consider MiMR, an example relevant to school psychologists. In our experience, most children with MiMR came to a clinic at age 6 years or younger. When we collected data on the age of diagnosis in a large sample of children, no child older than 8 years was first evaluated by us and ultimately found to have MiMR. Similarly, neither of us recalls ever participating in an evaluation of a child older than 10 years who was discovered for the first time to suffer MiMR. Therefore, one might assume that it is relatively unlikely that the underlying condition associated with school failure in a 15-year-old is MiMR. Of course, the past 30 years were a time in which IQ tests were routinely used with children who were failing to learn. Assessment practices that may be adopted today or tomorrow, which require no psychometric tests, such as RTI, might invalidate the usefulness of previously observed patterns. Nonetheless, if test data point in the direction of previously-undetected MiMR in a high school student, other possible explanations should be especially carefully explored before MiMR is ruled in.

Gender Ratios and Nature of Presenting Problem

Some of the same logic applies to gender ratios and presenting problems. It is known from clinic settings that some conditions are much more apt to present in boys (e.g., ADHD-C) than in girls; others are not. Never to be used in isolation, these facts can provide clues when used with other information. For example, fine-motor control problems that limit the ability to write (GU) were seen almost exclusively among boys in the clinic at Phoenix Children's Hospital. In contrast, an anxious, slow, and compulsive work style that limited work completion (CU) was seen just about as often in girls as in boys. Girls can present with GU, but when that seems like the explanation for slow work production, all possibilities, with careful vigilance to the probable ones such as CU (discussed in Chapter 4), must be considered.

Experienced practitioners recognize that teachers' (and parents') comments also are related to students' underlying problems. For example, teachers' dissatisfaction with a student's performance in all subject areas tends to be associated with IQ-related conditions, such as SL status (see Chapter 2). Poor across-the-board skills are much more rarely associated with narrow processing deficits, such as GU or phonological reading disorder (PRD), as seen in Chapter 3. On the other hand, relatively circumscribed complaints of poor oral reading are often associated with the narrow skill deficits in phonological processing (PRD). Thus, in order to help practitioners, we list the type of complaints commonly made by teachers for each condition. Of course, patterns vary from location to location. Collecting local information can be helpful in the decision-making process. Unfortunately, little research has been conducted on clinical decision making by school psychologists. What has been conducted suggests that decisions are sometimes vulnerable to faulty logic based on illusory associations between clinical signs and diagnoses (Gyns, Willis, & Faust, 1995). Collecting local information within clinical samples can help practitioners at their sites.

THIS SYSTEM'S COMPATIBILITY WITH RTI

A final word about RTI is in order at the conclusion of this chapter, which some may incorrectly view as antithetical with much of what is advocated in this book. Simply put, this book provides a method for detecting the types of learning problems commonly encountered by children, as well as an associated method (backed by empirical research where available) for selecting interventions. It is not intended to promote a single method of determining eligibility for special education services (indeed, our primary focus is not special education eligibility) or to discount the importance of the prereferral intervention process. In fact, we believe that RTI and our proposed system complement rather than contradict each other. Consider NASP's (2003) three-tier proposal for the identification and eligibility determination of students with specific learning disabilities. Briefly, tier one requires implementation of high-quality instruction and the use of behavioral supports for students in their existing general education setting. Tier two mandates prevention or intervention services for children whose skills are underdeveloped compared to same-grade peers. Tier three calls for "comprehensive evaluation by a multi-disciplinary team" to determine eligibility for services. This would include cognitive testing and review of health information. In addition, NASP emphasizes the need for assessments to identify children's unique strengths and weaknesses and to rule out competing diagnoses or "non-cognitive factors" as the central cause of the academic failure. Even outspoken proponents of RTI as the singular means of determining eligibility agree that standardized assessment may be necessary in some cases. For example, Fletcher and Reschly (2005) concede, "in-depth expensive assessments are required only if indicated by screening information. . . . If screening information suggests mental retardation, then in-depth cognitive assessments are appropriate" (p. 14). Our system demonstrates how these final tasks may be accomplished.

We concur with those who believe that RTI-related information can prove invaluable during the prereferral intervention and special education eligibility evaluation process. Furthermore, school-based professionals should reflect on the statements of Vaughn and Fuchs (2003). They assert that the RTI model has appeal because it *may* assist children at risk for failure (and not only those who have already failed), provide earlier interventions for students with learning disabilities, reduce bias in the referral process by targeting students at risk based on objective screening data, and directly connect assessment data with the construction and progress monitoring of interventions. Nonetheless, models of RTI appear to differ among themselves in the extent to which interventions are tailored to the individual student based on a problem-solving model versus prescribed based on the type of academic problem. Regardless of the RTI model, most emphasize students' engagement in effective instruction by a general education teacher, progress monitoring, changing instruction after a poor response and rechecking progress, and ultimate referral for further evaluation and possible special education eligibility for those who fail to respond (Fuchs, Mock, Morgan, & Young, 2003). In short, we contend that considerations related to RTI are often helpful during the course of prereferral intervention. However, learning problems resistant to intervention merit a closer look via an in-depth evaluation that includes a battery of standardized psychometric tools.

SUMMARY

This chapter presents an overview of a system designed to help school psychologists (and related professionals) recognize the nature of students' learning problems. It also provides a template for using this information to devise intervention recommendations. Our detailed system, which employs psychometric testing, is complementary to school-based informal and formal consultative approaches that should usually be used first. School psychologists are encouraged to recognize three broad problem types—IQ-related, narrow information-processing deficit-related, or performance-related—and to establish which subtype(s) of condition (recognizable pattern) is present. To work effectively, school psychologists are encouraged to conceive of the assessment task broadly and to use all sources of case information and psychometric data to understand and help students.

CHAPTER 2

◆◆◆

IQ-Related Conditions

◆

This chapter concerns academic problems that can be understood primarily by assessing the student's general cognitive ability (IQ). Three specific patterns (conditions) that are well known to or easily understood by school psychologists are described in this chapter. The first is mild mental retardation (MiMR). This condition is marked by IQ scores below 70 and significant adaptive behavior delays. The second condition is termed slow learner (SL) and is defined by relatively low IQ scores and commensurate academic achievement. The final condition is termed ability–expectation mismatch (AEM). Students with average IQ and achievement scores that attend school in very high-achieving school districts may be represented in this category. A detailed analysis of these IQ-related conditions appears later in this chapter.

Before addressing specific IQ-related conditions, however, a general discussion is needed. Some graduate students, especially those oriented toward applied behavior analysis, doubt the utility, if not the validity, of the very concept of IQ. For them, the notion seems entirely too mental and far too distant from the facts about the immediate behavioral contingencies that seem to influence better academic performance. For such skeptics, it is worth considering the hypothetical example of two fourth graders whose identical report cards comprise straight F's. The first was found to have a Full Scale IQ score of 68, the second of 138. Would anyone honestly contend that both youngsters should be approached in the same way? In other words, is it reasonable to conclude that both of these students warrant the same amount of follow-up assessment to understand why they are failing? Based on IQ scores alone, we have a strong suspicion why the first is failing but no idea why the second is doing so alarmingly poorly. Similarly, could interventions for each student possibly be the same? Extreme outlying scores like these may be the exception, but the underlying point raises a classic conclusion. Even nonpsychologists implicitly recognize that differences in ability matter in understanding why some students struggle and in establishing what can be done to help them. The question, of course, becomes one of when basic IQ differences are great enough to matter in the case of the individual struggling student. We present at least three situations where IQ matters a great deal.

In this chapter, the concern is with general cognitive ability. Most graduate students are aware that early research by Spearman and others demonstrated that IQ tests primarily measure a general cognitive ability, or *g*. This broad array of capabilities predicts, among many other things, substantial differences in the rate and ease with which students learn basic academic skills. Spearman's early findings (1904) have been consistently endorsed by research on subsequent editions of IQ tests suitable for school-age children. For example, contemporary psychometric researchers document the importance of *g* in basic academic tasks, such as reading (Flanagan, 2000), and the factor is present even in tests whose primary purpose is to assess relatively narrow cognitive capabilities (see Nyborg's [2003] comprehensive volume). The broader impact of this factor on school, vocational, and life performance has also been widely reported (e.g., Brody, 1997).

Although we contend that measuring IQ is essential because it represents the best predictor of many disparate academic tasks, we do not endorse the simplistic "jug and milk" principle espoused by Sir Cyril Burt (1937). This notion assumes that capacity (e.g., the size of a jug, or one's IQ) sets a rigid upper bound on the amount of content that can be acquired (i.e., the amount of milk, or a student's mastery of academic skills). We know from practical experience that many children achieve higher than their IQ scores would predict, and research indicates that many factors other than "g," such as attention, motivation, memory, motor, and phonological processing skills influence academic achievement beyond the effects of global IQ. Nonetheless, general cognitive ability is so directly related to so many classroom tasks (even borderline limitations in this ability constrain academic success in children without outstanding noncognitive factors) that measuring IQ is vital. Likewise, we do not quarrel with those who contend that IQ tests are too narrow to measure all actual aspects of intelligence (see Sternberg & Grigorenko, 2002). We simply contend that IQ scores, as indicators of general cognitive ability related to school learning, prove useful because of their strong relationship to many school subjects and to general school success (e.g., see Gottfredson, 1997, for a broad view; WISC-IV [Wechsler, 2003] manual for associations with specific academic domains).

MILD MENTAL RETARDATION

Criteria for Mild Mental Retardation

1. General cognitive delay, typically reflected by Full Scale IQ (and WISC-IV both Verbal Comprehension Index [VCI] and Perceptual Reasoning Index [PRI]) ≤ 70.
2. Concomitant adaptive delays (including academic performance).
3. Functioning above the level of moderate mental retardation.
4. Onset ≤ 18 years.

Note. Diagnosticians also should refer to local regulations, IDEA, or American Association on Mental Retardation criteria.

Common Presentation of Mild Mental Retardation

Frequent concern of teacher at time of referral	"Failing all subjects; not keeping up with classmates"
Typical grade of referral	Kindergarten or primary grades
Gender ratio	More boys than girls
Prevalence in referred sample	Common

Note. Estimates from clinic setting.

Manifestations

MiMR is a disorder marked by general cognitive and adaptive behavior delays that, according to the American Association on Mental Retardation (AAMR, 2002), manifests in functional limitations (i.e., specific performance impairments) and disabilities (i.e., the demonstration of performance impairments within a social/functional context) (see Table 2.1). Parents of children with MiMR have a sense early on that their child is not

TABLE 2.1. Common Special Education and American Association on Mental Retardation (2002) Levels of Mental Retardation

Common special education	
Level	Intellectual functioning and adaptive behavior
Mild mental retardation	Between two and three *SD*'s below the mean
Moderate mental retardation	Between three and four *SD*'s below the mean
Severe mental retardation	More than four *SD*'s below the mean

AAMR	
Level	Descriptor
Intermittent	Support is required if a need arises (e.g., job search, find housing, etc.).
Limited	Support is required for limited time periods (e.g., job training, learning mass transit system, etc.).
Extensive	Long-term support is required on a regular basis (e.g., ensuring hygiene, maintaining finances, etc.).
Pervasive	Intensive support is required across all environments (e.g., support is needed for feeding, toileting, ensuring safety, etc.).

Note. AAMR, American Association on Mental Retardation.

developing as quickly as other children. Commonly, it is late mastery of verbal and motor developmental milestones that raises parents' suspicions. For example, many parents report that their child with MiMR did not walk until after 16 months or did not express him- or herself with individual words until after 24 months of age. Parents may also experience a general sense that the child of concern was slower to acquire skills than his or her siblings, even if precise timelines cannot be recalled. For example, parents' concern about their young child's (7 years or younger) developmental status in dimensions like motor, language, and general cognition is fairly highly predictive of bona fide problems being found if the child is evaluated (Glascoe, 1997). Likewise, parents commonly describe their son or daughter as simply less quick to catch on, more concrete, and less mature than age-mates. Such a child may play with younger children and seem less curious than peers. As early as preschool, it may be observed that the youngster in question was less able than classmates to learn basic concepts. By the time school starts, it is common for children with cognitive delays to find most school subjects hard. Paradoxically, however, some children with MiMR may find some isolated academic tasks relatively easy. This appears to be the case on tasks that require less purely cognitive capability and concomitantly where splinter skills, such as intact fine-motor functioning or good rote linguistic memory, permit a degree of circumscribed success. In practice, one might find some children with MiMR to possess adequate penmanship, oral reading skills, or basic math skills, for example. Many children with MiMR, however, do not enjoy these isolated strengths. Unfortunately, among those with isolated intact skills, most find themselves encountering increasing school problems as the demands for high-level thinking increase with each passing year.

For children at the lower end of the MiMR continuum (e.g., those close to the range of moderate mental retardation), general impairment is typically quite obvious (see "Common Presentation" table on p. 34). However, children with less severe MiMR can be more difficult to identify in the classroom, and their accurate ultimate detection can be quite challenging without psychometric assistance. One reason that MiMR can be difficult to notice in preschool and early elementary settings is that the academic tasks being taught are simple in nature and can often be mastered by rote memorization. For example, in preschool and kindergarten children learn to identify colors, letters, and numbers. They also learn via direct practice and repetition of the sounds associated with letters so that they can decode words. It may not be until the requirements to comprehend passages and apply basic component skills arise that some children's problem-solving and reasoning deficits become obvious.

Typically, when complex problem-solving and reasoning skills are put at a premium, the student with MiMR will encounter academic difficulty. Reading comprehension, math reasoning, and written expression are generally of greatest difficulty; however, word decoding and math calculation can be areas of concern. Upon the initial diagnosis, parents are often fearful that their child will be incapable of being a fully functioning, independent adult. However, with well-planned special education interventions, the likelihood is increased that students with MiMR will attain adult vocational and living independence (Patton & Dunn, 1998; Patton, Polloway, & Smith, 2000), although continuing supports may be needed well into adulthood (Kiernan, 2000).

MiMR does not comprise just low IQ scores. For example, many children with MiMR experience comorbid psychiatric disorders that require treatment. One study found that 33% of participants with MiMR met International Classification of Diseases—Tenth Revision (ICD-10; World Health Organization, 1990) criteria for a psychiatric diagnosis, with the most common being hyperkinesias (i.e., hyperactivity–impulsivity; Stromme & Diseth, 2000). Other studies have examined the relationship between DSM-IV-TR diagnoses and mental retardation, concluding that approximately 25% of children with MiMR met criteria for a disruptive disorder, 22% for an anxiety disorder, and 4% for a mood disorder

(Dekker & Koot, 2003a). Furthermore, half of the children who met DSM-IV-TR criteria had severely impaired daily functioning, and 37% of the children met criteria for two or more disorders. A related study concluded that at greatest risk for a psychiatric disorder were children with MiMR who were socially incompetent, had underdeveloped daily living skills, experienced negative life events, and suffered heath conditions (Dekker & Koot, 2003b). Accordingly, school psychologists must be prepared to conduct comprehensive evaluations to assure that all aspects of functioning are considered when MiMR is at issue.

Not surprisingly, children with MiMR also lag behind peers in social skills (Freeman, 2000). The presence of social skill deficits is highly correlated with the degree of cognitive impairment. Early on, children with MiMR may engage in parallel play (i.e., play alongside peers) instead of reciprocal interactions with peers that might involve assigned roles, agreement of activities, and turn taking. This immature mode of interaction appears to derive from globally delayed play skills, not just limited understanding of the nature of a play activity (e.g., rules), insufficient communication skills, or inability to maintain interest in peers. As a result, parents and teachers commonly report that the child with MiMR plays alone or seems to prefer to play with younger children who are more easily directed and appear oblivious to social skills deficits or with older children and adults who will maintain the boundaries and responsibility for the social interaction. Unfortunately, therefore, same-age friends may be lacking, and it is for this reason that social skills training is often an important consideration for these children.

The category of MiMR is well known to psychologists who have taken basic intelligence assessment courses. Most practitioners recognize that the early history of mental testing by Simon and Binet in France resulted in the development of tests that constituted the first intelligence scales (see Schreerenberger, 1983, for a complete history of the concept of mental retardation dating from the Middle Ages). These tests were developed explicitly to establish which prospective students were likely to succeed in academic instruction and which were not (Sattler, 2001). The lowest performing of these children would now be considered to have mental retardation. The ability of IQ testing reasonably to predict student achievement has been repeatedly demonstrated, and the use of IQ tests in educational settings for this diagnostic purpose (i.e., to understand which students lack the ability to learn as well as their peers) continues to this day.

This category has direct legal and educational implications, as MiMR is one of the special education categories specified under IDEA. Children identified as meeting criteria for this condition almost universally receive special education services, and in many states, supplemental services through noneducational agencies afford parents support services and access to child advocates. For example, in Arizona, mental retardation is one of the categories served by the Department of Developmental Disabilities. Through assignment of a caseworker, families of children with this designation can obtain respite care, access to health-related services, and parent support to teach behavior management skills and to foster optimum child development.

Assessment Considerations

The first criterion of MiMR is delayed general cognitive development; therefore, IQ tests must be used if a diagnostician is to establish the presence of mental retardation. Delayed cognitive development has typically been defined in IQ terms as 2 standard deviations (*SD's*)below the mean (hence, WISC-IV Full Scale IQ [FSIQ] of 70 or less). Although the AAMR suggested a revision to IQs of 75 in 1992, and has subsequently reverted to 70 (2 *SD's*) with IQ scores as high as 75 in light of the standard error of measurement in 2002 guidelines, most state guidelines and the DSM-IV-TR call for IQ scores of 70 or less (AAMR, 2004c). The value of IQ notwithstanding, it is important to avoid too much emphasis on the overall IQ level. Diagnostic guidelines and best practice call for delayed general cognitive development, not just a single low IQ score.

For these reasons, the vast majority of school psychologists have long used the Wechsler IQ tests (Wodrich & Barry, 1991). One advantage of the Wechsler scales is that psychologists can examine the Verbal Comprehension Index (VCI) and Perceptual Reasoning Index (PRI) because these scores constitute the most distilled measures of verbal and nonverbal reasoning ability, respectively. Crucially, Harcourt Assessment, the publishers of the WISC-IV, now provides a means to calculate a General Ability Index (GAI) that is a composite of VCI and PRI scores without the influence of subtests tapping working memory and processing speed (Raiford, Weiss, Rolfhus, & Coalson, 2005). The GAI is probably more sensitive to cognitive delay than the FSIQ and it will prove a valuable supplement in clinical practice. All of these scores are an important feature of the WISC-IV vis-à-vis mental retardation's core notion, global impairment. Best practice would therefore dictate that if either VCI or PRI extends much above the 70 (or 75) IQ threshold, the diagnosis of mental retardation should be called into question.

A final level of analysis is also possible using Wechsler subtests. Again consistent with the notion of general and uniform cognitive impairment, children's profiles that are low at each subtest afford the most assurance that general ability is indeed markedly underdeveloped for the child being considered for MiMR designation. In other words, relatively high scale scores (e.g., scores of 8 or higher) on cognitively rich subtests such as Vocabulary, Similarities, or Block Design imply that an MiMR diagnosis may be questionable. For all of these reasons, during WISC-IV subtest comparisons diagnosticians must rely on their previously learned skills in making profile analyses to assure that they are interpreting differences that are indeed reliable.

Most school psychologists recognize that IQ scores should never be interpreted in isolation. This dictum is especially true when considering mental retardation within each child's particular situation (e.g., English-language learner (ELL), genetic syndrome with motor deficits, mental retardation with comorbid psychiatric disorder). VCI, for example, among students whose primary language is Spanish or who reside in bilingual environments, should generally be deemphasized when considering their general cognitive ability. Standards of practice, and even court decisions, suggest that nonverbal measures provide much more assured estimates of capability in these situations (e.g., see *Guadalupe v. Tempe Elementary School District*, 1978). In contrast, a child with longstanding low vision would have a better chance of showing her general cognitive ability on verbal measures. Similar interpretation practices, which deemphasize an area of deficit or lack of experience, would apply when school psychologists seek to determine general ability functioning, the construct of interest in MiMR. Although alternative methods of IQ assessment are available to school psychologists, it is for practical reasons mentioned above that Wechsler IQ tests have remained the gold standard when questions arise about general cognitive capability.

As seen in the case studies of Chapter 5, supplemental ability tests also provide estimates of cognitive capability, and they can help address important hypotheses that emerge during the assessment process. For example, a psychologist might entertain the hypothesis that a child earned a low VCI but might possess far better language skills than reflected in his or her WISC-IV scores. Receptive language tests such as the PPVT-III (Dunn & Dunn, 1997) or WISC-IV Integrated Picture Vocabulary Multiple Choice subtest (Wechsler et al., 2004) can be used to explore that hypothesis. Because both of these tests assess vocabulary knowledge without requiring the child to speak, normal range scores would add weight to the hypothesis that the obtained low VCI does not reflect general impairment, but rather signifies an inability to express in language what is truly known.

Parallel reasoning may lead diagnosticians to use supplemental nonverbal tests that eliminate motor (e.g., WISC-IV Integrated Block Design Multiple Choice subtest; Wechsler et al., 2004). In order to address and eliminate the prospect that apparently low IQ scores may be attributed to other factors, experienced diagnosticians develop sophisticated methods for adding to their core cognitive measures (often the Wechsler IQ test). To do so allows for the confident final diagnosis of MiMR. Beginning psychologists should receive intensive mentoring (case conference, examination of their reports) regarding how experienced psychologists select assessment instruments, refine their hypotheses, and arrive at final diagnostic conclusions. We provide case examples and a flowchart to facilitate development of these skills in Chapter 5.

Children considered for mental retardation designation must be assessed for adaptive functioning as well as IQ (general cognitive ability). This requirement is stipulated in the diagnostic criteria of mental retardation, and it is not optional. Adaptive behavior concerns the ability to meet life demands particular to a culture or setting. For the most part, this domain concerns non-school and nontest indices of functioning. AAMR's 2002 revised definition of mental retardation enumerated three broad areas of adaptive skills (conceptual reasoning, social skills, and practical skills) and provided many subskill examples (see Table 2.2). The current AAMR revision is an extension of earlier changes that supplanted the global notion of adaptive delay in favor of concern with relatively narrower adaptive skill strands. At the time that global concepts of adaptive behavior were leaving AAMR's definition in the 1990s, critics argued that there was no method of assessing each of these adaptive skill areas and that many of the areas are pertinent to adults but not children (Gresham, MacMillian, & Siperstein, 1995). These criticisms remain cogent. Furthermore, some classification systems embrace multiple spheres of adaptive functioning (e.g., DSM-IV-TR), but other guidelines (e.g., IDEA) specify only that adaptive delays exist. The latter position at least implicitly comports with the notion that adaptation is a global concept, not readily divided into meaningful components.

Practically speaking, most psychologists who assess adaptive functioning use standard psychometric techniques, and most of these provide a summary or composite scores that are of prime interest. By far the most common procedure is to interview parents and teachers using the Vineland Adaptive Behavior Scales, which is now available in a second edition (Sparrow, Cicchetti, & Balla, 2005). This procedure furnishes information about the child's development reflected in his or her daily behavior. Parents can provide information about their son or daughter's communication, daily living, and socialization (and motor for young children) levels. These can in turn be compared with age-mates using the familiar technique of converting raw scores to standard scores using the common IQ-like metric (mean = 100; SD = 15). Generally, however, diagnosticians look for adaptive scores roughly equivalent to IQ to rule in mental retardation (the 2002 AAMR, interestingly, suggests that adaptive behavior scores should be two SD's below average). Table 2.3 includes two commonly used adaptive behavior rating scales, as well the domain scores and subtests associated with each. We would also like to point out that the second edition of the Vineland Adaptive Behavior Scales includes a method to quantify adaptive behavior delays through the administration of rating scales.

TABLE 2.2. Examples of Adaptive Behavior According to the American Association on Mental Retardation (2002)

Broad skill areas	Specific examples of adaptive skills
Conceptual reasoning	◆ Receptive and expressive vocabulary ◆ Reading and writing ◆ Money concepts ◆ Self-direction
Social skills	◆ Interpersonal ◆ Responsibility ◆ Self-esteem ◆ Follows rules
Practical skills	◆ Activities of daily living (e.g., eating, dressing, managing money) ◆ Occupational skills ◆ Maintaining a safe environment

Supplemental information, such as social competence during assessment, observation or interaction with peers, and informal reports of parents, siblings, and teachers about the child can also be considered. Individual and group achievement test scores can also be reviewed, at least to help rule out a diagnosis of MiMR (see Chapter 6). Students who acquire skills approximately commensurate with classmates would be viewed suspiciously regarding mental retardation diagnosis. Although often not explicitly adaptive, academic skills are a developmental requirement of childhood and depend in part on intact cognitive functioning; satisfactory development here seems incompatible with mental retardation.

Other Possibilities

At the start of the evaluation process, those who know the child best typically agree that a learning problem is likely. The prime question is its nature and what to do about it. Figure 1.1/5.1 quickly guides the evaluating psychologist through alternative hypotheses about the type of problem, including some outcomes that suggest there is no recognizable problem at all. By the very process of determining that a child has very low VCI and PRI (as well as FSIQ or GAI), the prospect of narrow-band processing deficits or primarily performance-related condition can be ruled out. In other words, the first question is whether *general* ability is the core of the student's problem, and once this prospect is confirmed it is illogical to contend that the problem is a more circumscribed alternative, such as phonological

TABLE 2.3. Composition of Two Commonly Employed Adaptive Behavior Scales

Vineland Adaptive Behavior Scales—Second Edition[a]	Scales of Independent Behavior—Revised[b]
Communication	Support Score
Receptive	Broad independence (total)
Expressive	Motor skills
Written	Gross motor
Daily living skills	Fine motor
Personal	Social and communication skills
Domestic	Social interaction
Community	Language comprehension
Socialization	Language expression
Interpersonal relationships	Personal living skills
Play and leisure time	Eating and meal preparation
Coping skills	Toileting
Motor skills	Dressing
Gross	Personal self-care
Fine	Domestic skills
Adaptive Behavior Composite	Community
Maladaptive Behavior	Time and punctuality
	Money and value
	Work Skills
	Home/communication orientation
	Maladaptive behavior composite
	Internalized
	Hurts self
	Repetitive habits
	Withdrawn or inattentive
	Asocial
	Socially offensive
	Uncooperative
	Externalized
	Hurts others
	Destructive to Property
	Disruptive

[a]Sparrow et al. (2005). [b]Bruininks, Woodcock, Weatherman, and Hill (1996).

processing or ADHD. Of course, even after MiMR is ruled in, coexisting strengths and weaknesses still should be considered.

When behavioral or motivational factors appear to impede the ability or willingness of the child to participate in testing, it can be difficult to determine if a child does in fact have MiMR and/or a psychiatric disorder. Consider a child who has marked hyperactivity and only focuses for a couple of psychometric items at a time, a child who is inconsolable in the face of failure and extremely hesitant to guess, or a child who is absolutely noncompliant and confrontational. If they prove testable, many of these children may earn low IQ scores. In these situations, interviewing adults in the child's life and relying on adaptive behavior data is essential. For example, take a child who appears to have legitimate skill and knowledge deficits on those test items that she attempts, but who also expresses extreme frustration and ultimately refuses to guess. These observations provide a dilemma. Is anxiety negatively impacting the child's test performance and promoting excessively pessimistic scores? Alternatively, might she actually have MiMR with coexisting anxiety (perhaps amplified by failure and frustration)? We suggest that the evaluating psychologist look to adaptive behavior data, parent and teacher interviews, and school records (e.g., report cards, permanent products) to help solve problems like this. In this case, if it can be determined that the child met developmental milestones on time via clinical interview of parents and that global adaptive behavior delays are absent, then it is unlikely that the child has MiMR. Conversely, if global adaptive behavior delays are present, they would buttress the hypothesis that the child has MiMR.

Eligibility Issues

As will be true of all the conditions discussed in this book, consultation with relevant state regulations will be necessary when a team establishes eligibility for special services. This is because slight variations in special education eligibility criteria often exist. IDEA, upon which all state interpretations are based, defines mental retardation as "significantly subaverage general intellectual functioning, existing concurrently with deficits in adaptive behavior and manifested during the developmental period, that adversely affects a child's educational performance" (Federal Register, 1999). Note that this definition is composed of three critical components: impaired intellectual functioning, deficient adaptive behaviors, and educational need. Whereas the need for formal special education intervention is obvious if a child has MiMR, documenting educational need may be more difficult for other conditions presented in this book. This appears especially true of the performance-related conditions presented in Chapter 4.

It is standard practice to specify the degree of mental retardation present when determining eligibility for special education services. Although DSM-IV-TR and AAMR have outlined criteria for determining subtypes of mental retardation, special education service eligibility is governed by IDEA, which mirrors DSM-IV-TR criteria. IDEA defines MiMR as performance between 2 and 3 *SD*'s below the mean on measures of intelligence and adaptive behavior (see Table 2.1). Moderate mental retardation is defined as performance between 3 and 4 *SD*'s below the mean, and severe mental retardation as greater than 4 SD's below the mean on measures of intellectual functioning and adaptive behaviors. In contrast, AAMR (2002) makes reference to the intensity of supports needed by a child, as well as the length of time supports are required rather than levels of mental retardation. The descriptors used by AAMR include intermittent, limited, extensive, and pervasive and are reviewed in Table 2.1.

Lastly, IDEA dictates that all children with suspected disabilities are to be evaluated in all areas of concern. Therefore, the evaluating school psychologist should carefully consider the need for additional evaluation by related-service providers such as speech and language, occupational, and/or physical therapists, in addition to the data provided by the comprehensive evaluation. School psychologists may need to provide counseling services, assist in devising behavioral plans, or consult with outside mental health professionals in light of the high rate of behavioral/emotional difficulties children with MiMR experience. Related-service providers also share evaluation responsibilities in their disciplines and provide information to the evaluation team from which to make additional eligibility/treatment decisions. For example, a physical therapist might be needed to determine if a child has limited physical mobility to the extent that physical and/or occupational therapy services are required to make progress on individualized education program (IEP) goals.

Treatment Considerations

AAMR has been exceedingly active in advocating for the rights of children with mental retardation, and this includes a remarkable commitment to the needs of families. In fact, child- and family-focused intervention is a hallmark concept advocated by AAMR (2004). This philosophy asserts not only that the needs of the child should be addressed in the process of planning interventions, but so too must the needs of parents and siblings. Although family needs may receive greater emphasis in various governmental agencies (e.g., through state agencies), schools and school psychologists should also recognize the stressors families often face. Specifically, parents must manage the stress associated with learning they will care for a child with MiMR. They are charged with the task of wading through and making sense out of a seemingly endless volume of information (e.g., evaluation reports, suggested readings, Internet material); existing family resources may be strained (e.g., financial, time); and, finally, due to all of these stressors, effective parenting may be a challenge (Guralnick, 2000). Accordingly, even when it is impossible for school psychologists to intervene directly, they should strive to act compassionately and to help families access appropriate referrals.

Research suggests that children with MiMR are increasingly being educated within the general education setting with accommodations and modification to the curriculum, rather than in self-contained settings (Patton et al., 2000). This practice derives support from the extant literature. As a rule, children with mental retardation educated in general education settings enjoy higher academic achievement and better-developed social skills than their peers educated in self-contained settings (Freeman, 2000). In fact, after review of 36 studies on the topic, Freeman concluded that the more included a child is in the educational mainstream, the greater his or her academic and social gains. That is, in order to optimize outcome potential, a child with MiMR requires as much contact as possible with general education peers. To be successful and accepted by peers, however, a child must demonstrate positive social behaviors (Siperstein & Leffert, 1997). Those children with MiMR who lack requisite social skills are therefore candidates for social skills training. Regardless of educational setting, a student's intervention program should not just concern crystallized academic skills, but also should target current daily living capability, as well as mastery of those things that will be necessary ultimately to facilitate the transition from school to adult living.

Research suggests that children with MiMR are capable of benefiting from instructional practices that capitalize on existing higher level thinking skills (Butler, Miller, Lee, & Pierce, 2001; Wehmeyer, Sands, Knowlton, & Kozleski, 2002). Therefore, in inclusive classrooms, direct instruction is advocated that incorporates metacognitive activities (Wehmeyer et al., 2002). That is, focused instruction takes place with opportunities for practice and feedback, but wherein teachers challenge students to categorize, as well as to compare and contrast newly learned concepts with those previously learned. In a similar vain, peer-mediated instructional strategies, such as peer tutoring, cooperative learning, and reciprocal teaching (where children are paired and one acts as leader), have also been suggested (see Wehmeyer et al., 2002, for a review).

Unfortunately, a body of treatments with empirical support specific to children with MiMR does not yet appear to exist in the literature. Perhaps contributing to this fact, MiMR is one of the most heterogeneous of the many recognizable patterns presented in this book. Nonetheless, studies that have focused on the reading of children with moderate mental retardation concluded that the reading skills of such children can be maximized through programs based on a phonological approach to word decoding (see Chapter 3), rather than just a sight word program (Conners, 1992). Children with MiMR were found able to use mnemonic devices (in this case pictures of objects whose name begins with the same sound represented by the target letter) to enhance the ability to learn sound–symbol associations (Hetzroni & Shavit, 2002). Regarding mathematics, at least some evidence suggests that children with mild and moderate mental retardation benefit from basic skills tutoring, remedial drill, multisensory methods (e.g., TOUCH MATH; Bullock, Pierce, & McClellan, 1989), peer tutoring, use of technology (calculators), and self-regulatory methods like using student-produced reminders (Butler et al., 2001). Likewise, direct instruction that emphasizes specific goals, close monitoring and student feedback, controlled levels of success, and sufficient active practice would make sense for children with MiMR, as it does for all struggling learners (see Shapiro, 2004). Many teachers also recognize that simplified instruction helps. Simplification may involve elements such as slowed presentation and repetition, as well as drills to the point that skills are acquired at an automatic level.

As reviewed earlier, children with MiMR appear to be at risk for a variety of comorbid psychiatric conditions, including disruptive, anxiety, and mood disorders (Dekker, & Koot, 2003a; Stromme & Diseth, 2000). As is true of other conditions presented in this book, medication management may be necessary. Some studies, for example, have investigated the effects of methylphenidate on children with mental retardation and have found that this medication can effectively treat symptoms of ADHD (Pearson et al., 2003). Numerous case studies involving the use of psychotropic medication for children with MiMR are reported in sources such as the *Journal of the American Academy of Child and Adolescent Psychiatry*, although they are not organized by diagnosis (e.g., MiMR).

If problem behaviors are present, and prior to exploring medication management, applied behavior analysis that makes use of positive behavior supports should be implemented (Horner, 2000). Positive behavior supports are formulated via a functional analysis of behavior, reduce problem behaviors across settings, and serve to improve the general functioning of individuals (Horner, 2000). In addition to standard intervention techniques that include verbal praise and reinforcement of positive behaviors, research has shown, for example, that children with mental retardation can be taught to self-monitor their behavior and increase time spent on task. Brooks, Todd, Tofflemoyer, and Horner (2003) demonstrated that a child with Down syndrome and MiMR could be taught to self-monitor and increase his or her time spent on task by marking either a "+" or "0" when prompted via audiotape and headphones. Likewise, Firman, Beare, and Loyd (2002) found that students with moderate mental retardation could be successful even if they were not prompted to record their ratings of on-task behavior but merely recorded markings when they thought of it. Even though students who were prompted to record their markings increased on-task time the most, unprompted students improved as well. These studies demonstrate that positive behav-

---

**Box 2.1. Curriculum-Based Assessment,
Eschewing IQ Testing, and Mental Retardation**

Some professionals have decided that they will never perform IQ testing. This judgment often rests on the assumptions that such tests are incapable of providing information that aids in better instruction for students and/or that IQ scores may actually harm students. This way of thinking may be especially common among practitioners who suggest that students can best be understood by alternative assessment means, such as determining their skills vis-à-vis the curriculum (curriculum-based assessment; CBA), teacher interview, and observation. Forgoing IQ may be defensible if establishing the presence of an SLD is the only issue and a reliable method of categorizing students as with or without SLD can be devised (some proponents of CBA argue that this can be done, such as by use of the RTI model). With regard to RTI, various approaches are typically applied (especially those involving direct instruction in academics that are supported by empirical research) while students are carefully monitored for progress. Increasingly intensive and specialized services can be implemented until a level necessary to produce student success is reached. In fact, failure to progress with services less intensive than those of special education is typically the threshold for concluding that the student has a disability and requires special education and related services. Whether this system actually produces standardized results about who needs services seems less clearly demonstrated. Approaches that rely on CBA, RTI, and academic consultation, however, typically occur without consideration of students' cognitive differences. When psychologists are reluctant or refuse to attend to students' cognitive differences, an unspoken supposition is revealed: all students should be able (cognitively capable) to learn commensurate with the curricular demands (and their classmates). When failure occurs and a special education label is applied, it is almost always the SLD label. That is, it is assumed that this particular student is underachieving compared to his or her classmates because of "a disorder in one or more of the basic psychological processes" or that the student has a condition such as "perceptual handicaps, brain injury, minimal brain dysfunction, dyslexia, and developmental aphasia" (IDEA, 1997). Ignored is the prospect that he or she may be achieving poorly but actually learning at a rate matching IQ.

Without IQ testing (and supplemental use of adaptive behavior scales), there may be no method to rule out mental retardation. Although an individual teacher may not care whether a student's root problem is mental retardation, it is quite likely that a parent does. If parents express no desire to know that fact earlier (such as during first grade), they almost certainly will later (such as when the student is in high school). It is the unfortunate psychologist who finds him- or herself in the position of explaining to a parent that their son or daughter, a longtime recipient of special education SLD services (often with little progress) bears a mental retardation rather than an SLD label. Many parents would feel that such a student has received inappropriate instruction being focused exclusively on academic instruction rather than in a balanced program that included adaptive and life skills (typically provided to children with MiMR). Furthermore, parents may feel that their child missed otherwise necessary services (respite care, casework services through state agencies) and that they were denied essential information needed to plan for this youngster (estate and trust plans) and for subsequent ones (many forms of mental retardation are heritable, and subsequent pregnancies may need to be considered in this light). These events might occur if the diagnostic team (especially its psychologist) selected a particular philosophy of assessment that excluded IQ tests. One of the diagnoses we are obliged to assign is mental retardation, and the proper method of making that assignment involves IQ tests.

ioral interventions, with minimal support needed by the student, can be used to address the problem behaviors. Numerous case studies concerning children with MiMR are reported in sources such as the *Journal of Applied Behavior Analysis*, although material is not organized according to the classification system used here (i.e., separate sections do not exist for children with MiMR).

In summary, the literature currently appears to lack many treatments specific to children with MiMR that have clear empirical support. As a result, school psychologists often must rely on intervention studies aimed at low-achieving students (which will be discussed in the next section) or general treatments targeting children with specific learning disabilities, some of which are discussed in Chapter 3. For a case example of MiMR, see the information on Carmen in Chapter 5.

SLOW LEARNER

Criteria for Slow Learner

1. Full Scale IQ (or both WISC-IV VCI and PRI) $\leq$ 85
2. No VCI or PRI discrepancy expected
3. Most academic test scores statistically concomitant with Full Scale IQ
4. Primary deficit is not listed in Chapter 3 (i.e., specific language impairment, phonological reading disorder, nonverbal learning disability, graphomotor underproduction, or inconsistent performance with splinter skills)
5. Rule out mild mental retardation

Common Presentation of Slow Learner	
Frequent concern of teacher at time of referral	"Failing all subjects; not keeping up with classmates"
Typical grade of referral	Primary grades
Gender ratio	Roughly equal boys and girls
Prevalence in referred sample	Very common

Note. Estimates from clinic setting.

Manifestations

The pattern of children with slow learner (SL) status is often quite straightforward. These children possess general cognitive ability below many of their classmates, resulting in modest academic performance. These students have been denoted by the term SL for many years, although many students in this range may be referred to in DSM-IV-TR as having "borderline mental retardation" (i.e., if their IQ scores fall between 70 and 80).

Diagnosticians are sometimes too quick to disregard IQ if a student's score is above the 70 (or 75) cut-score necessary for MiMR. As previously stated, this can be a mistake. Even modest cognitive limitations, such as 1 or more SD's below the mean (i.e., IQ $\leq$ 85), are generally sufficient to make classroom learning relatively difficult. As might be expected, the academic problems associated with scores in the 70 to 85 IQ range are typically less incapacitating and less uniformly present than those experienced by students with MiMR. Given a generally linear relationship between IQ and achievement, children with the lowest IQ values on average perform most poorly on academic tasks. Students with IQ scores in the range of mental retardation (2 or more SD's below the mean) experience extreme academic problems. Those with IQs in the range from 1 to 2 SD's below the mean experience problems as well, but these are less pronounced. This latter group and their ensuing classroom problems are at issue in this discussion (see Table 2.1 for definition).

Parents and early elementary teachers may fail to notice problems for these students at the outset of formal schooling. For some children, however, problems are evident from the start. As a result, some students are held back in kindergarten or first grade. Others with this condition learn the basic academic skills taught during the primary grades reasonably well, although supplemental help from teachers, classmates, or parents may be required. Many of these children struggle when they attempt to generalize material that they have learned to new situations (Shaw, 2000a). Eventually, students with SL may be seen by their teachers as catching on more slowly, requiring more individual attention and repetition, and lacking the insight and level of reasoning possessed by classmates. Children with SL may possess the rote learning skills required for learning basic reading, spelling, and math facts, but struggle to move forward to mastery of higher academic tasks, as is done by most of their middle school peers. At this time, the emergent need for analysis, generation of ideas, and generalization of previously learned rote skills exposes learning problems where none were previously apparent. Thus, it is not uncommon for parents (or teachers) to complain about an onset of learning problems at this time as if something within the student had suddenly changed. In these instances, diagnosticians are encouraged to consider another possibility. Intensifying curricular demands, rather than student changes, may be responsible for seeming classroom declines.

Children with SL do not uniformly meet eligibility criteria for any special education services, nor are they generally seen as having a true disability (e.g., MiMR, SLD), leading one to wonder if students with SL escape the intense academic failure endured by students with formal disability labels and if qualitative differences distinguish the two groups. Some data suggest that there are few differences in the degree of deficits experienced by children with SL compared to those formally labeled with MiMR and SLD. For example, Gresham, MacMillan, and Bocian (1996) demonstrated that children with SLD, children with MiMR, and a third group with low achievement but no special services label (presumably including children with SL status) all displayed marked reading, math, and spelling delays, and teachers perceived all these students as experiencing similar academic struggles. Problems with the heterogeneous SLD administrative label notwithstanding, this information implies that some common elements may underlie most struggling students and that the body of empirically supported literature for students with SLD could also be applied to help those with the condition of SL.

In addition to academic struggles, and like children with MiMR and SLD labels, children with SL risk social skills deficits. A recent meta-analysis found that students with low achievement but access to special education services (presumably including many students with SL) experience social skills deficits and earn lower ratings of peer acceptance than children without learning problems (Nowicki, 2003). This matches reports of relatively low self-esteem and lower peer acceptance, plus increased levels of depression (Valas, 1999), risk of low self-esteem, and feelings of inadequacy (Masi, Marcheschi, & Pfanner, 1998) among children who experience academic failure. These studies suggest that the social–emotional functioning of children with SL should be assessed, and such children should be treated when necessary.

When conceptualizing the performance of a student with SL, Shaw (2000b) warned against reverse diagnostic overshadowing. "Diagnostic overshadowing" refers to the tendency to think of all problems experienced by a student as a manifestation of his or her particular disability. Among children diagnosed with ADHD, for example, it is common to attribute all problematic behavior to ADHD. The reverse is apt to occur in children with SL because the pervasive impact of borderline intelligence can be underappreciated. For example, it can be a mistake to consider genuine correlates of borderline intelligence, such as underdeveloped coping and social skills, lack of motivation, and academic failure, as distinct conditions and outside the context of borderline IQ (Shaw, 2000b). To do so would result in reverse diagnostic overshadowing.

Assessment Considerations

A minimal test battery consisting of a measure of general cognitive ability (IQ) and an individually administered achievement test is generally sufficient to establish the presence of SL. Tests that do a good job of measuring *g* are especially helpful. After ruling out MiMR, if the Full Scale IQ is below 85, a significant discrepancy between present nonverbal and verbal scores is not present, and commensurate academic delays are identified, SL is often the most compelling explanation for learning problems. Most children with this condition have a fairly uniform WISC-IV profile with measures of verbal and nonverbal reasoning falling in the borderline range, and no conspicuous linguistic or visual–spatial deficits apparent on testing (Hoskyn & Swanson, 2000). Still, additional tests may be administered to determine if relative strengths or weaknesses are present because their existence can be helpful during intervention planning (Shaw, 2001). Achievement testing typically produces a fairly uniform profile as well. The exceptions to this rule may be that less cognitively demanding academic skills are sometimes more readily mastered than those requiring complex analysis, good judgment, and application of existing skills. Learning straightforward academics may be easier because some children with SL possess relatively well-developed working memory and processing speed (despite weak scores on WISC-IV VCI and PRI). Likewise, word decoding, spelling, and computing may be more developed than reading comprehension and story writing, which might require organization, punctuation, and generation of detailed ideas.

Given the apparent risk of children with SL for social–emotional difficulties, including social skills deficits, it makes sense to assess personality, interpersonal, adjustment, behavioral, and emotional dimensions as part of a complete evaluation. Accordingly, clinical interview of parents, teachers, and student, behavior rating scales, and student observations are suggested as routine diagnostic practices. As will be reviewed in the next section, evaluation of social–emotional status is necessary to rule out competing psychiatric hypotheses, as well as to determine if supportive services are indicated.

Other Possibilities

The most common competing explanations for the school failure experienced by students with SL are quickly ruled out using the flowchart presented in Figure 1.1/5.1. MiMR and SLD can be ruled out as children with SL earn IQ scores above the range required for MiMR and a narrow information-processing deficit is not at issue because most of these children's problems are illuminated once it is clear that they lack general ability. The problem, again, is insufficient general cognitive ability, although there may be associated weaknesses in many other narrow skill areas (like students with PRD or GU). Weaknesses in information-processing skills, however, are generally no more pronounced than those of general ability, the root problem.

     As with all conditions, when evaluating children with suspected SL, test data must be carefully scrutinized, and clinical judgment must be applied when necessary. For example, sometimes it is difficult to determine if behavioral or motivational factors are impeding the ability, or willingness, of a child to participate in psychometric testing. Obviously, a child who is unwilling to engage fully in testing (e.g., due to marked hyperactivity or anxiety) may earn spuriously low IQ scores. In situations such as this, it is helpful to consider the attainment of developmental milestones, interview adults in the child's life (e.g., parents and teachers), and review school records (e.g., report cards, permanent products). Evidence that a child met all developmental milestones on time or early, is capable of producing grade-level work when motivated, and enjoys high adaptive skills should lead to questions about the validity of low IQ scores.

Eligibility Issues

Historically, children with SL status have typically not been able to access special education services, despite academic failure. According to the pre-2004 IDEA, composite diagnostic information on these students precludes the provision of services under the categories of MiMR (due to IQ scores above 70) and SLD (due to lack of meeting statutory definitional criteria, such as a disorder in one or more of the basic psychological processes and no evidence of ability–achievement discrepancy). Despite not meeting formal IDEA criteria, multidisciplinary evaluation teams apparently have sometimes deemed children with SL eligible for services under the category of Specific Learning Disability (MacMillan, Gresham, Bocian, & Lambros, 1998). Lack of service eligibility may be problematic for schools because approximately 14% of school-aged children may have SL based on the portion of students in the normal distribution with IQ scores below 85. Many of these children presumably endure academic problems. Thus, the number of school-age children with SL may be greater than the number of school-age children with MiMR, SLD, and autism combined (Shaw, 1999). Further compounding the pressure on schools, federal legislation (No Child Left Behind Act of 2001; Public Law 107-110) has challenged schools to improve the achievement of all students, including children with ability in the SL range (Shaw & Gouwens, 2002).

Although there are profound questions about the appropriateness of labeling them with a disability, some students with SL may receive services if evaluation teams use broadened elements in the newly revised IDEA definition of SLD. IDEA 2004 indicates that states may chose to forgo reliance on ability–achievement discrepancies (see Chapter 3) to identify those eligible for SLD services. Instead, states may now choose to document response to intervention (RTI) and use RTI to justify the need for more intensive services, ostensibly, through special education with SLD designation. This appears to be the method by which some children with SL will be found eligible for special education services. Thus, if a complete evaluation is not conducted, and students are simply identified based on RTI criteria, many students with SL may wind up in SLD programs. Some would question whether this is appropriate. Although students with SL status often struggle, and individualized accommodations and support may be warranted, these students arguably are not disabled. In other words, IQ in the low average or borderline range is not a disability. It is possible for schools to document ability in this range, recognize SL's potential impact on learning, and plan accordingly, but not provide specific learning disability services to students whose sole problem is ability in the SL range.

On the other hand, NASP's position on the reauthorization of IDEA appears to indicate that two criteria only are necessary for special services designation: significantly low achievement and insufficient RTI (plus the typical process of ruling out mental retardation and emotional and environmental/cultural factors). Likewise, Dombrowski, Kamphaus, and Reynolds (2004) propose emphasis on uniform procedures to identify children as eligible for special services, with an emphasis on low achievement scores (compared to national standards). Neither ability–achievement discrepancy nor, apparently, low IQ (above the range for mental retardation) will be exclusionary. Obviously, debate about how to handle children with SL will continue.

Treatment Considerations

According to IDEA's longstanding definition of disability, these students are not captured by an established disorder category, and they were unlikely to receive special services. Even with the reauthorization of IDEA, students with ability in the SL range, especially if they do not encounter severe academic problems, will probably continue to go without formal special education services. Thus, devising effective interventions and accomplishing their implementation can be challenging. As the student's core problem is lack of general cognitive ability, as reflected in Full Scale IQ, a logical question is what can be done to improve IQ. This question goes to the heart of the controversy over the malleability of IQ. The consensus of opinion is that IQ is not very malleable, especially as children age (e.g., see Brody, 1999; Kranzler, 1997). In other words, most of the school-age children who present with IQ scores in this range are unlikely quickly to realize average ability based on any available intervention. Accordingly, plans to promote success given the child's current complement of ability are needed rather than attempts to raise IQ. Fortunately, a set of general interventions that suit all learners can be used effectively with students in the SL range. These interventions are particularly important for students with ability in the SL range because such students lack surplus cognitive ability that might make up for suboptimal teaching. In order to succeed, student with ability in the SL range may need the very best educational practices available if they are to learn skills, complete classroom assignments, and score well enough on tests to advance from grade to grade and to pass high-stakes tests. Several suggestions for effective teaching are listed here.

Shaw (2000a) asserted that the learning potential of children with SL can best be maximized when teachers provide concrete descriptions and explanations of abstract concepts, use teaching methods that promote generalization of learning, and stress exercises that facilitate the automatic application of basic skills (e.g., math facts applied to money). Empirical support for these practices specifically applied to children with SL status, however, does not yet exist. For the best specific teaching strategies, one must turn to the more general literature on techniques with empirical support and speculate on which of these are suited for students with SL (based on the characteristics of research participants or on logical extrapolation of the techniques to situations in which children with SL are found). Fortunately, the school psychology literature provides substantial research on students who are experiencing varying degrees of academic failure (e.g., Rathvon, 1999; Shapiro, 2004). One of Rathvon's goals (1999), for example, is to describe detailed intervention protocols that can improve students' academic performance and behavior. An advantage of this intervention source is that the purpose, materials, outlined procedures, treatment evaluation methods, and literature sources associated with each intervention are clearly identified in a book targeted for school personnel, such as school psychologists. Other sources, like Shapiro (2004), include general intervention strategies that can be used to improve the performance of students experiencing academic problems, including students with SL, even though this subgroup of students is not explicitly identified as targets for his catalogued interventions.

Among the general categories of interventions with empirical support identified to assist students with learning difficulties are self-management strategies, peer tutoring, performance feedback, direct instruction, and cooperative learning groups (see Shapiro, 2004). These treatment domains, as reviewed by Shapiro, are briefly considered next. In some instances, studies have been added from our literature review to offer additional empirical support.

First, Shapiro (2004) advocates the development of self-management strategies to permit students with academic problems to learn to self-monitor and self-instruct. Self-monitoring interventions include techniques like those discussed in the MiMR section, which train students to monitor their own time spent engaged in assigned work (i.e., time on task). Improving time spent on task and engaged in academic performance is widely accepted as fostering positive student outcomes. Other strategies that fall under this broad area are cognitive-based interventions. Synthesizing his review of the literature, Shapiro advocates for self-instruction methods whereby teachers think aloud to model reasoning and problem-solving steps, students practice with teacher assistance while they (students) think aloud, and finally students complete tasks using private speech. Cue cards and other visual prompts may also be used during this procedure. Because SL status is presumed to be associated with deficits in metacognitive strategies and inefficient plan generation in academic settings and because these deficits may be causally linked to student failure, direct teaching of self-instruction techniques seems especially appropriate.

Mapping is another strategy that appears to fall under the category of cognitive-based interventions. Shapiro (2004) describes story mapping procedures that can be used to increase reading comprehension skills, as well as story webbing techniques to assist students in organizing thoughts and ideas to be communicated through writing. Data support not only the use of story mapping (e.g., Mathes, Fuchs, & Fuchs, 1997), but also mapping of content-specific concepts. For example, Guastello, Beasley, and Sinatra (2000) examined the effects of concept mapping on low-achieving seventh-grade students' comprehension of science-related concepts. The experimental group received instruction on how to represent concepts graphically according to major and minor associations and received teacher-led discussion. The control group received teacher-led discussion only. Although it is not particularly surprising that the concept mapping group earned significantly higher comprehension scores than its control group counterpart, the magnitude of group differences was quite surprising. Specifically, the concept mapping group of seventh graders enjoyed content-specific comprehension scores 6 SD's superior to the control group.

Next, Shapiro (2004) suggests the use of peer tutoring. Based on a review of the literature, programs that incorporate peers have earned widespread support. In fact, a recent meta-analysis of classroomwide peer-assisted learning (PAL) interventions determined that such programs result in significant achievement gains, especially in relatively young, urban, low-income, and minority children (Rohrbeck, Ginsburg-Block, Fantuzzo, & Miller, 2003). The researchers suggest PAL interventions are effective because their procedures often incorporate opportunities for students to act as natural teachers, tap methods that develop motivation to learn, increase students' engagement time and their prospects for feedback, and allow for students' autonomy. Clearly, PAL techniques can be implemented to address the needs of diverse groups of students in general educational settings (Maheady, Harper, & Mallette, 2001).

Given the effectiveness of PAL strategies, it makes sense to review briefly at least one PAL program that has been shown to improve the performance of students with low achievement (which presumably includes students with SL). Fuchs et al. (2001) reviewed reading peer-assisted learning strategies (PALS) and their implementation in kindergarten, elementary, and high school classrooms. Generally, a reading PALS program involved direct instruction provided by a teacher, student practice, and teacher feedback; reciprocal tutoring between pairs of students (one high-achieving and one low-achieving student); and points or rewards offered contingently for completing reading activities and demonstrating appropriate tutoring behavior. Three intervention activities took place during each PALS session. Partner reading involved high-achieving students reading to low-achieving students, and then the low-achieving student rereading the passage and engaging in story retelling. Paragraph shrinking helps develop reading comprehension skills by teaching students to identify main ideas in passages. Finally, the goal of prediction relay is to develop comprehension skills by prompting students to make predictions before reading, having students read the passage, and then discussing if the prereading predictions were found to be correct. These PALS procedures were awarded "best practice" status by the U.S. Department of Education Program Effectiveness Panel (Fuchs et al., 2001). Data indicate that PALS interventions can be effectively implemented across all grades and subject matter (e.g., Fuchs, Fuchs, & Kazdan, 1999; Fuchs, Fuchs, Mathes, & Simmons, 1997; Fuchs, Fuchs, Yazdian, & Powell, 2002; Mathes, Howard, Allen, & Fuchs, 1998; Rohrbeck et al., 2003). Again, the ease of implementation and the pervasive success of programs such as these are crucial in that many students with SL status will receive no instruction in special education settings.

Next, Shapiro (2004) argues that direct performance feedback can motivate students and promote skill development. Our review of the literature uncovered a recent meta-analysis that concerns teaching strategies to improve the mathematics skills of low-achieving students (potentially including students with SL). Interventions that enjoyed the greatest support not only included PAL and direct and explicit instruction (reviewed next), but also performance feedback offered directly to students, in addition to teachers and parents (Baker, Gersten, & Lee, 2002). Direct feedback appears to provide essential information on which areas require further work, and it serves as a motivator, spurring students to achieve.

Direct instruction is another widely accepted intervention strategy to be used with students with learning difficulties. Examples of direct instruction strategies include delivering scripted lessons, including exact words and presentation sequences, small-group instruction, asking students to respond in unison, use of signals (e.g., indicating when to respond), fast-paced instruction, prompt error correction, and praise of appropriate behavior (Shapiro, 2004). As previously mentioned, Baker et al. (2002) concluded that math instruction that incorporates explicit teaching of concepts, rules, and problem-solving strategies is highly successful.

Additionally, Shapiro (2004) argues that cooperative learning groups can be used to increase students' achievement. Cooperative learning groups may involve peer-assisted learning procedures (such as PALS); however, contingencies, such as the ability to take a final test or various types of rewards, are dependent on all group members demonstrating competent skills. Despite their advantages, cooperative learning groups should be used with caution if a student with SL is part of the class. Students with SL may have little to contribute and experience rejection by group members for preventing or delaying the group receiving its desired contingencies (Elliot, Busse, & Shapiro, 1999).

Finally, like their counterparts with ability–expectation mismatch (discussed next), many students with SL status benefit when teachers and parents develop reasonable and appropriate expectations. This is especially true for the subset of students who have been accused of laziness, irresponsibility, and lack of effort. For many students with SL status, these accusations arise when teachers and parents assume that the student enjoys skills and abilities that he or she in reality lacks. Consequently, understanding the exact academic and cognitive skills and strengths that a struggling student possesses can be helpful even if no changes in teaching occur. Likewise, as seen in the AEM discussion that follows, creating levelheaded expectations can prevent the search for nonexistent SLD and preclude recommendations for unneeded, and sometimes exotic, remedies. For a case example of SL, see the information on Todd in Chapter 5.

ABILITY–EXPECTATION MISMATCH

Criteria for Ability–Expectation Mismatch

1. Parental concerns are usually primary
2. Full Scale IQ (or both WISC-IV VCI and PRI) 15 or more points below estimated schoolwide or familywide Full Scale IQ
3. Discrepancy between student's achievement test scores and those of local school's
4. Most academic scores concomitant with (not significantly superior to) Full Scale IQ
5. No other condition present

Common Presentation of Ability–Expectation Mismatch

Frequent concern of parent at time of referral	From parents: "Isn't doing as well as siblings and classmates"
Typical grade of referral	Late elementary years and beyond
Gender ratio	Roughly equal boys and girls
Prevalence in referred sample	Varies by setting from common to virtually nonexistent

Note. Estimates from clinic setting.

Manifestations

Suggestions that a student with perfectly normal IQ, along with normal information-processing skills, is struggling because his or her IQ is too low may seem patently illogical. This possibility becomes plausible if the adequacy of IQ is considered in the context of expectations and classroom demands. Let us first consider the circumstances of the children in the preceding two categories (MiMR and SL). These students experience more problems than their classmates because they are less cognitively developed. As a result of their relative general cognitive deficits, they are unable to meet learning demands established in their classroom. Among students with this pattern that we have called ability–expectation mismatch (AEM), a similar discrepancy is evident, but the most salient factor is expectation, not IQ singularly. These students have average IQ scores, but their parents or teachers harbor unrealistically high expectations because most class-mates (or siblings) possess more developed cognitive abilities and enjoy generally unfettered academic success. To our knowledge, these children have not been fully reviewed in the school psychology/educational litera-ture. Because of this, the resulting discussion is largely based on our own professional experiences and a common-sense recognition that excessive expectations can sometimes cause myriad problems.

In clinic settings, we have found that these students are typically referred by their parents due to *perceived* academic shortcomings. Referrals are only occasionally initiated by schools or physicians, seemingly indicat-ing that these children are learning within normal limits. Referrals for these students are not evenly distributed across schools, but clustered in certain schools mostly comprising affluent families where significant educational attainment is taken for granted. We have spoken with school psychologists who have seen the same pattern in such diverse areas as wealthy Los Angeles suburbs, schools populated by children of scientists and academics in the Research Triangle of North Carolina, and neighborhoods filled with professional families in the Chicago metropolitan area. The problem may grow in scope as parents' and students' academic expectations ratchet up. Between 1982 and 2000, the number of high school graduates who had taken an honors English and an honors math course grew 2.5 and 1.5 times respectively, reaching a remarkable 34% and 45% of graduates nationwide by 2000 (Forum for Child and Family Statistics, 2004). Regardless of geo-graphic location, school psychologists should be sensitive to the needs of such children and recognize when to assist these generally well-intentioned, but frequently misguided, families.

Not surprisingly, family background and school placement are the key factors in understanding why these students present for evaluation. It is not uncommon for referrals to be launched by concerned parents, both of whom are professionals and with high-luster academic records. Often, these students attend the most competitive schools, and often their siblings attended the same school and succeeded there. Sadly, these children are sometimes taken from one medical, psychological, or educational profes-sional to the next in the hope that a definitive problem will be detected. Even more sadly, parents may have been offered any number of ad hoc explanations for why school is so hard (e.g., vision problems associated with fluorescent light, additives in junk food, failure to crawl before walk-ing). Even more frightening scenarios, such as the prospect of a brain tumor, have been invoked to explain school troubles, especially if grades have actually declined.

Some children with average ability will struggle in straightforward classroom competition if they are grouped with mostly well-above-average classmates. For many of these average students, school becomes increasingly difficult with each passing grade. Many are seen as scholastically adequate, or even above average, during the early elementary years, only to encounter problems later. Problems may not be evident if the average-IQ student is buffered by well-developed phonological processing, memory, and graphomotor skills. Therefore, early curriculum, which is dominated by rote learning, memorization, and pencil-and-paper work production, may prove relatively easy. When those students' academic status appears to decline as the years progress, it is probably attributable to stepped-up demands for higher-level thinking associated with advanced curriculum. These classroom demands are typically handled quite well by more gifted classmates, but students with average abilities may simply hit a wall of learning complexity when they reach junior high or high school. During interview, these students often report needing to study more than classmates and requiring tutoring just to keep pace with school demands. Even then, test grades are often poor.

Students with AEM appear particularly vulnerable in core academic classes like literature, composition, and mathematics. These are classes where abstract thinking, analysis, and judgment predominate and in which students with well-above-average skills often shine, dwarfing by comparison the performance of average students. On the other hand, classes such as government and health, which sometimes emphasize rote learning, can provide a more level playing field. We have found that success in these classes often helps preserve the average student's academic self-confidence and maintains his or her motivation to succeed. When questioned, average students who succeed in select classes often state that they suffer circumscribed subject matter weaknesses (e.g., "I am not good at math," or "I can't think of what to say when I write"). Few complain of global limitations (e.g., "School is not my thing," or "I am dumb").

Assessment Considerations

The majority of these students have straightforward profiles on psychometric tests and unremarkable developmental histories. Simply put, these students' information indicates healthy, average boys and girls (or young men and women) for whom expectations exceed their ability to perform. Most express roughly equivalent verbal and nonverbal skills on tests of cognitive ability such as the WISC-IV. On ability instruments that differentiate fluid and crystallized abilities (e.g., Woodcock–Johnson III Tests of Cognitive Abilities, Woodcock et al., 2001; Kaufman Adolescent and Adult Intelligence Test, Kaufman & Kaufman, 1993), these two cognitive factors

---

Box 2.2. Is It Possible to Be Too Smart for Your Own Good?

We have argued that greatly diminished general cognitive ability (MiMR) is important because it predicts significant and cross-subject academic problems. Likewise, slightly diminished general cognitive ability (SL) predicts mild cross-subject academic problems. Logically, then, having average or above-average ability must be an advantage for school learning. Indeed, students with IQ scores above 90 encounter academic failure at rates less than those with lower scores. Nonetheless, parents (especially fathers) sometimes contend that their children (often their sons) suffer school learning problems because they are bright. The line of reasoning is that the student catches on so quickly and absorbs material so well that he becomes bored by the curriculumÆs mundane nature. His gifted or near-gifted ability becomes a burden in the face of tedious work demands. Thus, work incompletion (i.e., a performance problem) is blamed on high IQ. Sometimes these same students also fail to acquire skills in reading, mathematics, or written expression; parents may similarly attribute this fact (a skill deficit) to high IQ status. If high IQ is a disadvantage in this way, this fact might be supported by evidence of a curvilinear relationship between IQ and achievement (i.e., increasing IQ predicts increasing achievement, but only up to a point at which further IQ increases predict declining achievement). Other evidence might be higher rates of attention problems or failure to complete work among students with high as compared to average IQ scores. We know of no empirical research that supports either of these contentions. When individual students suspected of high IQ–related attention problems are actually evaluated, in our experience they are often found to suffer genuine performance problems (e.g., ADHD) or narrow processing problems (e.g., GU). Often, their IQ scores are surprisingly close to average. At other times these students are the subject of poor teaching practices. Obviously, a complete evaluation is needed to identify (or rule out) any of these problems. Without such an evaluation, parents may resist abandoning their belief that unrecognized giftedness is the root of their child's school problems.

---

are typically equally developed or crystallized skills may be more advanced than fluid. Both, however, generally fall within the average range. So do scores on measures of information processing known to expose the underpinning of true SLD (e.g., phonological processing, memory, and visual–motor integration). Basic academic achievement (e.g., basic reading, spelling, computational mathematics) scores are equivalent and sometimes superior to measured abilities. Although still adequately developed, more conceptually demanding areas, such as reading comprehension or narrative writing, may be relatively less developed than students' skills in more rote school subjects. In sum, the psychometric pattern of these students is usually remarkably unexceptional.

Group-administered achievement tests are another source of data that should be considered as part of any comprehensive evaluation. For students with AEM, examining the results of group-administered achievement testing is particularly fruitful, especially if both national and local norms are provided. Students with AEM typically express average (and occasionally above-average) scores when national norms are considered, but low-average (or lower) scores when local norms are considered. In light of such evidence, and barring other referral concerns, a comprehensive evaluation may not be required. In other words, if a comprehensive history is collected, a group achievement local–national norm discrepancy is evident, then the school psychologist (or team) may suggest that no comprehensive evaluation is needed. Of course, many parents are insistent on a comprehensive evaluation if their child is earning low grades. As a result, a full evaluation may be indicated to convince parents that a serious undetected problem is not lurking and to set the stage for intervention planning.

Other Possibilities

A comprehensive evaluation can easily rule out competing explanations for low grades. Remember, for this learning pattern to be pinpointed, the student's profile must be marked by at least average performance across cognitive abilities and academic achievement as measured by individually administered tests. Such scores quickly rule out the presence of other IQ-related disorders (e.g., MiMR or SL) and learning disabilities attributable to narrow-band deficits (see Chapter 3). Ruling out a performance-based disorder like ADHD or an emotional disorder can be more difficult (see Chapter 4). Behavior rating scales from parents and teachers are generally needed in these situations. If an internalizing disorder is suspected, a thorough clinical interview of the child is also typically needed. Practically speaking, when a performance-based or emotional disorder is present, the primary complaint of those initiating the referral often includes inattention, work incompletion, or emotional dysregulation, in addition to academic failure. If conspicuous emotional and ADHD-related problems are confirmed during the course of the evaluation, the prospect of AEM mismatch is discounted. The presence of any of these conditions, however, does not conclusively rule out AEM. Emotional problems may be a consequence of longstanding frustration arising from the dynamics of AEM. Some students endure both AEM and a coexisting psychiatric disorder. Although children with AEM may experience a degree of discouragement and demoralization as a result of perceived school failure, depression is not considered the cause of these children's problems.

Eligibility Issues

If a student possesses cognitive abilities within normal limits, is free from narrow-band processing deficits and emotional problems, and can demonstrate academic skills commensurate to national standards (e.g., on a group achievement test), special education services clearly are not justified. Instead, interventions like the ones described in the SL section might be tried to help the student perform better. Concomitantly, parents and the student may be encouraged to avoid overreaction. One cautionary note is offered. With the reauthorization of IDEA, there is likely to be a greater emphasis on students' resistance to intervention as evidence that special education services are warranted. Although emphasizing poor response to intervention has a role in identifying students with SLD, singular focus on lack of responsiveness to intervention can be risky when a student with AEM is present.

Consider a 10-year-old girl referred to a student study team at a high-achieving school because her reading skills are lagging behind those of her classmates. As a first step, the team suggested additional tutoring and participation in a phonics-based remedial reading program. Although this intensive intervention caused her oral reading skills to improve, she continued to trail her classmates. Based on data documenting that she remains behind peers on curriculum-based measures and that her rate of skill acquisition is poorer than her classmates, some teams might conclude that she is entitled to special education services. Specifically, she might be deemed eligible for services in the SLD category as having demonstrated resistance to intervention and an academic discrepancy from peers. Such a conclusion is made more likely if both her parents and her current teacher insist that she is an outlier, has failed to respond, and can be adequately served only by the provision of special education services. However, through a comprehensive evaluation, it may be discovered that this student is of average ability, possesses adequate reading skills compared to the national normative sample, and performs in the classroom commensurate with her scores on standardized tests. This additional evaluation data would speak against SLD eligibility. For this reason, we advocate the use of academic assessment methods that allow for comparison against a national sample (also see Dombrowski et al., 2004). In addition to standardized, individually administered achievement tests like the WIAT-II and WJ III, national norms are also available for curriculum-based measurement technologies like AIMSweb (www.aimsweb.com).

Treatment Considerations

Parent–student feedback sessions can serve as a key intervention for students with AEM. Many students and parents experience relief and a sense of closure when they learn a disability is not present. The degree of relief seems proportionate to the length of the parents' search for the elusive cause of their child's low grades. It is often helpful to the child's morale to emphasize that he or she performed, across evaluation activities, at expected levels for a student of his or her age. The crux of intervention in the parent conference is adjustment of parental expectations. Accordingly, it must be made clear that for this student at this time, earning B's and C's may indicate reasonable learning and reflects the student's genuine best effort. To prove successful conferences need to provide clear and thorough information to convince parents that their child is problem free. A bottom-up interpretive conference (see Chapter 6) is typically needed.

Although comprehensive evaluations indicate uniformly normal functioning, some students with AEM have relative strengths or weaknesses that can be used for intervention planning. Take, for example, a male student who performs within the average range across all assessed domains with the exception of auditory memory, where he possesses above-average skills. His strengths may be capitalized on to promote learning. Specifically, a school psychologist may recommend adjusted learning and study strategies, such as taping class lectures and listening to the tapes at home, taping himself and listening to the tapes before tests, or requesting copies of the teacher's lecture notes so that time can be spent listening rather than partially focused on writing. Although a comprehensive evaluation in the school setting may not lead to special education eligibility, data gleaned from the evaluation may nonetheless be used to help each student capitalize on his or her strengths.

Of course, it is counterproductive to suggest remedial training in information processing for students with AEM. For example, training in phonological processing is unlikely to benefit a student who already has average phonological processing skills. On the other hand, general interventions suited for all students may be attempted. For example, study skills training may be in order to maximize the student's learning potential. Likewise, additional tutoring, and peer tutoring in particular, may be worth a try. We have encountered, unfortunately, parents who are determined to raise their child to the level of his or her classmates through seemingly endless repetition, drill, and tutoring. Often, this eventually takes a toll on a student's self-esteem and motivation to learn. Humane revision of parental expectations is the antidote to misguided and excessive drill.

For adolescents, guidance counselors can help students with AEM carefully select classes that capitalize on strengths and identify teachers who best match the student's learning style. Classes in which teachers award grades according to predetermined criteria, for example, may be well suited to students with AEM. Criterion-referenced tests (and grading standards) sometimes equal the playing field for these children because learning expectations are predetermined, and the individual child's performance is judged against that standard. In contrast, teachers who grade on a curve may inadvertently foster the perception that a disability is present and may need to be avoided.

SUMMARY

The information presented in this chapter suggests that using measures of general ability (IQ tests) is important in applied settings. School psychologists are likely to encounter many students whose problems (real or perceived) can be illuminated only by understanding their general ability status. Debate has swirled about whether ability assessments should focus primarily on overall capability with little emphasis on subtest patterns and intraindividual differences (e.g., Watkins, 2000; Watkins & Glutting, 2000) or on more narrow information processing skills (e.g., Schrank et al., 2002). It can be argued that this division is too simplistic and that compelling diagnosticians to think either about students' general ability or about their profile of strengths and weaknesses is too conceptually confining. In reality, it appears that a substantial group of students encounters difficulty with their overall levels of ability compared to peers. In cases where such general deficits may be at issue, it is imperative that psychologists use the best measures of *g* available to them.

Accordingly, in our clinic settings, the WISC-IV or WAIS-III is almost always used. This use is predicated on the notion that it is misguided to rely exclusively on instruments whose expressed purpose is to parse intellectual abilities into subabilities so that intraindividual differences can be detected (WJ III; Cognitive Assessment System [CAS], Naglieri, 1997; Kaufman Assessment Battery for Children–Second Edition [KABC-II]). One of the first steps in the comprehensive assessment of school-age children is to rule out general cognitive deficits as a factor (see Figure 1.1/5.1). This can be done only by appraising each child's general cognitive functioning. Subsequently, important (essential) information about processing weakness and strengths can be sought. Even here, however, narrow information-processing deficits can be understood only in light of each child's broad intellectual status. Leaving out assessment of *g* impairs our capability to understand, predict, and influence the development of students that we are committed to help.

CHAPTER 3

♦ ♦ ♦

Information-Processing-Related Conditions

♦

Unlike the children described in Chapter 2, these children possess IQs commensurate with their classmates. Their problems derive from narrow deficits in information-processing abilities rather than low IQ compared to classmates. Most are plagued by an inability to develop academic skills proportionate to their general cognitive ability. Most also have trouble with some, rather than all, academic subjects. Thus, intraindividual differences rather than interindividual differences characterize these children. Their ability configuration tends to be uneven, and it is the nature and depth of the low points of their irregular development (viz., deficits) that predict classroom problems.

Many children described in this chapter meet the legal criteria for SLD. It is essential to remember, however, that the SLD designation is an administrative rather than a clinical one. For administrative reasons, it is important to determine whether the students described in this chapter meet criteria for special services. For clinical reasons it is important to determine what underlies their problems. The conditions described in this chapter, in contrast to the SLD classification, are relatively homogeneous clinical entities. As such, each provides enhanced potential to understand how school functioning might be affected and to make adjustments to optimize success.

As we work with teams, it is important for psychologists to indicate the potential educational impact associated with conditions contained here. In this sense, the conditions outlined in this chapter represent information-processing problems that may interfere with academic skill acquisition; they may also disrupt classroom functioning. It is helpful in planning for students to make clear that a condition like an SLI, for example, jeopardizes all language arts subjects and threatens the ability to follow spoken directions. Special education and related services may be warranted, but a determination of eligibility and an accompanying need for services occurs in a legally prescribed set of procedures apart from the type of evaluations discussed here.

SPECIFIC LANGUAGE IMPAIRMENT

Criteria for Specific Language Impairment

1. WISC-IV VCI < PRI
2. Typically has at least two of the following: (1) linguistic milestones more delayed than motoric; (2) reading, spelling, or written expression scores < computational arithmetic score at statistically significant level; (3) parent or teacher reports of problems with understanding directions and/or expressing self; (4) parent or teacher reports of conversational skills less developed than age-mates'.
3. The language problems are not due primarily to sensory (hearing) or bilingualism.
4. May have coexisting phonological reading disorder.

Common Presentation of Specific Language Impairment

Frequent concern of teacher at time of referral	"Poor reader; doesn't understand directions; doesn't talk as well as others"
Typical grade of referral	Elementary grades
Gender ratio	More boys than girls
Prevalence in referred sample	Common

Note. Estimates from clinic setting.

Manifestations

Students with limited ability to understand and speak their native language and to communicate effectively with classmates are apt to struggle in school, even when their nonverbal abilities are adequate. Language's pivotal status in learning failure was codified when the U.S. government defined SLD as "a disorder in one or more of the basic psychological processes involved *in understanding or using language*" (IDEA, 1997). Instruction in school is inextricably tied to presentation of verbal material through auditory means. For students in general, verbal abilities are strongly correlated with school grades and teachers' ratings of performance; this is especially true for success in reading comprehension (Flanagan, 2000).

Two types of language problems that can affect students' classroom functioning are often cited. DSM-IV-TR distinguishes children with limitations in understanding spoken language (receptive problem) from those who struggle to speak or express themselves verbally (expressive problem). At school, children with receptive language delays often appear confused and unable to follow directions, especially those with multiple steps. On the other side, children with expressive language deficits often have poor word choice, small vocabulary, inappropriate grammar and syntax, and an inability effectively to explain themselves in general. Children with either problem may reveal themselves in underdeveloped reading comprehension and written expression skills in class. Not surprisingly, many students have generalized language problems characterized by both problems in understanding *and* expressing, as well as limitations on vocabulary size, language concepts, and language-based knowledge, such as appreciation of current events. Of course, in the larger population of students, it is common for children to have relatively well-developed receptive language skills in comparison to expressive language skills. This pattern follows the maturation of language skills from infancy, as receptive language skills develop more quickly than expressive skills.

When general language deficits are present, and nonverbal deficits are not, specific language impairment (SLI) is the preferred terminology (Schuele, 2004). Children with SLI are a heterogeneous group and do not all display the same deficits. That is, children with SLI may display degrees of impairment in phonology, morphology, syntax, semantics, and pragmatics (Botting & Conti-Ramsden, 2004), as well as underlying skills like productive vocabulary, rapid naming, and verbal memory (Morris et al., 1998) that are related to disabled reading (Mann, 2003). Deficits in these critical areas can cause reading and writing and math dysfunction, as well as impaired communication. As they learn to read for meaning, children with SLI often experience problems understanding the literal meaning of passages and additional trouble with inferential comprehension of text; they are similarly constrained in the use of context clues to help decoding (Bishop & Snowling, 2004). The association of SLI and poor reading shows up, for example, in high rates of comorbid reading problems among elementary students with SLI (41.8% among second graders and 35.9% among fourth graders; Catts, Fey, & Tomblin, 2002).

Many experts argue that most children with SLI do not simply display delayed language skills, but dysfunctional language skills. The term "delayed" implies a late beginning with normal development from that point forward (Leonard, 1998). Instead, children with SLI are characterized by a late start and a slower than expected rate of subsequent language development (Leonard, 1998). Additionally, along the way, abnormal error patterns and profiles of language skills are generally present. Furthermore, children with SLI often suffer language deficits into adulthood (Young, et al., 2002), and, for that reason, many children with SLI cannot be considered delayed because they never actually attained a level of mastery (or caught up).

There is an interesting relationship between phonological deficits and general verbal problems regarding the process of learning to read. As is seen in the section regarding PRD, the sound or phonology aspect of language is crucial to early reading success because it supports word decoding and oral reading. However, general language competency, especially related to vocabulary and understanding (semantics), is essential to reading comprehension (Jitendra, Edwards, Sacks, & Jacobson, 2004; Snow, 2002). Accordingly, research confirms that both phonological awareness and general verbal abilities are related to the development of children's reading skills (Lewis, Freebairn, & Taylor, 2000; Lewis, Freebairn, & Taylor, 2002; Morris et al., 1998; Poe, Burchinal, & Roberts, 2004; Schuele, 2004).

Nonetheless, debate continues regarding the extent to which phonological knowledge and general language skills each contribute to reading difficulties. When the role of each was examined in high-risk children from pre-K through second grade, it appeared that general language skills better predicted reading achievement (including reading comprehension; Poe et al., 2004) than phonological knowledge. Other studies (Lewis et al., 2000, 2002) have shown that children with generalized language weakness in addition to a phonological disorder are at much greater risk for word reading, reading comprehension, and spelling disorders. For example, word reading, reading comprehension, and spelling disorders were present in 4%, 4%, and 30% of the children with phonological disorders, respectively, compared to 46%, 25%, and 55% of the children with phonological and language disorders. In short, a body of research indicates that SLI is related to greater difficulties in language-based academic skills areas than a phonological disorder alone (Jitendra et al., 2004; Snow, 2002).

Although for clinical utility we address the notion of global language problems here, literature supports the existence of various subtypes of language-related learning disabilities. For example, Morris et al. (1998) conducted a statistically sophisticated study to identify precise subtypes of reading disabilities. Cluster analysis yielded seven subtypes, all of which involved phonological awareness deficits. However, two subtypes were characterized by global language deficiencies. Furthermore, four more sub-types were marked not only by poor phonological awareness but also by deficits in rapid naming and verbal short-term memory. Comprehensive evaluations of students with learning problems, especially if reading and spelling deficits are present, should include assessment of language skills.

Children with SLI often, but not always, are noted by parents to speak later and to be less interested in communication than their peers. This is especially true if no other family members experienced language problems and if the child's primary cultural and family group values communication and language skills. For some children, however, concerns arise only after they start formal schooling, such as at the beginning of kindergarten. For a few, especially if they learned to read adequately during the primary grades, SLI may be unnoticed until the demands to understand unfamiliar concepts, such as in science and social studies, appear during the later elementary years or junior high school.

Regardless of how fluently a student reads orally, reading comprehension depends on vocabulary, linguistic conceptual development, and one's store of crystallized knowledge. Without these general verbal skills, some students during the primary grades become effective "word callers," only later to encounter noteworthy problems with reading comprehension. This is especially true when junior high or high school students must read and understand material from several subject matters each night. Consider how difficult a passage from a biology text might be for a student with limited language skills and few background science ideas. A child with SLI may be able to decode the word "cardiac" (due to one-to-one letter–sound corre-spondence) in the text but have no idea what the word means or that it refers to the human heart. This student similarly would be at risk for prob-lems on writing assignments that call for elaboration of ideas or sophisti-cated and clear expression. Writing samples taken from students with SLI often are directly stated but sparse and simplistic. Obviously, teacher and parents benefit by appreciating that such limited written output may have less to do with laziness than limited vocabulary and a dearth of language concepts to write about.

Beyond basic literacy, children with SLI risk other problems at school. If teachers' instructions are spoken quickly or contain even moderately sophisticated words and ideas, then direction following may be con-strained, assignments may be started incorrectly, and learning opportuni-ties may be missed. Class discussions are often hard to follow. Oral reports or participation in classroom discussion can be embarrassing. Such stu-dents often live in fear of extemporaneous speaking, and they may find ways to avoid being called on to participate in class.

Likewise, social interaction can be affected as some children with SLI also suffer deficits in pragmatic language (i.e., use of language in a social context, such as a conversation; Bishop, 2000). This is important because even young children establish and maintain relations with peers through verbal exchange that depends upon (although it is not limited to) possessing adequate understanding of words and their meanings. Language competence is even more crucial for socialization among middle school and older students as conversation over a mutually engaged activity (e.g., games) plays a central role in interactions. Characteristics of pragmatic language impairment seen in some children with SLI are verbosity, comprehension deficits, trouble finding words, unusual word choices, poor conversational skills, talking to no one in particular, poor topic maintenance, and irrelevant responses to questions (Rapin, 1996). Reviews of the literature have also identified poor prosody and misinterpretation of nonverbal cues, such as gestures and facial expressions (Bishop, 2000), as characteristics. As a result, children with SLI and coexisting pragmatic language deficits may find it hard to hold conversations with classmates, and they may struggle to make friends (Van Balkom & Verhoeven, 2004). Children with SLI often display poor social skills, appear socially awkward, and seem generally out of step, but even more worrisome, they may also suffer diminished self-esteem and ultimately encounter demoralization or even frank depression (American Academy of Child and Adolescent Psychiatry, 1998a). Even as preschoolers, children with SLI have problems with assertiveness and frustration tolerance and tend to be dependent and isolated in the classroom (McCabe, 2005). Indeed, studies working in complementary directions document the same strong association. A review of 26 studies found that 71% of children with emotional-behavioral diagnoses suffered significant language deficits, and 57% of children with language deficits were diagnosed with coexisting emotional-behavioral disorders (Benner, Nelson, & Epstein, 2002).

Assessment Considerations

As is true for all the clinical conditions listed in this chapter, an early step in assessment is to rule out general cognitive delays (i.e., low IQ). To accomplish this, the practitioner should use Figure 1.1/5.1. For children in the SLI category in particular, an instrument that measures nonverbal reasoning and problem solving is required. Among the very first patterns to be affirmed as associated with school failure and SLI was lower WISC-IV VCI than PRI (on the preceding WISC versions Verbal IQ lower than Performing IQ). It is almost always true that composite IQ scores, such as the Wechsler Full Scale IQ (FSIQ) score, underestimate the capability of these children because composite IQ scores are computed by averaging the child's performance on tasks that are vulnerable to the disability (in this case language) with his or her intact functioning (in this case nonverbal reasoning). Consider the subtests that make up the WISC-IV Verbal Comprehension Index: measures of language-related knowledge, conceptual abilities, vocabulary skills, and lexical capabilities. All are assessed via verbal questions and answers. Children with SLI produce low overall scores across these subtests. These children, compared to their classmates, know fewer facts, struggle to discern relationships among language concepts, problem-solve more slowly and inefficiently when presented with verbal tasks, and fail to appreciate meaning and interrelationship of words and categories of concepts. In contrast, the WISC-IV PRI taps visual–spatial analysis, judgment, and reasoning abilities, and it imposes few overt language demands. As a result, the thinking ability of children with SLI is apparent without the contaminating influences of verbal tasks.

To adopt the PRI over FSIQ or GAI, a statistically significant discrepancy between the child's verbal and nonverbal abilities must be uncovered. If this is so, standard practice is that the higher of the two scores can be used as the best estimate of ability (Sattler, 2001). However, diagnosticians must follow standard psychometric rules to assure that verbal/nonverbal differences are statistically reliable before adopting the nonverbal score as a better indication of cognitive functioning.

After it is clear that the child has adequate nonverbal capability (i.e., MiMR and SL problems are ruled out), the scope and severity of language problems are explored. Initial evaluation of language is often undertaken by a school psychologist; however, the assistance of a speech–language pathologist may be ultimately necessary, especially if speech and language therapy services are to be considered. A detailed examination of language skills typically involves assessing the child's receptive and expressive skills. Receptive language can be informally assessed in the classroom by noting requests for repetition and poor direction following (assuming that the child is paying adequate attention). Informal assessment of expressive language in the classroom includes observation of limited output and trouble explaining oneself (i.e., restricted quality and quantity of speech). Psychometric techniques are also available. Some instruments that assess language skills, such as the Clinical Evaluation of Language Fundamentals–4th Edition (CELF-4; Semel, Wiig, & Secord, 2003), are almost exclusively administered by speech–language pathologists. This test aims to measure expressive and receptive language, language structure, content, and memory, as well as phonological awareness, rapid naming, sequences, and word associations. A school psychologist's primary task is to identify patterns outlined in this book so that plans can be made; more fine-grained language assessment is not addressed here. The following discussion concerns instruments often administered by psychologists to help confirm SLI.

As supplements to the WISC-IV, first consider instruments designed to assess receptive language and direction following. A classic example is the Peabody Picture Vocabulary Test–Third Edition (PPVT-III; Dunn & Dunn, 1997), an instrument designed to tap receptive vocabulary by asking a child to point at which of four pictures matches a vocabulary word spoken by the examiner. Another means to assess receptive language requires that simple directions be followed. The Comprehension of Instructions subtest of the NEPSY (closely related to the Token Test) requires the examinee to point to different designs (which vary in color and shape) in a particular sequence. We have occasionally identified children with receptive language deficits who had good expressive skills using these instruments. More often, these instruments have confirmed that an apparent general SLI is not, in fact, a mere expressive problem. That is, when a child with low VCI is unable to score well on the PPVT-III, his language weakness is unlikely to be confined to problems with verbal output. A low score on the PPVT-III, thus, can substantiate that both expressive and a receptive problems are present in a constellation of deficits that is best characterized simply as SLI.

Expressive language tests are equally plentiful for school psychologists. A simple index of vocabulary (expressive) can be obtained from the Expressive Vocabulary Test (EVT; Williams, 1997), which requires the child to express a word that matches a picture card. A similar option is available on the WJ III Picture Vocabulary subtest. Expression is also measured via a test of fluency (e.g., NEPSY Word Fluency), which requires the child to produce as many words as possible that belong to a specified category (or begin with a certain letter). Another option is a test of speeded naming (e.g., NEPSY Speeded Naming). Although it taps expression, Word Fluency also requires planning and maintenance of a response set (executive functions). Speed Naming requires rapid access of lexical and phonemic material, rather than vocabulary knowledge. Other vehicles for detecting expressive language deficits are the WISC-IV and the WISC-IV Integrated. When the WISC-IV is supplemented with the WISC-IV Integrated, it is possible to determine if poor performance on verbal subtests, like Vocabulary or Information, is due to poor general knowledge or expressive language difficulties. The WISC-IV Integrated offers supplemental multiple-choice or picture formats for these subtests for Vocabulary and Information. When standard scores for the conventional Vocabulary or Information subtests are compared with their WISC-IV Integrated counterparts, and the former only are poor, an expressive problem may exist. If the child performs equally poorly on standard and supplemental subtests, a global language problem, and not an expressive problem alone, is presumably present. On the other hand, superiority on standard WISC-IV subtests, which require more spoken answers, implies a language problem's basis may be relatively receptive in nature.

If an SLI is present, low scores on measures of verbal memory may also be uncovered. Research has related verbal short-term memory deficits to reading disability in particular (Morris et al., 1998). Verbal memory is typically assessed by orally presenting a long list of words to recall (e.g., California Verbal Learning Test—Children's Version [CVLT-C], NEPSY List Learning), sentences to repeat (NEPSY Repetition of Sentences), and/or stories to retell (e.g., NEPSY Narrative Memory, Wide Range Assessment of Memory and Learning–2 [WRAML-2] Stories). After a trial(s) of independent recall, many instruments also provide a recognition trial(s) in which the child receives cues (e.g., responding "yes" or "no" if a word was on a list, or pointing to choices rather than verbatim recall). If the child is able to perform adequately with cues or can recognize but not recall, adequate memory encoding presumably took place. The underpinning of poor performance in these instances may be limited ability to retrieve, a paucity of strategies, or faulty attention. Of course, low scores on memory tests that use words or stories often arise from simple general language weakness for children with SLI. Individual diagnosticians, or diagnostic teams, must decide how much detail to include in their linguistic evaluations. For many students, simple recognition of SLI's presence is sufficient to permit formulation of an effective intervention plan.

Other Possibilities

Although general verbal weakness occurs in isolation, it may also be present as part of other developmental disorders (e.g., MiMR or autistic spectrum disorder), neurological disease, or significant hearing loss. The evaluation process, including review of health history and audiometric screening, can rule out the presence of a greater medical concern (e.g., a developmental syndrome or a chronic health condition). For preschoolers, it is sometimes difficult to determine if speech delays exist in isolation or within the context of greater developmental delay. Because the preschool years are a time of rapid development, it can be challenging to predict if a delay is destined to become a chronic deficit or will be subject to a sudden developmental spurt. Still, if a child has obvious speech and language delays, and especially if adaptive deficits coexist, regardless of age, the prospect of mental retardation needs to be eliminated. As referenced in Chapter 2, mental retardation involves global delays in areas beyond language, specifically general cognitive ability and adaptive behavior. On the other hand, general language delays are sometimes attributed to poor classroom attention (such as when a student who cannot follow directions is held to be "inattentive") or to social skills deficits (such as when a student lacks the basic language skills necessary for reciprocal interaction). Figure 1.1/5.1 assists school psychologists in determining if the referral concerns are due to a language deficit in isolation (SLI), a more pervasive developmental disability (e.g., mental retardation), or some other condition.

Speech and language delays are also hallmarks of autism and related disorders. As will be reviewed later (see Table 3.6, p. 102), autistic-spectrum disorders are marked by significant delays in social interaction, communication skills, and atypical behavior (e.g., preoccupations, marked inflexibility, stereotyped behaviors, and fascination with parts of objects). Some children with SLI may display deficits in social interaction and communication due to disordered language skills, but they typically do not engage in behaviors reminiscent of an autistic spectrum disorder. Furthermore, children with SLI alone have normal interests in social interaction. If atypical behavior is present to the extent that it is the focus of clinical attention, disorders beyond SLI should be considered.

Finally, SLI (and learning disorders generally) can co-occur with and be mistaken for a variety of developmental disabilities and genetic and psychiatric conditions. Possibilities besides mental retardation are disorders of motor skills, ADHD, mood disorders, anxiety disorders, and medical/neurological conditions like fetal alcohol and fragile X syndrome (American Academy of Child and Adolescent Psychiatry, 1998a). The flowchart presented as Figure 1.1/5.1 should help school psychologists rule out conditions such as these and help assure that SLI is present. Nonetheless, familiarity with DSM-IV-TR and other user-friendly medical resources (see Chapter 1) may also be required.

Eligibility Issues

Two special education categories have traditionally served students with SLI. The category most familiar to school psychologists is SLD. Before reauthorization of IDEA in December 2004, most states required a significant discrepancy between the best estimate of a student's cognitive abilities and his or her performance on an individually administered achievement test, along with demonstrated academic need, to qualify for special education support. If using the discrepancy model for a student with SLI, the best estimate of cognitive abilities is typically performance on a nonverbal ability measure (e.g., WISC-IV PRI). Subsequent to determining cognitive ability, the next step would be comparison of ability and achievement, especially scores on individual achievement tests. The student would be considered to have an SLD if any one of seven achievement areas (oral expression, listening comprehension, written expression, basic reading skill, reading comprehension, mathematics calculation, and mathematics reasoning) is significantly discrepant from ability and educational need exists (plus emotional, sensory, motor, and significant experiential factors are eliminated). An alternative method might be used after the reauthorization of IDEA. Using such a procedure, most children with SLI would receive intensive language and reading treatment during an intervention period, those who failed to respond might then be deemed eligible for special education services.

Like those with PRD, children with SLI commonly experience oral reading deficits. Unlike children with PRD alone, children with SLI have general language deficits that often manifest in compromised reading comprehension, written expression, listening comprehension, and oral expression skills, all of which have historically been considered as potential areas of underachievement suitable for SLD documentation. Therefore, children with SLI may qualify for SLD special education services. In our experience, school-based teams feel most comfortable identifying SLD in the core academic areas of basic reading, reading comprehension, and written expression, while leaving evaluation directly related to language functioning to speech–language pathologists. It is for that reason, we believe, that the areas of listening comprehension and oral expression SLD historically have been underutilized in student identification. Assigning listening comprehension and oral expression SLD status is beneficial for many students in that the nature of the disorder (e.g., expressive language disorder) is directly related to difficulty learning in class. In other words, an SLD designation often refocuses the IEP team on classroom manifestations of SLI.

A child with SLI may also qualify for special education services under the IDEA category of speech and language impairment (see Table 3.1 for the IDEA definition). School psychologists may provide valuable data to be included when making an eligibility determination under this category. However, a speech–language pathologist is almost always responsible for conducting the in-depth evaluation needed to authorize services in this area.

Treatment Considerations

If a student with SLI is eligible for speech and language therapy services, a speech–language pathologist probably will be the primary provider of services (Owens, 2004). However, not all students with SLI receive school-

TABLE 3.1. Individuals with Disabilities Education Act Definition of Speech or Language Impairment

Speech or language impairment means a communication disorder such as stuttering, impaired articulation, a language impairment, or voice impairment that adversely affects a child's educational performance.

Note. From *Federal Register* (1999).

based speech and language therapy services. Those for whom SLI causes reading and spelling problems may work with a resource special education teacher, not a speech–language pathologist. Some students will work with both. We reviewed the literature for techniques commonly employed by speech–language pathologists so that information could be shared with school psychologists, educators, and parents. Especially useful are two literature reviews that outline interventions with empirical support to develop vocabulary skills and general verbal skills of children with SLI. Given their complexity, the two sources themselves may need to be reviewed by interested readers.

Jitendra et al. (2004) outlined five general techniques to improve vocabulary of students with learning disabilities. However, they indicated that research does not yet support any specific method (over direct instruction). Mnemonic strategies, such as presenting a new vocabulary word and linking it with a visual image, have been shown to aid vocabulary development. So has cognitive strategy instruction. Cognitive strategy instruction involves activities such as mapping out interrelated concepts, predicting relationships between new and previously acquired knowledge, attempting to define unknown words from reading passages, and engaging in cloze activities using concept maps. Direct instruction is well known to psychologists and teachers alike. This method comprises teacher-guided presentation of vocabulary words and their meanings and checking to assure understanding. The constant time delay technique is characterized by an instructor presenting a vocabulary word and then immediately offering its definition. The instructor then presents the vocabulary word, and waits a pre-established amount of time (i.e., a few seconds) before asking the student to recount the definition. If an incorrect definition is given, the instructor repeats the word and once again states the correct definition. Finally, activity-based methods also target vocabulary development. This method requires students to be engaged in concrete, hands-on learning tasks that incorporate new vocabulary words. For example, for the word "malleable," the teacher might provide modeling clay as the definition of malleable is discussed.

Other reviews also concern intervention approaches commonly used to treat children with SLI. Leonard (1998) summarized six approaches to treat children with SLI; again, the original source should be consulted for details. Like Jitendra et al. (2004), Leonard suggested that clearly preferred methods of intervention have not yet been established by empirical research. Imitation-based approaches are characterized by the therapist or teacher producing an utterance, or demonstrating a skill, and then requiring the student to reproduce *exactly* what was said or done. Modeling techniques require the student to observe a model producing an utterance or speaking in a certain manner; the student is then prompted to produce a different utterance that displays the target behavior. Leonard explains that the rationale for this method is that the problem solving necessary for the student to generate (not exactly imitate) an appropriate utterance is therapeutically valuable. In both of the previous two treatments, the child's attention is drawn to what the model is demonstrating. Focused stimulation as a treatment approach differs from imitation-based methods as the child's attention is not drawn to the purpose of intervention. Rather, targets of intervention are embedded within activities (e.g., stories or play). For example, a story is read that repeatedly uses a new vocabulary word. Milieu teaching primarily occurs in play situations where the child is free to select an activity and the therapist or teacher responds when a target behavior is demonstrated. For example, the therapist might only respond when the child provides eye contact. Conversational recasting strategies also typically occur during the course of natural activities. When the child engages the therapist or teacher, he or she responds to the child by demonstrating target behavior. For example, if a target of treatment is using the word *I*, the therapist might respond to the child with an utterance like, "Yes. *I* would like a drink." Of note, data exist to demonstrate that emphatic stress on a target word leads to enhanced vocabulary development (Weismer, 1997). Finally, the expansion approach involves others responding to a child's brief utterance (e.g., "Mommy up") with a more complete utterance (e.g., "Mom, will you pick me up? Yes, I will.").

In sum, interventions that engage children in activities (naturally occurring or contrived) appear to be effective in developing language skills for children with SLI, including expanding vocabulary size. As stated earlier, mnemonic strategies have been shown to develop further the vocabularies of children with SLI. It appears the same is true for receptive language skills. For example, Gill, Klecan-Aker, Roberts, and Fredenburg (2003) studied the ability of children with SLI to follow directions before and after treatment. Three treatment groups comprised children who were taught rehearsal strategies, children taught rehearsal and visualization strategies, and children receiving traditional therapy alone. Children in the visualization condition were trained to visualize that they were performing an action as the therapist stated instructions. Results demonstrated that children who received rehearsal training and rehearsal/visualization instruction outperformed children in the traditional therapy group. Additionally, 8 months after treatment, the rehearsal/visualization group maintained their advantage over the traditional therapy group.

Perhaps the greatest challenge to language intervention for students with SLI is ensuring the generalization of treatment gains (Owens, 2004). The functional approach to language intervention, as proposed by Owens, involves engaging students in treatment activities that directly transfer to classroom and community settings. Owens proposes that treatment should also occur within the context in which the problem arises to assure the greatest chance of generalization. For example, vocabulary building exercises might be devised that would develop a student's ability to follow classroom directions, ask questions and check for understanding when confused, participate in classroom discussions, or socialize with peers.

To this point, the interventions discussed are more apt to be used by speech–language specialists, and perhaps parents after training, than teachers. Although many of these methods may help resource teachers bolster the language of their students with SLI, and thus improve general academic and social functioning, additional strategies are nonetheless available that target reading comprehension. One such example is from Blachowicz and Ogle (2001), who outlined reading comprehension interventions usable by classroom teachers. Acknowledging that word exposure and knowledge is key to reading for meaning, these authors suggested several routine classroom activities. These include repeated readings and words on walls, to provide extensive exposure to words, as well as word games that actively engage students in learning. Examples of word games include matching word cards by synonyms, matching word card memory games, word bingo, 20 questions, or a word of the day.

Blachowicz and Ogle (2001) also suggested several strategies to help students learn and retain unknown words and concepts. For example, word logs and concept mapping require students to identify new words or concepts (or frequently misinterpreted words or concepts) and organize them visually for subsequent study. Word logs require students to divide blank paper into three columns labeled "word," "page," and "interpretation and sentence." Next, in the first two columns, students write the new word and the page number on which it is found. In the third column, students write the definition of the word or a synonym that is easily remembered, write a sentence using the word, and can even include a picture or drawing to represent the word.

Concept mapping or story mapping strategies are also suggested for children with reading comprehension difficulties (Blachowicz & Ogle, 2001). Concept mapping was also a recommended strategy for children with IQ-related disorders in Chapter 2. Concept mapping is a visual organization technique that requires students to consider a new word, determine in which category it belongs, and list related characteristics of the word, or even how this new word may be related to other words or concepts. For example, if the new word were hockey, students may discover that hockey is a sport, more specifically an ice sport. Subsequently, students would be prompted to map characteristics related to hockey, such as team sport, puck, stick, and goal. Similar to the method depicted in Figure 3.1,

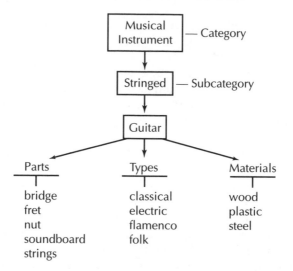

FIGURE 3.1. Diagram of a concept map for the word *guitar*. From Blachowicz and Ogle (2001, p. 183). Copyright 2001 by The Guilford Press. Reprinted by permission.

story mapping requires students visually to organize information learned in a story for later study. As an example, a map of a fictional story might include the location of the story, its time period, characters and their ages, and relationships among characters. A story map for nonfiction material might include much more detail in terms of timeline and factual information.

Because reading problems often accompany SLI, generalization of language training gains to actual reading is a critical issue. There is some evidence that spoken language training transfers to reading skills. For example, Gillon and Dodd (1995) followed a small group of disabled readers, who as a group had relative language delays, over several years of standard reading intervention, followed by language intervention addressing semantic and syntactic processing and language intervention addressing phonological processing. The semantic and syntactic processing portion of training consisted of assistance from a speech–language pathologist regarding formulating, reducing, combining, and expanding sentences orally and enhancing vocabulary via oral drills. Phonological process training involved elements of the Auditory Discrimination in Depth program (addressed in the PRD section of this chapter). Crucially to students with SLI and reading problems, children, then ages 8–13 years, showed statistically significant acceleration in both reading accuracy (1.6 years) and reading comprehension (2 years) during a 6-

month semantic and syntactic training interval. Some children, such as those suffering extreme problems with word identification (and coexisting phonological processing problems), however, experienced relatively little growth in reading comprehension from oral language instruction (without additional assistance in phonological processing). Thus, it appears that for some children with severe reading problems, development of both general language abilities and specific phonological processing skills may be needed to permit reading improvement (see the next section in this book). Crucially, children with SLI alone benefit greatly from direct language instruction.

Aside from activities specifically designed to improve the language of children with SLI, interventions presented in Chapter 2 should also be considered. As an example, a PALS program whereby students are engaged in explicit instruction, as well as peer-assisted learning, makes a great deal of sense when language problems constrain academic progress. Furthermore, assistive technology tools are available to students with SLI and reading difficulties. Computer software (e.g., Kurzweil 3000) has been developed that allows students to scan text into a computer and easily access definitions of unknown words, thereby improving comprehension of classroom material. Unfortunately, when general language problems (SLI) are present, these techniques may be less valuable than when a student is merely a poor reader (e.g., PRD). For a case example of SLI, see the information on Brody in Chapter 5.

PHONOLOGICAL READING DISORDER

Criteria for Phonological Reading Disorder

1. Reading standard scores discrepant from IQ at statistically significant levels.
2. The following pattern found among reading subtest scores: nonsense words (e.g., WIAT-II Pseudoword Decoding; WJ III Word Attack) < words-in-isolation (e.g., WIAT-II Word Reading) < reading comprehension.
3. Low scores reaching statistically significant levels on tests that measure phonological processing (e.g., NEPSY Phonological Processing, Memory for Names, Repetition of Nonsense Words or WRAML-2 Sound Symbol subtest).
4. Developmental history that typically includes one or more of the following: (1) articulation problems during the preschool years, (2) name finding problems, (3) problems remembering verbal sequences (e.g., phone number, address, months).
5. Family history of reading and/or spelling problems.

Common Presentation of Phonological Reading Disorder	
Frequent concern of teacher at time of referral	"Reads slowly, with many mistakes; fails to sound out unknown words; poor speller"
Typical grade of referral	Kindergarten or primary grades
Gender ratio	More boys than girls
Prevalence in referred sample	Common

Note. Estimates from clinic setting.

Manifestations

Although researchers debate exactly which deficits cause reading failure, phonological awareness has been identified as the hallmark of deficient word reading, or the inability to use phonics skills to decode words (Morris et al., 1998; Shaywitz, 2003). This is a prime source of reading disability. Phonological awareness is defined as "the ability to notice, identify, and manipulate the individual sounds—phonemes—in spoken words" (Shaywitz, 2003, p. 51). Becoming a phonologically competent child in the English language is especially difficult because there are 44 identifiable phonemes, or basic sound elements. Phonemes may be represented by individual consonants (e.g., /b/ or /g/) or vowels (e.g., /a/ or /e/) with one-to-one sound to letter correspondence or by multiple letters (e.g., /sh/ or /ea/) in which each letter is not represented by an individual sound. Furthermore, sounds represented by letters are sometimes dependent on the remaining letters in a word (e.g., *mad* as compared to *made*) and are the result of unconventional letter–phoneme correspondence schemes (e.g., knight). Patterns of association between phonemes and symbols (printed text) obviously exist, but there are many exceptions to the rules for associations. These complex rules make it difficult for children with PRD to learn to read (Torgeson & Mathes, 2000; Gillon, 2004).

Overall, children with poor phonological awareness fail to recognize words rapidly and reliably by their phonic signature (Gillon, 2004). Early in reading training, most children with poor phonological awareness will encounter difficulty naming letters presented in print and producing the sounds associated with individual letters (Shaywitz, 2003). Later in training, segmenting words into separate sound elements, blending sounds to form words, and manipulating individual sounds (e.g., as in pig latin) are all difficult for children with this disorder (Torgesen & Mathes, 2000).

Efficiently learning the relationships between phonemes and letters is essential in order to become a competent reader (Share & Stanovich, 1995); without integrity in the key ability to process sounds, the child with PRD is destined to struggle and may require supplemental help.

Decoding to identify words and comprehension to derive meaning from text are both required for reading. Children with PRD alone have poor decoding skills but intact comprehension (see Shaywitz, 2003, for a review). In theory, then, if a child with pure PRD were able to decode, reading comprehension should be adequate. However, if a student is able to decode words well but lacks adequate reading comprehension, an SLI affecting overall language competency may be hypothesized (see previous section). For the same reason, the interplay of comprehension and decoding can render a student with SLI poor at both oral reading (i.e., is weak at decoding) and reading comprehension because he or she is unable to understand what is read due to limited vocabulary and general language development and may lack other language-dependent strategies (e.g., use of context to aid in decoding). Of course, a student with PRD may also be poor at both oral reading (cannot sound out unknown words) and reading comprehension (cannot decode words in a passage and thus cannot understand the passage's meaning).

Besides oral reading difficulty, other academic problems may be expected of a child with PRD. It has been known for some time that performance on word decoding and spelling are highly correlated and that phonological awareness is a skill set both share. For example, Juel, Griffith, and Gough (1986) found a .84 correlation between word reading and spelling. Many children with PRD are both poor readers and poor spellers. If severe PRD is present, spelling patterns often reflect extremely poor correspondence of sounds and symbols (e.g., *ast* for *cat*). On the other hand, less severe PRD may manifest in spelling errors that seem to be phonologically based and are discernible to most readers (e.g., *fon* for *phone*). Boder and Jarrico (1982) developed a system for recognizing dyphonetic spelling patterns more than 20 years ago that is still instructive. As noted in the previous section, however, it can be difficult to separate the impact of phonics-related deficits from SLI. Children with pure phonics-related deficits are at great risk for spelling disorder, and it appears that word decoding and reading comprehension impairment exists to the extent that SLI is also present (Lewis et al., 2000, 2002; Schuele, 2004).

Assessment Considerations

The pattern associated with PRD is most clearly seen in information-processing (i.e., phonological-processing) and academic (i.e., oral reading and spelling) tests when administered in tandem. Like all other conditions in this chapter, however, global cognitive delays must be ruled out first (see Figure 1.1/5.1). That being said, there is a body of evidence to suggest that many children with reading disabilities have lower verbal reasoning than nonverbal reasoning skills, especially as measured by the WISC-IV (i.e., VCI < PRI; Wechsler, 2003). If one is using an ability instrument other than the WISC-IV, such as the WJ III, verbal ability may be relatively low. At the subtest level, on the WJ III, one might expect a child with PRD to have greater difficulty on Verbal Comprehension, which requires verbal reasoning and judgment, as compared to Concept Formation, which requires nonverbal analysis and rule formation. When ruling out general cognitive problems, intact abilities, as reflected in high index scores, may be a fairer appraisal than composite scores (such as FSIQ), which average in low subtest scores that are negatively affected by a disabled student's processing deficits. In other words, the intellectual ability of a child with a reading problem may be better recognized by his WISC-IV PRI than by his FSIQ, which for many poor readers includes low VCI and Working Memory Index (WMI) scores.

After general cognitive weakness is ruled out, one examines performance on subtests that specifically measure phonological processing. As the Wechsler Scales and many other tests of cognitive ability (e.g., CAS; Naglieri, 1997) lack such measures, school psychologists are encouraged to add supplemental tests (or subtests) to their batteries when a referral for a reading problem is made. Measures of phonological awareness and related constructs are included in Table 3.2. These include measures of letter and sound identification, sound blending, and sound–symbol associations (e.g., NEPSY Memory for Names; WRAML-2 Sound–Symbol Subtest).

Phonological processing is tapped by at least one test able to measure general cognitive ability. Designed to measure abilities according to a specific theoretical model (the Cattell–Horn–Carroll [CHC] model), the WJ III's authors have nonetheless labeled an interpretable cluster Phonemic Awareness that involves the "ability to perceive separate units of speech sounds in order to analyze and synthesize those units" (Floyd, Shaver, & McGrew, 2003, p. 26) This is equivalent to the factor called auditory processing, or (Ga) in the CHC model. The standard battery includes two subtests that are related to phonological awareness (Sound Blending and Incomplete Words), and the extended battery includes one more (Auditory Attention). Also of potential interest, the standard battery includes a subtest called Visual–Auditory Learning that tests the child's ability to develop associations between words and symbols (a task that is in some ways analogous to learning to read).

Similarly, the NEPSY includes two subtests that directly evaluate phonological processing. The first is called Phonological Processing and

TABLE 3.2. Measures of Phonological Processing and Related Psychometric Techniques That May Be Sensitive to Phonological-Processing Deficits

- Comprehensive Test of Phonological Processing (CTOPP; Wagner, Torgesen, & Rashotte, 1999)
- Phonological Awareness Test (PAT; Robertson & Salter, 1997)
- Test of Phonological Awareness (TOPA; Torgesen & Bryant, 1994)
- Dynamic Indicators of Basic Early Literacy Skills (DIBELS, 6th ed.; Good & Kaminski, 2002)
- A Developmental Neuropsychological Assessment (NEPSY; Korkman et al., 1998)
    Phonological Processing
    Nonsense Word Repetition
    Memory for Names
- Wide Range Assessment of Memory and Learning–2 (WRAML-2; Adams & Sheslow, 2003)
    Sound–Symbol subtest
- Woodcock–Johnson III, Tests of Cognitive Abilities (WJ III; Woodcock et al., 2001)
    Phonemic Awareness
    Sound Blending
    Incomplete Words
    Visual–Auditory Learning
- Woodcock–Johnson III Tests of Achievement (WJ III; Woodcock et al., 2001)
    Letter–Word Identification
    Word Attack
- Wechsler Individual Achievement Test—Second Edition (WIAT-II; The Psychological Corporation, 2002; Wechsler, 2002)
    Word Reading
    Pseudoword Decoding

requires the child to delete a phoneme(s) from a verbally presented word, insert a new phoneme, and then state the new word. The other subtest measures the ability of the child to repeat nonsense words presented via audiotape (Repetition of Nonsense Words). The NEPSY includes a subtest (Memory for Names) that may be used to assess the child's ability to learn names (which include phonemes) associated with faces. Even though this is not a pure measure of phonological processing, if PRD is present, the child may have substandard performance. In fact, a recent study discovered that this subtest discriminated children referred for evaluation due to academic failure, especially in reading (who had mean scaled score of 6.8), from children in a control group (who had a mean scaled score of 9.9). Differences in the two groups remained even after the effect of WISC-III FSIQ was removed (Schmitt & Wodrich, 2004). In part because they can be easily administered and scored, the NEPSY subtests related to phonological processing may become increasingly popular among school psychologists.

For school psychologists seeking a more in-depth evaluation of phonological processing, test batteries to measure phonological processing have been expressly designed. Based on extensive work in this area, Wagner,

Torgesen, and Rashotte (1999) developed a 12-subtest Comprehensive Test of Phonological Processing. Besides basic phonemic awareness and sound blending, this test contains measures of auditory memory and rapid naming, which have been found to predict phonics-based oral reading deficits. Although not always necessary, in-depth measures of phonological processing can be used to confirm an underlying problem in the face of diagnostic uncertainty or to explore fully the nature of suspected phonological deficits (e.g., distinguish deficits in rapid accessing of phonemes from limited awareness of phonemes).

Patterns on achievement tests can also help document PRD. This is especially true of individual achievement tests that measure several aspects of reading. For example, both the WIAT-II and WJ III contain subtests requiring decoding of nonsense words, decoding of individual real words, and reading sentences or passages for meaning (reading comprehension). The first subtest does not allow the reader to rely on previously learned patterns of phoneme combinations or instant recognition of the printed matter as a "sight word." That is, nonsense words can be decoded only by using phonics strategies. Consequently, reading nonsense words proves extremely hard for a child with PRD as the word can only be expressed by producing sounds. Children with PRD often make extreme errors or are unable even to generate a guess. Relatively easier for the student with PRD is the task of reading single (real) words. Here, students may tap their phonics skills and their ability to recognize words from prior practice. Reading comprehension is often easiest for children with PRD because here individuals are not actually appraised for their oral reading skills, only for deriving meaning from the text.

The ability of the child with PRD to comprehend what was read is dependent, at least to some extent, on the degree to which effective decoding actually took place. Absent a general language delay or SLI, if the child is able to decode the text, he or she can understand. Reading comprehension, however, tends to be compromised to a greater extent as the complexity of the material increases or as topics become unfamiliar to the reader. This is because the child with PRD often relies on context clues to compensate for inefficient decoding skills when unsure. When the passage content is unfamiliar, context is blocked as a decoding strategy.

Diagnosticians are encouraged to use judgment as they plan the components necessary to examine each child. When the chief complaint is oral reading, and especially if the student is in elementary school, then measures of phonological processing are justified (e.g., NEPSY or WJ III). However, clues from the student's history can also help. In large-scale studies in Colorado, researchers found developmental variation strongly predictive of PRD. Among the most potent predictors were (1) articulation problems during the preschool years, (2) name-finding problems, and (3) problems remembering verbal sequences (e.g., phone number, address, months). Researchers also found a moderately heritable component for phonological-processing deficits and for the reading problems associated with them (Olson, Forsberg, Wise, & Rack, 1994; Pennington, 2002). The presence of male relatives predicted such problems in probands; a positive family history of reading and/or spelling problems was found to add to the predictive power of the problems with articulation and auditory rote memory noted above.

Other Possibilities

Of course, poor oral reading, including limited phonics competence, can occur for many reasons. Some children lack adequate engagement in reading and consequently never develop adequate skills. Others fail to receive instruction that involves teaching phonics and word attack strategies. Because general language ability is so important to oral reading, and because deficits in it can cause or contribute to poor reading (Morris et al., 1998; Schuele, 2004), care should be taken fully to investigate general language development. When several measures of language functioning are found to be low (or there is a low general language index, such as the WISC-IV VCI), and nonverbal functioning is average, general verbal delay or SLI may be present. The presence of SLI has important implications for treatment as language skills other than phonological awareness, such as vocabulary, syntax, and pragmatics, generally should be targets of intervention in such instances. Literature reviews have also suggested there is a comorbidity rate of 10–59% between ADHD and language disorders (e.g., Riccio & Hynd, 1993). Furthermore, ratings of attention significantly predict response to early reading intervention (Stage, Abbott, Jenkins, & Berninger, 2003; Torgesen et al., 1999). Accordingly, it makes sense to rule out the presence of significant attention difficulties that may hamper the acquisition of phonics and reading skills, as well undermine even a well-conceived and consistently implemented reading intervention program.

Visual–spatial and visual–perceptual deficits have long been thought to cause dyslexia or severe reading problems with a presumptive neurological basis. Research suggests that relatively few reading problems arise from such underlying difficulties (see, instead, the array of academic problems that accompany NLD in subsequent sections of this book). Nonetheless, visual–perception problems may contribute to reading and spelling failure in some students.

Eligibility Issues

As the regulations supporting changes in IDEA's definition of SLD are promulgated (which is the case as this book goes to press), school psychologists are advised to reflect on the statutory definition of SLD. Particularly pertinent is the phrase that calls SLD "a disorder in one or more of the basic psychological processes ... involved in language" and "imperfect ability to read, write, spell" (see Table 3.3). Whether some states continue to employ procedures for SLD identification that require an ability–achievement discrepancy or some other procedure, it is easy to see how many children with significant PRD would qualify for SLD services. Using the traditional ability–achievement discrepancy approach, ability is typically measured by performance on an IQ test and estimates of academic achievement are generally obtained from individually administered achievement tests. If a significant discrepancy between the best estimate of a child's intelligence and, in this case, reading skills is present, an important requirement for eligibility for SLD services is satisfied. For PRD, it is essential that reading skills be assessed fully. It has been up to the individual state to decide the method by which a severe discrepancy is identified. Some states employed a regression procedure whereby a statistically significant discrepancy between a child's actual achievement test scores and scores predicted by a child's IQ were utilized. Other states used a simple difference method where the discrepancy between ability and achievement measures is determined by a preestablished number of standard scores, or standard deviations, between the two values. With the reauthorization of IDEA, states are experimenting with a procedure that requires progress monitoring of interventions and limited RTI as the basis for eligibility for special education services. If RTI is the preferred method of the evaluation team for establishing eligibility for services, a comprehensive evaluation should take place in order fully to understand the nature of the learning difficulty (Kavale, Kaufman, Naglieri, & Hale, 2005). In the case of a student with PRD, detecting the underlying

TABLE 3.3. Individuals with Disabilities Education Act Statutory Definition of Specific Learning Disability

---

... a disorder in one or more of the basic psychological processes involved in understanding or in using language, spoken or written, that may manifest itself in an imperfect ability to listen, think, speak, read, write, spell, or do mathematical calculations, including conditions such as perceptual disabilities, brain injury, minimal brain dysfunction, and developmental dyslexia. The term does not include learning problems that are primarily the result of visual, hearing, motor disabilities, of mental retardation, of emotional disturbance, or of environmental, cultural or economic disadvantage.

Note. From Federal Register (1999).

problem may be impossible if curriculum-based assessment, progress monitoring, and consultation alone are used.

Besides SLD, speech and language services may also be appropriate for some students with PRD. Speech and language therapy can be used to improve the child's phonological awareness and word decoding skills, as well as articulation problems that sometimes accompany phonological deficits. Many of the treatments discussed in the next section can be reinforced via speech and language therapy. The IDEA definition of SLD is included in Table 3.3. The IDEA definition of speech and language impairment was reviewed in the previous section.

Treatment Considerations

The typical treatment for a student identified with a significant reading disability, (regardless if it is due to PRD, SLI, or some undetermined information-processing deficit) is to provide additional instruction in a special education resource setting. Resource assistance generally assures the student instructional material that precisely matches his or her reading level and a degree of individualized attention often impossible in a regular classroom. Despite the advantages associated with resource services, some research exists to suggest that resource intervention does little to get reading-disabled students caught up with their non-reading-disabled classmates. For example, Hanushek, Kain, and Rivkin (1998) and Zigmond et al. (1995) found resource programming was unable to close the gap in reading skills between students with reading disabilities and their typically reading peers. However, resource intervention did succeed in preventing a widening gap in reading skills compared to peers. Other studies paint a more negative picture of special education support, unless services include systematic instruction in phonological awareness. At least one longitudinal study concluded that average reading standard scores of children in special education decline over the elementary years, thereby suggesting the gulf between disabled and their non-disabled peers expands (McKinney, 1990). It appears as though direct, programmatic instruction in phonological awareness is required to improve significantly the reading skills of children with disabilities (see Swanson, 1999, for review of meta-analysis). Furthermore, the National Reading Panel also conducted a meta-analysis of 52 studies that validated phonological awareness training's role in improving word decoding, spelling, and reading comprehension (Ehri et al., 2001).

Goals of training in phonological awareness include teaching the child with PRD to make associations between the printed letters of the alphabet and the sounds in words, while directly linking spoken language and print

TABLE 3.4. Principles of Effective Phonological Awareness Training

1. Phonological awareness training should be integrated with the general curriculum, and teachers should speak slowly and clearly so that individual sounds in words are obvious.
2. Phonological awareness training should be connected to letter-sound association training.
3. The link between speech and print should be made explicit.
4. Phonological awareness training should start at the phoneme level.
5. Individual and/or small group instruction may be necessary in order to maximize outcomes.
6. The training program should be flexibly administered and tailored to the individual student's skill sets and needs because response rates vary.
7. Phonological awareness training preceded by general language instruction is most effective.
8. Phonological awareness exercises should be fun for teachers and students so that all are engaged in the process.

Note. Data from Gillon (2004) and Torgesen and Mathes (2000).

(Gillon, 2004; Torgesen & Mathes, 2000) (see Table 3.4). Most phonological awareness programs—whether implemented in the classroom, introduced in a small group setting, or presented on computer—seem to acknowledge and incorporate both components. The phonological awareness programs that Gillon (2004) and Torgesen and Mathes (2000) outline include activities that target skill sets such as general listening skills, perception of sounds, rhyming, blending of phonemes, segmenting words into phonemes, connecting letters and words to spoken language, and recognition and naming of letters and words. Similarities of program focus aside, the methods by which these skill sets are taught vary from program to program. Table 3.4 outlines the principles of effective phonological awareness training.

A recent study compared the effectiveness of two programs geared to improve the reading skills of children with previously-identified reading learning disabilities, presumably including many children with underlying PRD (Torgesen et al., 2001). At the time of the investigation, the first program was called Auditory Discrimination in Depth. The program has since been revised and renamed the Lindamood Phoneme Sequencing Program for Reading, Spelling, and Speech (Lindamood & Lindamood, 1998). The goals of this program are threefold: (1) develop the ability of the child to discriminate between phonemes by training him or her to recognize the unique kinesthetic, auditory, and visual (mouth form) characteristics of all phonemes; (2) teach the child to recognize and track sound sequences that constitute spoken syllables; and (3) teach the child self-monitoring of him pr her reading (Torgesen et al., 2001). Hallmark activities of the Lindamood method include making the child cognizant of mouth movements associated with spoken phonemes through the use of mouth forms. Phonemes are associated with mouth forms and then with actual letters. As used in this study, the Lindamood condition spent 95% of its time on facilitating phonemic awareness and recognizing words in isolation and 5% of its time on reading text developed specifically for this program.

A second program, Embedded Phonics, was developed for this study. In this program, students spent a greater percentage of time engaging in reading and spelling activities, as well as direct instruction in phonemic decoding. Students participated in this program for two 50-minute sessions per day. Activities included practice reading sight words, spelling, word games, direct phonics instruction, oral reading, and writing activities. Torgesen et al. (2001) summarized that the first condition (newly termed Lindamood method) devoted 5% of the time to reading and comprehending text, 85% to receiving phonemic decoding training, and 10% to learning sight words, whereas the Embedded Phonics program spent 50%, 20%, and 30% of intervention time on these same activities, respectively. Although the two programs differed greatly in their treatment approach, their outcomes were found to be equally positive. In fact, the children that participated in these two programs not only improved their reading skills, but also closed the gap between themselves and their nondisabled peers. Both were found to improve significantly the reading skills of children to the extent that special education services were not required within 1 year after the intervention period for 40% of participants.

Other intervention programs with empirical support also exist. The underlying commonality among effective treatments appears to be the development of sound–symbol relationships, among other phonemic awareness-related skills (e.g., Byrne, & Fielding-Barnsley, 1991; Rashotte et al., 2001). As another example, Rashotte, MacPhee, & Torgesen (2001) demonstrated that the Spell Read P.A.T. (Phonological Auditory Training) program improved the performance of poor readers (again, presumably including those with PRD) via small group intervention. Children across grade levels were selected for this study based on underdeveloped phonetic decoding and work reading skills. The complete program consists of 140 lessons and three phases of treatment. This study primarily led students though the first phase of intervention, which included daily 50-minute sessions comprising phonemic awareness, shared reading, and free writing activities, in addition to group instruction. Phonemic activities included using sounds to build syllables, blending consonants and vowels, and isolating individual sounds that make up syllables. The performance of the treatment group was then compared to control participants, who also demonstrated pretreatment phonological and word decoding deficits. Children who completed the program outperformed controls on measures of phonological awareness, word decoding, reading accuracy, reading comprehension, and spelling. Level of pretreatment deficits and grade level were unrelated to outcome, suggesting that Spell Read P.A.T. may be appropriate for children of all grades and levels of reading difficulty.

Many remedial programs require a long period of intervention (more than 100 hours of instructional time) and intensively trained instructors, excluding numerous special education resource teachers. Nonetheless, some programs show impact on phonological-processing deficits in as few as 20 hours of work, with improvements reportedly generalizing to reading accuracy and comprehension (Gillon & Dodd, 1995, 1997). As special education teachers increase their familiarity with the role of phonological deficits in reading and acquaint themselves with available intervention programs, instruction with a strong phonological process core many become increasingly available for students with PRD.

In addition to remedial instruction, various classroom accommodations may help students with PRD succeed and bolster their academic self-concept. That is, many students require a dual approach of accommodation and direct instruction. Examples of accommodation are books on tape, which may benefit students with PRD who enjoy adequate verbal knowledge and intact general language skills. It is easy to understand how a poor reader would gain information from tapes in subject areas (e.g., science, social studies) that would be unavailable if he or she were merely given standard textbooks. With respect to accommodating for poor spelling, access to spell checkers (word processing) and/or a scribe (such as when students work in teams, and one student writes) allows a student with limited spelling skills to demonstrate his or her knowledge without frustration or embarrassment.

Computerized assistive technology now provides exciting opportunities previously unavailable to students with reading disabilities, such as those with severe PRD who have failed to become proficient readers even with intensive instruction. For example, Kurzweil 3000 is a computer software package that circumvents decoding by scanning text into a computer that then reads aloud to a student. What makes this package so interesting is that almost all text printed in standard fonts can be scanned into it. The computer can even read to the child in a dialect of his or her choice. Furthermore, the text scanned into the program appears on the computer screen and is highlighted as the voice system reads the words. Other programs provide dictation software. We have seen children with PRD and intact verbal knowledge flourish with this software. In fact, some middle school and high school students acquire a degree of academic independence that seemed impossible prior to the development and deployment of the software. For a case example of PRD, see the information on Daniel in Chapter 5.

NONVERBAL LEARNING DISABILITY

Criteria for Nonverbal Learning Disability

1. WISC-IV PRI < VCI at statistically significant level.
2. Visual–perceptual deficits that may be evident on copying tasks (e.g., VMI; NEPSY Design Copying, Rey Complex Figure Test).
3. Social problems, such as lack of appreciation of social cues, limited pragmatic language or communications skills, inflexibility in play situations, avoidance of or confusion in dealing with novelty.
4. Motor clumsiness, tactile perceptual deficits.
5. Problems with computational arithmetic, later reading comprehension, sci-

Common Presentation of Nonverbal Learning Disability

Frequent concern of teacher at time of referral	Poor math performance; sloppy handwriting; overly literal"
Typical grade of referral	Elementary
Gender ratio	More boys than girls
Prevalence in referred sample	Rare

Note. Estimates from clinic setting.

Manifestations

Nonverbal learning disability (NLD) is a syndrome often cited in the psychology, neuropsychology, and psychiatry literature, but one that may be unfamiliar to educators (Telzrow & Bonar, 2002; Roman, 1998). NLD was originally described in great detail by Byron Rourke (see Rourke 1989, 1995, for an exhaustive review), and its formulation arose largely from his empirical work. Rourke, a neuropsychologist, presents a rationale for his contention that NLD is associated with right-hemisphere dysfunction (but not necessarily frank damage) that manifests in a seemingly diverse array of academic, adaptive, and interpersonal problems. More recently, Telzrow and Bonar (2002) reviewed seven primary deficits endured by children with NLD. Perhaps the hallmark of NLD is relative deficits in nonverbal as opposed to verbal skills (Rourke et al., 2002, provide a specific and detailed set of research criteria more extensive than those that may be used in clinical practice). Indeed, studies show that children with NLD have difficulty with nonverbal reasoning as evidenced by depressed Performance IQ on earlier versions of the WISC, and presumably relatively low PRI on the WISC-IV, plus impairments in visual attention and memory and in making effective inferences about spatial relationships (e.g., Cornoldi, Rigoni, Tressoldi, & Vio, 1999; Telzrow & Bonar, 2002; Worling, Humphries, & Tannock, 1999). Likewise, children with NVLD often have poor problem-solving capabilities that are especially evident on novel and complex tasks. Changes in routine often prove difficult, as an inflexible and rigid response style may predominate. In contrast, rote memory is usually intact and con-stitutes a relative strength, which often facilitates mastery of routine, con-vergent, and rote academic skills (e.g., phonological awareness, word decoding, and mastery of math facts) subsequent to their repeated practice. However, children with NVLD prove concrete, and conceptually complex tasks that require analysis and judgment often are difficult. Consequently, some of the problem-solving difficulties of children with NVLD derive in part from limited inferential ability (Worling et al., 1999).

Most children with NLD also display a recognizable profile of aca-demic strengths and weaknesses. These children often excel on school tasks that require rote learning, but founder as task demands step up in complexity. For example, well-developed word decoding and spelling skills are commonly seen in the face of math deficits, a hallmark of NLD. Children with NLD often have difficulty learning time, money skills, and measurement (Roman, 1998), in addition to aligning numbers, attending to math signs, and working with spatial concepts (Frankenberger, 2005). However, problem-solving demands and the need for judgment and infer-ences also make reading comprehension and math reasoning daunting tasks (Stein, Klin, & Miller, 2004; Roman, 1998). Frankenberger (2005), in a non-reviewed source, argues that poor understanding of cause and effect relationships and subtleties of language and concrete interpreta-tions negatively affect reading comprehension. Written expression may also be difficult due to poor handwriting and limited organization of ideas (Stein et al., 2004). Classes like science may prove difficult to the extent that complex reasoning is required (Rourke, 1989; Williams, Richman, & Yarbrough, 1992).

True to the nonverbal descriptor, NLD is often associated with motor deficits. Thus, a child with NLD may appear physically awkward and encounter delayed acquisition of motor skills (Telzrow & Bonar, 2002). In class, motor incoordination may result in sloppy handwriting and difficulty completing paper-and-pencil tasks, such as coloring and drawing, and forming letters and numbers (Frankenberger, 2005).

Sometimes most concerning to parents, impaired social skills are com-mon and may result in isolation from peers due to misinterpretation of nonverbal cues and pragmatic language deficits. Children with NLD overrely on verbally mediated and rote interpersonal behaviors (e.g., greet all people with the same phrase); they seem to lack social intuition and appear to be quite literal, socially naïve, and slow to respond in interpersonal situations (Stein et al., 2004). Missed or misinterpreted social cues especially involve body language, facial expressions, and tone of voice (Roman, 1998). Regarding language pragmatics, children with NLD may have atypical prosody (the patterns of stress and intonation in language) and engage others in conversation on topics that are not of mutual interest. Impaired pragmatic language skills, limited eye contact, insensitivity to social feedback, "cocktail party" speech (e.g., speaking excessively on a topic not of great interest to others), and difficulty maintaining reciprocal verbal interactions often lead to peer rejection (Little, 2001).

Given all of the forgoing, striking social–emotional difficulties, including social skiFll impairment, are also common. Rourke (1989, 1995) attributes difficulties in these areas to problems adapting to novel situations, impaired social judgment and interaction skills that lead to withdrawal, and the presence of "internalized" psychopathology. Children with NLD appear to have twice the risk of internalizing disorders of children without NLD (Petti, Voelker, Shore, & Hayman-Abello, 2003), perhaps because they are less accurate than children with verbal learning disabilities at interpreting the facial expressions and gestures of adults. Likewise, children with NLD may be mistaken as merely hyperactive during early childhood. In fact, it is not uncommon for the diagnosis of ADHD to be mistakenly applied, especially if a child has not undergone a full evaluation. Little (2001) also documented that children with Asperger's disorder and/or NLD are at significant risk for peer rejection and peer victimization. Perhaps as a result, children and adults with NLD are at particularly high risk for suicide (Bigler, 1989; Fletcher, 1989; Rourke, Young, & Leenaars, 1989).

As would be expected given right-hemisphere involvement, math learning disability, including poor mechanical arithmetic and math reasoning, is also typically present (Rourke, 1989, 1995; Rourke & Conway, 1997). Strictly speaking, a math learning disability is a separate entity from NLD. Nonetheless, it is likely that math deficits experienced by children with NLD match some of what is already generally known about failure to develop math competencies among otherwise cognitively able students. For example, procedural and visual–spatial subtypes of math problems, as described by Geary (2003), seem to apply directly to children with NLD. The procedural subtype is marked by developmentally immature calculation procedures, underdeveloped understanding of the concepts behind mathematical procedures, and difficulty completing complex mathematical procedures requiring sequencing of multiple steps (e.g., the steps involved in long division). Geary argues that this subtype is best thought of as a developmental delay (i.e., presenting features are similar to those of a younger age), and the deficit often improves with time and math experience.

The visual–spatial subtype of arithmetic disability seems to arise mostly from right-hemisphere dysfunction (Geary, 2003). This subtype is marked by misanalysis of information presented spatially and impaired ability of the child spatially to represent mathematical information for analysis. Although this subtype is not thought to be related to reading disorders, it is commonly seen in children with genetic disorders, like Turner syndrome (46 XO) resulting in short stature and spatial and mathematical deficits (Mazzocco, 2001).

Assessment Considerations

IQ testing plays a crucial role in the diagnosis of NLD. If NLD is present, the child should possess verbal problem-solving skills superior to nonverbal problem-solving skills (Rourke, 1989, 1995; Telzrow & Bonar, 2002). This direct comparison can be made with use of the WISC-IV. On the WISC-IV, one would expect to find PRI to be significantly lower than VCI. Psychologists should also keep in mind that other verbal subtests, like Comprehension, also seem to tap social problem solving, which is a processing capability thought to be deficient in children with NLD. Therefore, even the VCI composite score may artificially lower estimates of verbal problem solving. Incidentally, the seminal research on NLD used WISC, WISC-R, and WISC-III to detect Verbal IQ versus Performance IQ differences. The sensitivity of the WISC-IV PRI, which has abandoned manipulative and spatially demanding subtests like Object Assembly, for NLD-type deficits is unknown at present.

Many children with NLD produce severe distortions on drawing tasks, especially those that require pattern recognition (see Figure 3.2). Because children with NLD also suffer visual memory deficits (Rourke et al., 2002) they may produce poor reproductions after a delay. Accordingly, straightforward copying tasks (e.g., NEPSY Design Copying, VMI, Bender–Gestalt–2) all may have value. The Rey Complex Figure Test, which may include a delayed memory task, is sometimes especially distorted for these children and teenagers.

Tests of executive function, which require flexibility and sensitivity to feedback in the presence of novel stimuli, are often helpful when testing children suspected of having NLD. However, school psychologists may not always have such instruments at their disposal. Children with NLD have difficulty approaching and mastering novel tasks (especially when presented in nonverbal modalities) and shifting responses according to changing task demands (Fisher, DeLuca, & Rourke, 1997). Examples of tests that reveal these deficits are the Children's Category Test (Boll, 1993), the

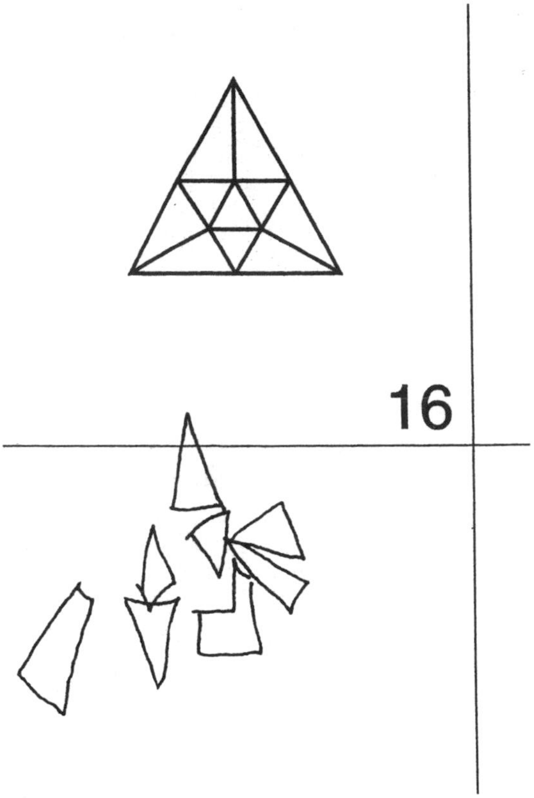

FIGURE 3.2. Child's drawing of one figure from the NEPSY Design Copy subtest. From Korkman, Kirk, and Kemp (1998). Reprinted by permission of the author.

Wisconsin Card Sorting Test (Heaton et al., 1993), and, perhaps, selected subtests of the NEPSY, such as Tower (Korkman et al., 1998). The Category Test and Wisconsin Card Sorting Test require children to learn a rule for solving a problem of a nonverbal nature based on feedback from the examiner. After each item, the examiner tells the child if he or she is "right" or "wrong." However, at predetermined points within the test, the rules change, and the child must conform, flexibly, to the new rule. Children with NLD are slow to catch on to the rules of the game, and once established, they are given to perseveration and inefficiency shifting their previously successful response set.

Motor impairment and poor tactile perception are also hallmark deficits of NLD. Tactile and motor function can easily be assessed via Sensorimotor subtests of the NEPSY if the child is 12 years or younger. If the NEPSY is utilized, the psychologist can gain access to subtests such as Fingertip Tapping, Imitating Hand Positions, Finger Discrimination, Visuomotor Precision, and Design Copying that allow for analysis of tactile perception, fine-motor skills, and visual–motor integration. Rourke (1989) has suggested that, consistent with the right-hemisphere dysfunction notion, left-hand motor speed and tactile scores are usually inferior to right-hand scores (the pattern reflecting the contralateral organization of most sensory and motor pathways between the cerebral cortex and extremities).

Given the prospect of pragmatic language and social skills deficiencies, as well as social-emotional maladjustment, examination of the child's social–emotional functioning is indicated. Although behavior rating scales such as the BASC-2 or Child Behavior Checklist may be used to screen for the presence of maladjustment, and especially internalizing disorders, clinical interviews and observations may prove more helpful for the purposes of intervention planning. Many school psychologists are extremely knowledgeable regarding language patterns and social skills typical of children at various stages of development and should therefore trust their judgment. It is of great importance to examine, through clinical interview or observation, the appropriateness of pragmatic language skills (e.g., eye contact, prosody, ability to read nonverbal cues and maintain a reciprocal interaction), complex social skills (e.g., greeting a friend, asking children to play, turn taking, etc.), the child's subjective reports of happiness and emotional functioning, and his or her personal reports of daily functioning (e.g., some children report getting easily lost). Given apparent high risk for suicide, an assessment in this area is also warranted.

Finally, academic function should be carefully assessed. Although math dysfunction is of special interest, broad-band psychometric measures of math calculation and reasoning skills, as can be provided by the WIAT-II or WJ III Tests of Achievement, should typically find use.

Other Possibilities

Rourke (1995) identified a multitude of medical conditions/diseases with neuropsychological sequelae similar to those of NLD. Most of these involve right-hemisphere dysfunction and/or abnormalities of white matter (relatively long, myelinated axons, which are thought to be especially prevalent in the right cerebral hemisphere). Examples familiar to school psychologists might include hydrocephalus, fetal alcohol syndrome, multiple sclerosis, traumatic brain injury, Turner syndrome, and Williams syndrome. Obviously, although psychologists may be involved in documenting the cognitive, behavioral, and academic manifestations of these disorders, diagnoses such as these are made by physicians.

One syndrome with characteristics that overlap with NLD is Asperger syndrome (referred to in DSM-IV-TR as Asperger's disorder), a diagnosis in the autism/PDD spectrum that has increased dramatically in prevalence during the past decade. DSM-IV-TR criteria for Asperger's disorder appear in Table 3.5. Proper detection of Asperger's, versus NLD, may depend on school psychologists more than medical professionals. In a case study format, Stein et al. (2004) reviewed similarities of and differences between NLD and Asperger's disorder. Both include well-developed verbal skills but impairments in motor and social skills. Furthermore, both have pragmatic language deficits that interfere with social interactions (e.g., impaired eye contact and uses of facial expression, body postures, and gestures to regulate social interaction), failure to form developmentally appropriate friendships, and lack of social reciprocity. In addition, aversion to novelty and adherence to routines are found in both. The crucial difference is that

---

TABLE 3.5. DSM-IV-TR Diagnostic Criteria for Asperger's Disorder

A. Qualitative impairment in social interaction, as manifested by at least two of the following:
  (1) marked impairment in the use of multiple nonverbal behaviors such as eye-to-eye gaze, facial expression, body postures, and gestures to regulate social interaction
  (2) failure to develop peer relationships appropriate to developmental level
  (3) a lack of spontaneous seeking to share enjoyment, interests, or achievements with other people (e.g., by a lack of showing, bringing, or pointing out objects of interest to other people)
  (4) lack of social or emotional reciprocity

B. Restricted repetitive and stereotyped patterns of behavior, interests, and activities, as manifested by at least one of the following:
  (1) encompassing preoccupation with one or more stereotyped and restricted patterns of interest that is abnormal either in intensity or focus
  (2) apparently inflexible adherence to specific, nonfunctional routines or rituals
  (3) stereotyped and repetitive motor mannerisms (e.g., hand or finger flapping or twisting, or complex whole-body movements)
  (4) persistent preoccupation with parts of objects

C. The disturbance causes clinically significant impairment in social, occupational, or other important areas of functioning.

D. There is no clinically significant general delay in language (e.g., single words used age 2 years, communicative phrases used by age 3 years).

E. There is no clinically significant delay in cognitive development or in the development of age-appropriate self-help skills, adaptive behavior (other than in social interaction), and curiosity about the environment in childhood.

F. Criteria are not met for another specific Pervasive Developmental Disorder or Schizophrenia.

Note. From American Psychiatric Association (2000). Copyright 2000 by the American Psychiatric Association. Reprinted by permission.

Asperger's disorder mandates the presence of unusual, restricted, repetitive, and stereotyped patterns of behavior, interests, and activities that typically are not seen in NLD (Stein et al., 2004). A child with Asperger's is typically the "little professor" who talks ad infinitum on arcane topics of his or her own selection.

ADHD is often on the minds of parents and school staff early in the evaluation process of children with NLD, and hyperactivity is indeed often seen in the early history of such children (Telzrow & Bonar, 2002). ADHD may seem like a plausible diagnostic alternative, especially given the comorbidity between ADHD, motor output dysfunction, and social skills deficits. Behavioral observations and a thorough functional analysis of behavior should be sufficient to determine if the scope and severity of the inattentive behavior constitutes a dual or alternative diagnosis of ADHD.

Eligibility Issues

NLD is a quite complex syndrome with symptoms in a variety of domains (e.g., academic, social, adaptive behavior, etc.), but it is not a learning disability in the legal or administrative sense. It is a label that denotes a clinical syndrome, and there is no specific IDEA category that fully encompasses the syndrome of NLD. When making eligibility decisions, the school-based evaluation team determines which behaviors are most salient and in need of specialized intervention and lets those conclusions guide the team toward specific eligibility categories. Given this fact, it is important that the evaluation process illuminate all the children's needs so that they are targeted for intervention (i.e., spelled out in an IEP for children found to be service eligible). For example, pragmatic language skills and social skills may be addressed along with academic skills.

Roman (1998) suggests a child with NLD be considered for special education services as a student with SLD (most likely math) or emotional disturbance (ED). Occupational therapy services, due to motor deficits, may also be considered. In some instances, internalizing symptoms, extreme responses to novelty in the environment, and/or impaired social skills, may lead the team to find the child with NLD eligible for special education service under the category of ED. ED as a category of eligibility will be discussed in greater detail in the ADHD-C section of the next chapter. Finally, to the extent that impaired pragmatic language affects the ability to socialize with peers and to function in the broad school context (e.g., socially, academically), speech and language therapy eligibility may also be considered.

Treatment Considerations

The overwhelming majority of intervention techniques garnered from our review of the literature arise from the clinical judgment of professionals familiar with the disorder rather than empirical comparisons of treatments. For example, a long list of treatment considerations has been compiled by Rourke (1995). These reinforce the need to capitalize on the verbal strengths of children with NLD, while providing explicit, step-by-step instruction with respect to interpretation of nonverbal stimuli, development of motor abilities, and complex academic tasks (e.g., mathematics, reading comprehension, and writing). Others who have written on NLD echo the need to compensate for nonverbal deficits and capitalize on verbal strengths, while fostering the problem-solving abilities and skills needed for complex academic activities, appropriate social interactions, and social-emotional well-being (Roman, 1998; Telzrow & Bonar, 2002).

Telzrow and Bonar (2002) have also compiled a list of suggestions for children with NLD to address psychomotor, arithmetic, problem-solving, and social skills deficits, in addition to social-emotional problems (see Table 3.6). These are arranged as remedial interventions (which involve skill practice), compensatory interventions that bypass the skills deficits, and specific instructional/therapeutic techniques to develop target areas.

One empirically validated treatment for NLD is cognitive-behavioral modification (Meichenbaum, 1985). The purpose of cognitive-behavioral modification is to assist the child in using verbally mediated means to analyze and judge nonverbal stimuli or to complete an academic task. Specifically, the child is taught to engage in private speech in order to initiate, direct, or maintain a behavior. Williams et al. (1992) taught children with NLD verbally to negotiate/analyze a visual–spatial task. The 20-minute treatment consisted of an examiner talking aloud in order to demonstrate how verbally to reason through a visual–spatial task, talking out loud while a child completed the task, requiring the child to complete the visual–spatial task while he or she talked aloud, and then having him or her perform the task while engaging in private speech. Interestingly, at posttest, the visual–spatial performance of children with NLD significantly improved from pretest levels, suggesting that children with NLD can draw upon verbal strengths effectively to engage in visual–spatial problem solving. This finding leads one to infer that when a nonverbal deficit is uncovered, teaching the child to verbally mediate a response has a certain likelihood of success. Obviously, expanded research involving many more subjects and measuring persistence and generalization of findings would be necessary before this approach could be considered to enjoy empirical support. For a case example of NLD, see the information on Mona in Chapter 5.

TABLE 3.6. Remedial, Compensatory, and Instructional/Therapeutic Interventions for Children with Nonverbal Learning Disability by Deficit Area

Psychomotor and perceptual interventions

Remedial
  Handwriting practice and training
  Explicit instruction in functional perceptual skills like understanding facial
    expressions and gestures
Compensatory
  Extended time to complete academic tasks
  Assistive technology like use of a word processor or scribe
  Use of multiple-choice exams rather than essay formats
  Minimize note taking by providing lecture outlines
  Provide oral directions
Instructional/therapeutic
  Training in keyboarding skills
  Occupational therapy to develop psychomotor skills

Arithmetic interventions

Remedial
  Instruction in verbal mediation
  Graph paper to align columns
  Use of calculator
  Rhymes/memory aids to learn math facts
  Instruction of checking strategies
Compensatory
  Rehearsal strategies that make use of mnemonic devices
Instructional/therapeutic
  Teach use of graphic organizers

Problem-solving interventions

Remedial
  Practice appropriate actions in response to various situations
Compensatory
  Prompt reference to "rules" to guide behavior
Instructional/therapeutic
  Explicit problem-solving instruction

Social skills interventions

Remedial
  Teach pragmatic language skills
  Teach social skills necessary to make and keep friends
Compensatory
  Vocational guidance toward careers with minimal social skill demands
  Avoid unstructured, large-group activities in favor of individual, structured activities
Instructional/therapeutic
  Social skills training
  Pragmatic language therapy

Social–emotional interventions

Remedial
  Self-monitoring of behavior

(continued)

TABLE 3.6. *(continued)*

Compensatory
  Psychoeducation regarding NLD
Compensatory
  Relaxation skills when anxious
  Engaging in pleasant events and activities
Instructional/therapeutic
  Psychoeducation regarding risk for depression and suicide
  Insight counseling
  Cognitive-behavioral therapy to improve self-esteem and address cognitive
    distortions (if present)

GRAPHOMOTOR UNDERPRODUCTION

Criteria for Graphomotor Underproduction

1. Teacher concerns about poor handwriting, especially if it is associated with extreme difficulty completing written work.
2. Standardized scores on tests of copying (e.g., NEPSY Design Copying, WRAVMA, Copying, VMI) or graphomotor speed and accuracy (e.g., NEPSY Visuomotor Precision) poorer than VCI, PRI, or FSIQ.
3. May have coexisting NLD, ADHD-C, or ADHD-I.
4. Rule out frank neurological disease, such as cerebral palsy.

Common Presentation of Graphomotor Underproduction

Frequent concern of teacher at time of referral	"Slow to get work done; sloppy handwriting"
Typical grade of referral	Primary grades
Gender ratio	More boys than girls
Prevalence in referred sample	Common

Note. Estimates from clinic setting.

Manifestations

In many classrooms, especially at the K–3 level, students spend much of their time using a pencil to complete worksheets or copy material. It is easy, then, to understand how a student lacking precise motor control or needing to work slowly with a pencil would be constrained in work completion. The primary pattern here is poor handwriting that results in handwritten work that is completed with great effort, of poor quality, or both. Thus, a common complaint is that these students do not finish their worksheets. Poor penmanship is generally easily recognized, and both teachers and parents are apt to complain about a long history of sloppy handwriting or illegible arithmetic papers. Such children may produce drastically inconsistent written work, although overall its quality tends to be poor. Letters may be irregular in size and shape and slanted in unusual ways. Spacing is often a problem. Older children with graphomotor underproduction (GU) may fluctuate randomly between cursive and manuscript writing. Their papers may appear smudged and disarrayed.

Not surprisingly, many students develop coping behavior in attempts to correct the problem or to minimize their suffering. For example, some students resort to extremely slow letter production to compensate for poor fine-motor control. Others may work at the upper level of efficiency for a while, only ultimately to lapse into slapdash rapid responding. Given the subjective distress that many students report in association with their writing, it is easy to see how their careless responding can be maintained by negative reinforcement (i.e., fast writing hastens the end of the unpleasant tedium of writing). That graphomotor problems sometimes occur within the more general context of fine-motor incoordination or clumsiness might go unrecognized. On close observation, however, many students with poor handwriting have cramped or unusual pencil grips (such as holding the thumb over two fingers and then writing with wrist movements). Many of them also have a hard time with other hands-on activity, such as arts and crafts projects. Students who lack dexterity with a pencil and compensate by writing slowly may be misjudged to be inattentive, lazy, or obstinate.

Berninger (2004) presented an excellent review of the literature discussing motor processes involved in handwriting (see Berninger, 2004, for a review), which includes important information for school psychologists. For example, there is evidence of a wide degree of variation in how students grip their pencils and that pencil grip is seemingly unrelated to handwriting quality and speed (Berninger et al., 1997; Graham & Weintraub, 1996). Therefore, it seems that handwriting quality itself, rather than attempting to change a child's grip, should be the target of intervention. It is also important to realize that graphomotor problems manifest not only in poor handwriting, but also in compromised composition fluency, such as how much can be written in a given period of time (Berninger, 1994, 2000), and quality of writing content and its organization (Graham, Berninger, Abbott, Abbott, & Whitaker, 1997). Interestingly, among normally developing children, visual–motor integration is not correlated with handwriting quality (Graham & Weintraub, 1996). Nonetheless—and this makes intuitive sense—among children with notable handwriting problems, there is an association with impaired visual–

motor integration (Weintraub & Graham, 2000). Because we are concerned with those children expressing poor handwriting and slow work completion, accompanying visual–motor deficits are often found.

Assessment Considerations

As is true throughout this chapter, identifying children with GU requires establishment of overall developmental level, requiring IQ testing. It is common for WISC-IV FSIQ to underestimate these children's cognitive levels, as poor Processing Speed Index, or PSI (comprising the Coding and Symbol Search subtests), often results from the very same motor or hand–eye problems that cause graphomotor problems themselves. This was also true on the WISC-III, which contained several tasks requiring manipulation and rewarded speedy performance, more than on the WISC-IV PRI. Nonetheless, on both Wechsler IQ tests, a common pattern may be nonverbal performance poorer than verbal, though this is not universally so. The PSI is generally the poorest index score on the WISC-IV.

Beyond IQ scores, it is necessary to document genuine deficits in the quality of visual–motor coordination on tasks such as copying (NEPSY Design Copying, Test of Visual Motor Integration, Bender–Gestalt-2) or speed with a pencil on time tasks (NEPSY Visuomotor Precision composite score for constituent scores of "speed" or "accuracy") to rule in this condition. As many of these visual–motor and fine-motor subtests are unreliable, it is best to rely on those with recent norms, clear scoring criteria, and clearly reported standard errors of measurement. Psychologists are cautioned that poor scores on these tests alone, even if dramatically poor, do not demonstrate the presence of GU. Like all the conditions discussed here, it is essential to rely upon multiple information sources and to require that data converge to support the presence of any type of problem. Thus, it is almost always necessary to detect a history of teachers' complaints; likewise, contemporary work samples can almost invariably be used quickly to confirm that pencil-and-paper work is inferior to that of classmates'.

Other Possibilities

As is true when considering other narrow information-processing disorders reviewed in this chapter, before GU can be ruled in, other problems must be ruled out. As always, following the flowchart in Figure 1.1/5.1 can be helpful. For all the conditions listed in this chapter, the first step is to ensure that general cognitive delays do not exist. This can be accomplished by reviewing developmental information and performance in other school areas or by IQ testing. If either verbal or composite cognitive functioning falls into the average range, then general cognitive delays can be rejected.

As the hypothesis favoring the presence of GU gains strength, eliminating other problems besides general ability impairments is the next requirement. Because graphomotor problems comprise difficulty using motor movements and vision together, it is essential to confirm that visual acuity is intact. Typically, this can be accomplished with a simple vision screening, which takes place for most students annually in their local school. More detailed vision evaluations are controversial. Likewise, pathological motor problems need to be ruled out. Some children present with both fine-motor, including graphomotor, and gross-motor deficits. If these are pronounced, include abnormalities of muscle tone, or affect one side of the body more than another, then cerebral palsy needs to be ruled out (Pellegrino, 2002). As cerebral palsy need not always present with conspicuous symptoms such as altered gait, it is important for school psychologists to be vigilant for the possibility that this condition exists in subtle form when assessing children, especially those with potential graphomotor problems. Discussing observations with those who familiar with motor assessments (e.g., a physical therapist or occupational therapist) or reviewing suspicious findings with the child's primary care physician makes sense.

For all of the conditions listed in this book, it is important to make sure that the child's performance in class and on standardized measures is not merely a reflection of problems with inattention or hyperactivity–impulsivity. Ruling out ADHD is especially relevant regarding GU. This is so because some extremely impulsive students fail pencil-and-paper tasks because they either give up quickly or turn in poor-quality scribbles. The same student may fail to pay close attention on copying tasks during standardized testing. We are accustomed to seeing students rush wildly through the race tracks that make up the Visuomotor Precision subtest of the NEPSY (see Figure 3.3), yielding scores that indicate impulsive responding rather than true motor impairment. Accordingly, school psychologists must collect detailed historical information. Parents and previous teachers can almost always provide information about impulse control, attention to detail, and effort; it is quite likely that their reports would contain references to such problems if ADHD were the true problem. Similarly, standardized behavior rating scales provide abundant data, including objective indices of hyperactivity–impulsivity and inattention. We typically use either the BASC-2 (Reynolds & Kamphaus, 2004) or the Child Behavior Checklist (Achenbach & Rescorla, 2001). Further, it is easy to see flagrant ADHD symptoms during standardized testing. For example, the student with poor scores on the VMI or NEPSY Visuomotor arising from rapid or careless responding can be detected by even casual observation. We encourage psychologists to report unflinchingly ADHD symptoms when they see them. Underreporting can lay the foundation for flawed conclusions, which sometimes harms children.

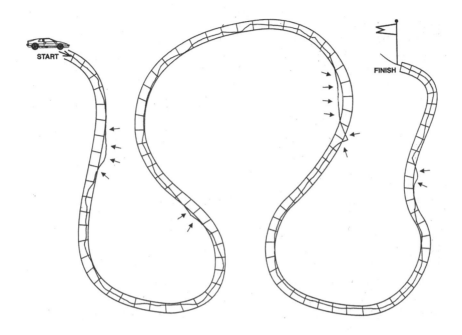

FIGURE 3.3. Child's response to one portion of the NEPSY Visuomotor Precision subtext. From Korkman et al. (1998). Reprinted by permission of the authors.

Children with graphomotor problems may also meet criteria for an NLD. If this is true, then recognizing the presence of both conditions can help in planning for the student's future and determining which interventions are needed now. It is unknown how often children with either of these conditions express the associated nonverbal problem, but in our experience it appears to be true in only a minority of instances.

Eligibility Issues

Poor handwriting, even when it is so severe that there are major problems getting work done, typically does not compel eligibility for special education services. It is essential to analyze carefully the nature of these students' poor classroom performance. If the concern derives mostly from failure to complete work, then it is necessary to establish whether the demand to write is the limiting factor. If it is, then accommodations may be sufficient to allow the student to be successful without recourse to special services. Furthermore, if the student fails to advance because of frank motor problems, he or she typically would not be eligible for SLD designation. The

IDEA definition for SLD requires that motor handicaps are not the primary cause of learning problems (see SLD definition in Table 3.3). In addition, if motor problems beyond those associated with hand–eye coordination and graphomotor control are at issue, school psychologists should probably seek information from professional colleagues. As legal requirements dictate a team evaluation regarding questions of special education eligibility, it is suggested that school-based occupational or physical therapy staff participate or that a clinic-based physician serve as an ad hoc team member (e.g., examine the student and prepare a report that can be used by the team).

In other instances, some students' graphomotor deficits derail their broad ability to communicate in writing. In other words, these students endure problems far greater than poor handwriting and completing written assignments on time. A variety of higher-order writing assignments are failed, such as narrative composition, preparation of answers to reading comprehension questions, or coherent written answers to social studies or science assignments. This is true even if teachers disregard poor penmanship and a plodding pace of written production. These students have been unable to master the key writing ("written expression") tasks expected at their grade level on dimensions such as the ability to develop ideas in writing, organize their writing with unity and coherence, and produce sentences that form paragraphs with acceptable grammar, punctuation, capitalization, and variety. Because such skills are instrumental in high school and college success, it is important that additional instructional help is provided.

When it appears that a written expression like that mentioned above is at issue, then additional assessment by a school psychologist or someone working with him or her is typically called for. Besides collecting work samples and interviewing teachers, parents, and student, standardized measures of written expression can be administered. Individually administered achievement tests such as the WIAT-II, the WJ III Tests of Achievement, and the Test of Written Language–3 (Hammill & Larson, 1996) provide detailed, multiple-component tests of written expression. As written expression is one of the academic areas in which students with SLD can manifest underachievement or prove refractory to intervention (might be deemed eligible for services based on poor RTI), difficulty in this area and a supporting history can be used to qualify students for special services. The necessary rule outs of sensory, cultural–experiential, emotional, and mental retardation issues must be addressed any time that a student is considered for SLD designation.

When special education eligibility is deliberated, it is important that a fair appraisal of the student's cognitive ability is conducted to rule out mental retardation or if an ability–achievement discrepancy is part of the qualifying process. Because of the effect of slow and inaccurate pencil control, Full Scale scores from the WISC-IV are sometimes quite depressed for these children (i.e., a low PSI depresses FSIQ). A better appraisal of nonverbal ability on the WISC-IV is often the PRI or VCI for language-based reasoning abilities. The WISC-IV GAI, which excludes both WMI and PSI subtests, may need to be considered.

Treatment Considerations

Three lines of intervention are suggested for students with this condition: (1) circumvent the weakness and require the student to write less; (2) provide the student alternative ways to write (i.e., keyboarding); or (3) intervene to teach the student better, more efficient handwriting.

Regarding accommodations, it appears intuitively obvious that circumventing pencil-and-paper work may benefit these students. If writing is made less essential in the execution of daily classwork, these students are less likely to be impaired by their graphomotor deficits. Among the accommodations suggested, although not empirically verified, are (1) changing the rate at which written results are expected, (2) reducing the volume of written work, (3) simplifying writing requirements, (4) providing tools to aid writing, and (5) providing a format that minimizes writing problems (see Jones, 1999, for a more extensive list). Consistent with these ideas, teachers might review each seatwork task to determine how much writing is required. If demands appear to be excessive, adjustment can be made before tasks are assigned. Copying from the blackboard might be replaced by giving the student a written copy of material in advance. Mandatory full-sentence responses in social studies might be supplanted by short answers or multiple-choice options, which could allow the student merely to circle his or her choice.

If the assessment verifies that language functioning is intact (i.e., language is a relative strength), then oral communication can sometimes replace a portion of written requirements. Group projects can be devised that permit all students to respond verbally but require only one student (i.e., never the one with GU) to write the group's responses. Tasks involving copious writing can be revised to permit students to submit an outline and accompanying audiotape recording (especially for students who are in junior high or high school) in lieu of a full written report. Some researchers have advocated use of dictation and accompanying voice recognition devices, in addition to training students to develop, evaluate, and organize their ideas (De la Paz & Graham, 1997). These researchers compared the performance of students who received planning training to those who received more traditional writing instruction (e.g., were taught essay structure, revised samples, composed and shared writings with peers). Additionally, half the students in each study condition dictated required essays, and half wrote the required essays. In support of the use of assistive technology, dictation coupled with planning training maximized writing quality as compared to the other treatment conditions.

Although empirical backing for accommodations of the type mentioned in this chapter is modest, it certainly makes sense to embrace them on an individual case basis. It is easy to see how astute psychologists or educators could use the basic notion of accommodation as a springboard for functional behavioral analysis (Kazdin, 2001). For example, assume that a student with a documented graphomotor problem struggles in one academic setting but flourishes in another. Following functional behavior analysis tenets, classroom observations could be conducted to determine if tasks characterized by heavy writing demands were completed more slowly and less accurately than equivalent tasks free of such demands. Similarly, if classroom conduct was at issue, the conditional probabilities for disruption or defiance in the presence of written versus oral demands could be investigated. Proceeding logically, if intense writing demands represented an antecedent condition for poor productivity, then an initial intervention to reduce writing could be implemented. If successful in the short term, this intervention could be adopted for long-term use. Although it is true that such functional behavior analyses can be conducted earlier in the evaluation process and often without psychometric testing, at times a salient antecedent condition is lacking until a more comprehensive evaluation, including psychometric testing, reveals the antecedent dimension(s) most important in the analysis.

A variation on the accommodation theme involves replacing handwriting with typing or keyboarding. The logic is that the motor requirements associated with typing are simpler and less effortful than equivalent printing or writing. Furthermore, the finished product derived from use of a word processing program, once it is printed, is uniformly legible. With the advent of relatively inexpensive, highly portable laptop computers, students can easily carry with them the material necessary to word process. The challenge, of course, is to teach the student to type efficiently. Software tutorial programs, such as Mavis Beacon Teaches Typing (available through Broderbund products) and MicroType Pro (available through Thomson Learning College), are available. When it is best to launch such programs with younger students is unknown. Because it is important for students to learn the most effective long-term approach, it seems logical to insist that touch typing is taught systematically rather than letting the student find his or her way via a trial-and-error, hunt and peck system. This means that a formal course or several months of structured practice may be needed before typing becomes more efficient than handwriting. Accordingly, we rarely suggest that a switch be made during the school year. A summer program to learn typing, when the demands for other work production have waned, is usually suggested. However, if a formal school-based keyboarding course is unavailable and the student's schedule can tolerate such demands, then learning the proper way to keyboard during the school year can sometimes be accomplished.

Whether switching from handwriting to use of a laptop computer influences long-term success is not clear from the literature. For example, there is some short-term evidence in favor of keyboarding regarding spelling, although the research contains possible confounds (Margalit & Roth, 1989). Also, writing accuracy appears to be improved but not ease of recording written material, writing quality, or attitude toward writing (Lewis, Graves, Ashton, & Kieley, 1998). Similarly, when typing on a computer was pitted against handwriting, use of the computer resulted in more words and sentences written, but there was no difference between the two approaches regarding amount of time off-task. In most of these investigations, the groups of children studied appeared quite heterogeneous. Thus the data, fail to speak to the precise effect that might occur when these techniques are applied to children with significant and circumscribed graphomotor impairments.

A third option is to attempt direct improvement of the student's handwriting. One could argue that such attempts do not tackle academic skills directly and accordingly risk the fallacy of attempting to remedy the processing problems underlying crystallized academic products (see Chapter 1). It is important, however, to distinguish efforts to remedy handwriting from those designed to remedy fine-motor control per se. In the former, it is the academic product of writing that is addressed; in the latter, the goal is to improve a core neurocognitive deficit associated with all types of hand–eye coordination and manual dexterity problems. Thus, the former approach makes more sense than the latter. Indeed, there appears to be both logical and empirical evidence for remedial handwriting drills but not for fine-motor proficiency training.

For example, Graham, Harris, and Fink (2000) provide a practice-based treatment program (see Graham, Harris, & Fink, 2000, for a full review). The treatment program implemented by this group required first-grade students with handwriting difficulties to participate in 27 lessons composed of letter-identification activities, tracing and evaluation exercises, sentence copying under timed conditions, and unusual letter-writing activities like writing letters with exaggerated strokes or writing letters to look like a familiar object (e.g., an *s* into a snake). Similar to the intervention discussed next, this program improved the handwriting and writing fluency performance of children who participated in the program above control students who received phonological awareness instruction alone.

Likewise, Berninger et al.'s (1997) treatment also presents suitably clear guidelines that its key components can be readily put into operation. Moreover, empirical research has documented that the overall intervention is effective and that the critical training elements are use of visual cues and memory retrieval drills. Visual cueing comprises marking lower-case letters with numbered arrows that depict the proper order and direction of pencil strokes. Memory retrieval involves studying the letters' appearances, followed by covering and writing from memory. Over a series of lessons, the interval between covering and writing increases from 1 to 9 seconds. At the conclusion of approximately 22 training sessions, first graders with graphomotor problems who received the program's most effective elements improved the quality of their handwriting and compositional fluency (i.e., composing within time limits).

Interventions like this set the stage for subsequent progress in written expression. There may be a necessary but sufficient relationship between automaticity of writing and the ability to develop written expression skills. In other words, without the ability to write letters quickly, efficiently, and with little conscious thought, students find it quite difficult to spell adequately and to put their thoughts down on paper. Efficient and automatic writing alone, however, fail to guarantee good written expressive skills. Indeed, even among young children (first graders), Jones and Christensen (1999) found that orthographic (specific visual representation of specific symbols, letters, or groups of letters) and fine-motor integration explained 67% of the variance in written expression after other literacy variables were controlled. When children, especially young ones, struggle to write legibly, seldom complete written assignments, or are slow to develop higher-level writing language skills, GU may be the core problem and direct intervention may be required. For a case example of GU, see the information on Jeremy in Chapter 5.

INCONSISTENT SUCCESS WITH SPLINTER SKILLS

Criteria for Inconsistent Success with Splinter Skills

1. Either a history of adequate school performance during a portion of the primary grades or currently adequate performance in some subjects only (e.g., those emphasizing work production or rote memorization); poor performance in other subjects (e.g., those requiring analysis and judgment).
2. Scores on measures of clerical skills (e.g., WISC-IV Processing Speed, copying, graphomotor speed and accuracy) and/or rote learning (e.g., memory) superior to Full Scale IQ scores (or WISC-IV VCI and PRI).
3. Full Scale IQ (or WISC-IV VCI and PRI) $\leq$ 90 or substantially poorer than estimated average IQ of classmates.
4. One or more academic areas (either indexed by individual achievement test scores or subject area report card marks) may exceed IQ scores.
5. Parents or teachers report poor judgment or application of some academic skills.
6. Unusual or intense interests may be present (e.g., military history, stock exchange).

Common Presentation of Inconsistent Success with Splinter Skills	
Frequent concern of teacher at time of referral	"Confused why student is struggling because he or she does some things very well"
Typical grade of referral	Varies
Gender ratio	Unknown
Prevalence in referred sample	Very rare

Note. Estimates from clinic setting.

Manifestations

To this point, we have presented patterns recognizable by broad (e.g., IQ) and narrow (e.g., phonological processing) deficits. The concept of inconsistent success with splinter skills (ISSS) is somewhat different. Although there may be identifiable cognitive deficits, this pattern's hallmark is the presence of one or more intact or even very advanced "splinter skills" in a student who otherwise struggles in school. Of course, most school psychologists associate splinter skills with the savant capabilities sometimes reported in autism or other pervasive developmental disorder (PDD), such as Asperger syndrome. However, in our experience, children with mental retardation, formal learning disabilities, and even performance-based deficits (ADHD) sometimes show well-developed, narrow-band cognitive skills without PDD presentations. Children with ISSS are thus quite heterogeneous in terms of general cognitive development and splinter skill(s) expressed and, as a result, their presentation is the most varied of all conditions listed in this book. The occasional appearance of this pattern and the fact that it puzzles graduate students and colleagues prompted its inclusion in this book. How useful the notion of ISSS proves to be in practice is not yet known.

Two characteristics these children share are (1) some degree of academic failure (which is why they were referred for evaluation) and (2) a splinter skill that may or may not buffer the effects of a larger problem. For example, we have seen many early elementary children who were referred for academic failure in one or more school subjects. Surprisingly, some of these children actually possessed a nice complement of rote academic skills in letter and number recognition, phonemic awareness, math fact retrieval, or sight word vocabulary. The complaint, however, was that these students failed to perform higher-order thinking commensurate with their rote skills. Evaluations may show a student with PDD at one end of the cognitive impairment continuum and one with SL status at the other end. This often comes as a surprise to parents and teachers who assumed the child was much brighter than objective evaluation results indicate. In other words, composite IQ (especially WISC-IV GAI), executive function, or adaptive behavior scores for children with ISSS typically are low, or at least lower than parents and teachers assumed.

The heterogeneous make up of ISSS means that many types of children fall within this category. Some children with ISSS may have very well-developed verbal and/or social skills. When spoken to, they may respond appropriately with adequate vocabulary and language pragmatics. This would lead even seasoned psychologists to believe they possess adequate general cognitive ability. But testing may reveal that their social skill development is remarkable in the face of other significant impairments, such as IQ in the SL range. Such low IQ, of course, may underlie academic failure. Other children with ISSS may be hyperverbal, yet lack true social competence. Thus, there may be some overlap with NLD, although we have seen children like this with ISSS who cannot satisfy NLD criteria.

Graphomotor/visual–spatial development is another potential splinter skill. Precocious graphomotor skills can have considerable mitigating effect on weak cognition during the early school years when classroom tasks emphasize copying shapes and printing of numerals and letters. Cognitive deficits may go unappreciated until later school years when the student is asked to write independently or construct lengthy narratives that must be filled with ideas. Alternatively, we have found that some motorically advanced adolescents successfully complete vocational training and go on to enjoy success in occupations that emphasize graphomotor/visual–spatial skill, even if they have only modest cognitive ability. The hands-on jobs that are used in the arts or mechanics are often preferred.

Children along the continuum of PDD often display splinter skills, plus impaired social skills and/or focused interests. Furthermore, some children with ISSS have unusual interests for their age. For example, we have assessed first and second graders with obsessive interests in the stock exchange or naval history. Parents and teachers often comment on the child's mature interests and vast store of facts without fully appreciating (1) their detrimental effects on peer relationships and social skills and (2) accompanying cognitive deficits that may eventually lead to academic failure if knowledge and skill development are confined to a single, overly developed topic. Social skill intervention, or at least promotion of contact with peers, is often necessary, as these children may have much greater comfort with adults than with peers (see Safran, Safran, & Ellis, 2003; Tsatsanis, Foley, & Donehower, 2004).

In the extreme form, children with ISSS may appear like those with specific genetic or developmental syndromes who suffer overall cognitive impairment but retain narrow splinter skills. For example, many children with Williams syndrome possess well-developed expressive language (e.g., they may be able to recount complex stories clearly and coherently), but many have mental retardation (Mervis, 2003). Children with Prader-Willi syndrome, including those with mental retardation, commonly have "spared" visual–spatial skills (e.g., ability to locate words embedded in a matrix, ability to do jigsaw puzzles), some of which exceed the skills of their normal age-mates (Dykens, 2002). Likewise, children with hyperlexia have advanced ability to read words concomitant with cognitive and social impairments, some of which are quite severe (Grigorenko et al., 2002). In these cases, assuming that the student can achieve commensurate with his or her highest splinter skill leads to unreasonable expectations. Level of general cognitive ability, not that of isolated splinter skill, often predicts ultimate academic success. Although ISSS is heterogeneous and of unknown etiology, subtle syndrome-like nervous system differences may be present for some children with ISSS, even when their problems are relatively mild and there is no evidence that they suffer a specific syndrome.

Assessment Considerations

As for most conditions, the WISC-IV is a good place to start psychometric testing. A child with ISSS tends to have FSIQ scores below 90 or IQ scores substantially lower than the estimated average of classmates. Although many of these children also have lower WISC-IV VCI than PRI, most striking is an oft-seen decrement in scores as analysis and judgment are increasingly tapped. For example, on the verbal side, children with ISSS may excel on relatively rote subtests, like Information, then falter on subtests requiring abstraction and reasoning, like Similarities and Comprehension. Similarly, on the nonverbal side, difficulty often occurs on subtests requiring complex problem solving, like Block Design, compared to Picture Completion. That is, *g* or fluid-ability tasks often reveal surprising deficits in the presence of better (sometimes excellent) crystallized, perceptual, or rote memory skills.

Like the other conditions covered in this chapter, a comprehensive evaluation is necessary with ISSS to document which skills are present. For example, we found that simple processing speed, graphomotor skills, rote memory, phonological awareness, and academic skills subject to memorization (e.g., math facts) are common splinter skills. We have seen several children who performed excellently on the PSI of the WISC-IV but who had substandard scores on indices more closely related to *g* (e.g., FSIQ, VCI, PRI). We also found some children with ISSS who displayed excellent drawing and/or fine-motor skills. Select subtests of the NEPSY, especially those in the Sensorimotor Domain, are helpful in locating these strengths (e.g., Fingertip Tapping, Imitating Hand Positions, Visuomotor Precision, and Design Copying).

Despite low overall ability, standardized measures of simple visual and/or verbal learning (e.g., recognition of faces and list learning) may reveal learning strengths that were previously unappreciated. At the same time, well-developed rote memory skills sometimes also lead to unexpectedly solid academic capabilities, such as letter and number identification, acquisition of math facts, mastery of sound–symbol associations and phonological awareness skills, and grade-level word decoding. Thus, in the academic realm, WJ III subtests like Reading Fluency, Writing Fluency, and Math Fluency, as well as measures of math calculation, word decoding, and phonological awareness may detect narrow competencies.

Other Possibilities

Besides appearing in its own right, ISSS may also coexist with other recognizable patterns discussed in this book. However, in order to be considered splinter, a skill must be clearly superior to general cognitive development. As mentioned earlier, we sometimes find advanced clerical skills in children with mild cognitive impairment. The comprehensive nature of the psychological evaluation is sufficient to identify the presence of learning problems related to intelligence factors. Of course, more than standardized testing may be required in order to rule out the presence of other developmental disorders, namely PDD and Asperger syndrome.

To be clear, we are not suggesting that children with ISSS are in a continuum of PDD. Nonetheless, sporadic high achievement and splinter skills do occur in PDD, a group of conditions outside the scope of this book. Thus, when academic failure, unusual interests, underdeveloped social skills, clear-cut splinter skills appear, the psychologist should explore possibilities beyond the learning disorders in this book by consulting DSM-IV-TR. Specifically, Asperger syndrome might be considered under these circumstances (see diagnostic criteria in Table 3.5). Differential diagnosis can be difficult, as children with PDD spectrum disorders, which are often conceptualized as emotional/psychiatric disorders, sometimes look like children with NLD or SLI. In some ways, the distinction between emotional/psychiatric disorders and learning disorders is artificial, as either class of disorder can manifest in both bothersome interpersonal and learning problems.

Eligibility Issues

Detecting a pattern consistent with ISSS is one thing and, even more than for the other conditions of this chapter, determining special education eligibility is quite another. Accordingly, the school psychologist may have to lead the evaluation team through the process of considering a categorical disability (e.g., MiMR, SLD, etc.) that would entitle the child with ISSS to special education services. ISSS is listed here primarily for its heuristic value. Its presence may help psychologists, teachers, and parents better understand some perplexing children, but ISSS does not lead to Section 504 services under the Rehabilitation Act of 1973 (Public Law 93-112), as it is not a condition codified elsewhere.

Nonetheless, two special education eligibility categories may have direct application for children with ISSS: emotional disturbance (ED) and autism. Remember that a few children with ISSS have intensely focused and deeply refined interests, impaired social skills, and academic failure. Some of these children meet ED eligibility criteria. The formal IDEA definition of ED will be reviewed in greater detail in Chapter 4; however, it is worth mentioning here that inability to build or maintain satisfactory interpersonal relationships with peers and teachers and/or displaying inappropriate types of behavior or feelings under normal circumstances (affecting educational performance) may qualify a student as ED. On the other hand, if an underlying syndrome like autism is identified, the evaluation team may consider eligibility for special education services under the category of autism (see Table 3.7 for the IDEA definition of autism). The diagnosis of autism comes loaded with a host of preconceived notions regarding course and treatment. Therefore, parents in particular may be unsettled to learn that the school is proposing services under this eligibility category. Parents who are resistant to their child being evaluated may need to be reminded that eligibility for services depends upon being evaluated and meeting criteria for at least one category of service. Children with Asperger's disorder (or PDD, NOS) do not routinely meet IDEA criteria for autism (although there is debate about whether Asperger's disorder is synonymous with high-functioning autism; Safran, 2001); however, they may be eligible for Section 504 accommodations.

Treatment Considerations

The uncovering of splinter skills and recognition that general abilities may be weak can facilitate treatment planning. That is, the discovery can provide insight as to how the child might best learn. This prospect is especially valuable if the splinter skill is identified in the presence of general cognitive impairment. When a splinter skill gives the impression that the child is more cognitively sophisticated than is true, expectations need to be recalibrated (just as is true for AEM). Take the example of a fourth-grade female who is quite verbally and socially skilled, yet struggles academically. Her academic failure may confuse parents and teachers

TABLE 3.7. Individuals with Disabilities Education Act Definition of Autism

(i) *Autism* means a developmental disability significantly affecting verbal and nonverbal communication and social interaction, generally evident before age 3, that adversely affects a child's educational performance. Other characteristics often associated with autism are engagement in repetitive activities and stereotyped movements, resistance to environmental change or change in daily routines, and unusual responses to sensory experiences. The term does not apply if a child's educational performance is adversely affected primarily because the child has an emotional disturbance, as defined in paragraph (b)(4) of this section.

(ii) A child who manifests the characteristics of "autism" after age 3 could be diagnosed as having "autism" if the criteria in paragraph (c)(1)(i) of this section are satisfied.

because it appears that she is quite bright, judged by conversational skills. Those who know the child wonder if she lacks motivation or if she has an unidentified disability. Upon evaluation, it is found that she possesses both general cognitive abilities and most academic skills in the low-average range. Such information and recognition of ISSS status reveals that the child may indeed be performing commensurate with her capabilities. Accordingly, a shift in expectations is in order. The psychologist can work with teachers and parents to explain that the girl's conversational skills led to a false impression of substantial overall ability. Thus, there are reasons for psychologists to stay involved as consultants because many parents and teachers misunderstand IQ scores and how to calibrate expectations. The school psychologist also may help assure that any academic failure is not due to lack of effort or laziness. CBA in each academic domain may be needed. By using her isolated conversational skills, the child may be able to shine in some social situations or, for example, during classroom dramatizations.

Additionally, consider an 8-year-old boy whose evaluation documents cognitive abilities in the MiMR range. Paradoxically, he has strikingly well-developed rote memory skills, as established by list learning and visual recognition tasks, and he can read a grade-level list of words quickly and accurately. As a result of conducting a detailed evaluation, the psychologist has some promising news for the school-based team, including the child's parents, and some information with potential value in planning. Confirmation that the child is able to learn rote information efficiently can be provided, thereby raising adults' expectations for the child (if they were low). By making sure that the student has a routine chance to show off his oral reading skills, a sense of pride and self-confidence might be instilled. Furthermore, given adequate recognition memory, multiple-choice testing also may be a sensible classroom accommodation. For a case example of ISSS, see the information on Carlos in Chapter 5.

Box 3.1. What about Other Narrow Deficits?

This system does not provide a complete listing of potential patterns. Although it is not exhaustive, definitive, or final, our list should prove helpful. What about other patterns of narrow processing deficits that might exist, and why were they not included here? We list three possibilities here (there certainly are more) and explain why they were left out of the present classification scheme.

DEFICIT IN PROCESSING SPEED

Speed of processing is known to relate to success in reading (Catts, Gillespie, Leonard, Kail, & Miller, 2002) and to general cognitive development (Kail, 2000). Diagnosticians working in clinical settings probably find that some children score poorly only on tasks that tap speed and efficiency (i.e., those who are bright but fail speed tasks). For example, such a student might produce low WISC-IV Coding and Symbol Search scores (PSI Index) but average scores on all other WISC-IV subtests (and have average VCI, PRI, and WMI scores). Other children may be very slow on speeded naming tasks. If the same student scored worse on, for example, Reading Fluency than Letter–Word Identification and worse on lower Math Fluency than Calculations on the WJ III Tests of Achievement, the hypothesis of slow processing speed would be strengthened (Reading and Math Fluency reward fast responding; the others are untimed, "power" tests). Further substantiation might come from the classroom, such as teacher reports of a plodding work tempo. Cumulatively, this evidence would suggest a pervasive inability to process information rapidly, and that deficit might be the keystone explanation for a struggling student's poor performance. On other hand, the same facts might be explained by a more familiar pattern obviating the need to resort to (or add to this scheme) another condition (viz., speed deficit disorder). Specifically, low WISC-IV PSI and work incompletion may arise from lack of ability to work quickly with a pencil (GU), a limitation that appears because the student is poor on fine-motor tasks (see Feldman, Kelly, & Diehl, 2004). Alternatively, the same presenting pattern might be better explained by problems with attention (ADHD-I) in a student who cannot sustain effort on any tedious task, whether timed or not. Another possibility is a student who has a generally overly cautious response style (CU), who may respond slowly on Coding and Symbol Search because of repeated checking of his or her responses. When associated with poor reading, slow processing speed may be indicative of an underlying phonological processing problem. For these reasons, and pending expanded publications on processing speed as an impairment to learning, we chose not to include it. Nonetheless, our system is not exhaustive, and many children will not be classified if it is used exclusively. Psychologists may have times when the most cogent explanation is that an individual student works slowly and fails to acquire skills at an automatic level, with no other, better overarching explanation available. Under those circumstances, there is no reason to avoid conceptualizing the problem as one of processing speed. Indeed, both of us have occasionally used such explanations.

DEFICIT IN EXECUTIVE FUNCTIONS

There is no more frequently discussed psychological construct today than executive function. Executive function is a set of metacognitive abilities related to planning, organization, and mental flexibility (Denkla, 1994). Executive functions are independent of specific modalities of information processing (e.g., linguistic or visual–spatial). Accordingly, an impairment of these abilities is hypothesized to affect performance across settings whenever individual component skills must be coordinated and flexibly applied. Many children referred for evaluation are described by parents and teachers as lacking these very abilities. Psychometric measures of executive function have existed in neuropsychological batteries for some time and are now readily available in the form of standardized instruments with good psychometric properties (e.g., Delis–Kaplan Executive Function System; Delis et al., 2001). Patterns characterized by primary deficits in executive measures certainly are seen when children's test scores are scrutinized. For example, many children referred for evaluation score poorly on tests like Trail Making (Reitan & Wolfson, 1992; which requires rapid responding, attention to detail, retaining rules in working memory, and avoiding mental rigidity) or NEPSY Tower (which requires developing a mental plan, retaining the plan in memory, and executing it without becoming distracted). However, children with low scores on tasks like these often match patterns already included in this text. For example, such children often satisfy the criteria for ADHD-I or ADHD-C. Other children who are suspected of executive dysfunction because of poor judgment actually have low IQ scores (e.g., in the SL range). For these reasons, we did not include executive dysfunction as a separate disorder. Nonetheless, psychologists can benefit for recognizing the executive function construct and appreciating its contribution to school learning. At times, executive dysfunction may be legitimately used as the best explanation for the existing findings (see Anderson, 2002).

MEMORY DEFICIT

Teachers and parents sometimes indicate that a student is unable to remember what he or she has learned; accordingly, memory is thought to be the core problem limiting school success. Memory is a complicated set of interrelated functions, not a single ability (see Squire & Schacter, 2003). Most commonly used cognitive tests, such as the WISC-IV, assess short-term or working memory. Many neuropsychological tests measure memory encoding, consolidation, and retrieval of long-term declarative or explicit memory (e.g., the ability to remember a long list of words after immediate exposure[s] and again after a 30-minute delay). For example, the CVLT-C (Delis et al., 1994), the NEPSY (List Learning subtest), and the WRAML-2 contain such tasks. Parallel visual tasks exist in many of these tests as well. Long-term memory problems may appear to be key for struggling students, but closer investigation often detects other problems that are more directly explanatory. Although long-term memory impairments are rampant among children with acquired central nervous system disease or injury (e.g., traumatic brain injury, CNS radiation to treat leukemia or brain tumors), their presence is not widely documented in experimental studies as the prime deficit among children with simple developmental or learning problems. Apparent memory problems often turn out not to be memory problems at all or at least not declarative memory per se. For example, among poor readers, suspected memory problems often relate more to limitation of encoding, registration, and organization (skills that are at least in part extra-memory) than to retrieval (Howe, Bigler, Lawson, & Burlingame, 1999). Absent a history of nervous system disease, memory complaints (such as inability to retain previously mastered spelling words) are often attributable to underlying general cognitive (SL) status. Low general ability may prevent the generation of effective strategies when material is present (thus it is not recalled later) or preclude adequate background ideas to provide scaffolding to support memory (i.e., the ideas presented for memorization are too novel to be remembered well). Obviously, deficits in general language function (SLI) also limit recall of verbal material. Complaints of forgetfulness are often ascribed to attention problems (e.g., see Baron, 2000). Accordingly, we did not include memory deficit among our listed conditions. Once again, this does not mean that memory deficit never represents the best explanation for school learning problems. A thorough evaluation, which may include measures of working and long-term memory, can sometimes help discover the root of classroom learning problems.

CHAPTER 4

◆ ◆ ◆

Performance-Related Conditions

◆

The conditions described in this chapter (ADHD, combined type [ADHD-C], and ADHD, inattentive type [ADHD-I]; and compulsive underproduction [CU]) are distinct from those discussed in the two previous chapters that came before, but they share certain essential diagnostic steps. Performance-related conditions are distinctive in that each of them is principally a failure to use academic skills that have been acquired, rather than primarily a failure to acquire these skills. Nonetheless, they are similar to the other conditions in this book in that a thorough evaluation is generally required to assure that a performance-related condition (rather than some other condition or no condition at all) is present.

As seen in the case studies of Chapter 5 (and flowchart Figure 5.1), two points merge in diagnosticians' practices and conceptualizations. First, diagnosticians must establish as a logical first step that there are no problems with general cognition (IQ) or narrow information processing. Second, diagnosticians must determine that the student possesses basic academic skills roughly equivalent to those of his or her classmates. With these preconditions met, the supposition is that the student has a performance, but not a skill-related, problem. In light of the fact that the student was referred for evaluation and generally has gone through a process of problem solving by a school-based prereferral team, it is likely that a problem exists with skill application. Thus, the diagnostic search narrows to the three conditions presented in this chapter.

Of course, other possibilities exist. The student, for example, may have no problem with either skills or performance. Once a detailed evaluation is conducted, this fact often becomes obvious (although the prereferral process should detect most students who are truly free of academic impairments and prevent their subsequent referral for a full evaluation). It may also be true that a performance problem other than one of the three in this chapter is present. Many children with adequately developed academic skills underperform at school because of psychiatric problems, environmental stresses, lack of support at home, or inadequate instruction. Accordingly, use of behavior consultation at school, especially if both teachers and parents participate, may be necessary (see Sheridan, Eagle, Cowan, & Mickelson, 2001). That is, there may be nothing to be added by placing the child in this classification system; likewise, there may be no disorder-specific interventions for the school psychologist to offer.

ATTENTION-DEFICIT/HYPERACTIVITY DISORDER, COMBINED TYPE

Criteria for Attention-Deficit/Hyperactivity Disorder, Combined Type

1. DSM-IV-TR criteria for ADHD-C or ADHD, predominately hyperactive–impulsive type (although hyperactivity–impulsivity symptoms rarely appear among school-age children without accompanying symptoms of inattention).
2. As discussed here, concerns children with academic performance deficits or, more rarely, frank academic skill deficits.

Common Presentation of Attention-Deficit/Hyperactivity Disorder, Combined Type

Frequent concern of teacher at time of referral	"Doesn't finish work; disrupts other students"
Typical grade of referral	Elementary grades
Gender ratio	More boys than girls
Prevalence in referred sample	Very common

Note. Estimates from clinic setting.

Manifestations

ADHD is among the most widely recognized of all the conditions listed in this book and the most controversial. The number of schoolchildren assigned ADHD diagnoses (e.g., see Harpaz-Rotem & Rosenheck, 2004) and treated with stimulant medication (e.g., see Lin, Crawford, & Lurvey, 2005) such as methylphendiate (e.g., trade name Ritalin) has increased dramatically in recent decades. Much of the national controversy likely arises from these facts. ADHD can be even more disquieting for school-based psychologists who carry certification from state departments of education but not licensure for independent practice. Teachers are more likely than parents or physicians first to mention the prospect of ADHD (Sax & Kautz, 2004) and this may place school psychologists on the front line of diagnosis. On the other hand, many individuals in and outside of the educational system appear to believe that ADHD should be identified by medical doctors and licensed psychologists, not school-based professionals such as school psychologists (U.S. Department of Education, 2003).

Much of the public appears to view ADHD as a medical condition, perhaps because of its widespread treatment with stimulant medication and because the majority of ADHD diagnoses are established by physicians. Related to this assertion is a recent survey of school psychologists in which 60.8% believed ADHD diagnoses should be provided in school settings, yet only 31.6% actually indicated diagnosing ADHD themselves. Nonetheless, there is nothing more inherently medical about ADHD than other diagnoses listed in DSM-IV-TR, such as depression or mental retardation. It is true that the pediatric organizations have produced practice guidelines for diagnosing ADHD (e.g., American Academy of Pediatrics, 2001a), but it is false that the guidelines' key provisions are medical or that pediatricians are better prepared than psychologists to confirm the behaviors necessary to establish the diagnosis (and rule out competing psychiatric diagnoses). In one sense, physician involvement is required in order to rule out low-frequency health conditions that mimic ADHD, such as the rare instance of unrecognized seizure disorder (Wodrich & Kaplan, 2005), but not to document inattention, hyperactivity–impulsivity, or both (i.e., the hallmarks of ADHD) that impairs functioning. It is beyond the scope of this book to resolve these issues of professional responsibility and interprofessional boundaries, but school psychologists are encouraged to refrain from downplaying their considerable diagnostic skills.

In this section we address ADHD, combined type, children who have prominent symptoms of hyperactivity–impulsivity and inattention. DSM-IV-TR does recognize ADHD, predominately hyperactive–impulsive type, but these children rarely appear during the school years (Biederman et al., 1997), hence the ADHD-C designation is used throughout this section. Furthermore, when either the combined or hyperactive–impulsive type is present, it is the dysregulated symptoms common to both types that warrant the most treatment consideration; therefore, discussing hyperactive–impulsive behavior while considering the combined type is germane. In addition, our concern is with the impact of ADHD-C on classroom productivity and learning, not on core symptoms per se or their impact on social function or conduct.

Nonetheless, regarding ADHD itself, the symptoms of hyperactivity and impulsivity are perhaps the most troubling aspect for parents, teachers, and classmates. Hyperactivity is characterized by excessive, seemingly purposeless body movements that often possess a driven quality. Classroom manifestations of hyperactivity appear directly in DSM-IV-TR (see Table 4.1). Behavior like fidgeting, leaving one's seat, and excessive talking obviously can disrupt classroom instruction and frustrate parents, teachers, and fellow students. Beyond annoying others, this type of behavior may be incompatible with work completion for the affected student. Chronic underproduction is therefore a common manifestation of ADHD-C (Barkley, 2006; DeShazo-Barry, Lyman, & Grofer-Klinger, 2002; Hechtman, Abikoff, Klein, Weiss et al., 2004; Rapport, Denney, DuPaul, & Gardner, 1994), as is delayed acquisition of academic skills (DuPaul et al., 2004). Work may be left incomplete, or completed in a hasty manner near deadlines because so much time is spent engaging in restless and driven actions (e.g., trips to the bathroom, talking with peers). Completing and submitting homework can also prove difficult when impulsive actions lead to underregulated engagement in activities of interest (e.g., socializing with peers) instead of attention to assigned tasks. Accordingly, teachers frequently describe these children as not only failing to complete homework assignments, but also lacking time management skills and acting so disorganized that they do not track the location of study materials between school and home and back to school again. Teachers' complaints may include, for example, "Michael did not turn in his math assignment, but when I went through his backpack at the end of the day, his assignment was in the front of his folder." This array of troubling behaviors seems to imply that cognitive deficits are a root problem of ADHD. This does not appear to be the case, however, as disruptive and other task-irrelevant actions are found to predict academic underachievement better in children with ADHD than cognitive deficits such as executive dysfunction or limited general cognitive ability (DeShazo-Barry et al., 2002; Rabiner, Malone, & the Conduct Problems Prevention Research Group, 2004).

Impulsivity, an underdeveloped ability to inhibit responses (especially pre-potent ones) is closely related to hyperactivity. Barkley (1997a; 2006) described children with impulse control problems as generally underregulated, unable to delay responses, and incapable of deferring gratification. As might be expected at school, the child with ADHD often acts without thinking and with little regard for consequences for him- or herself and classmates. This manner of responding can be especially aggravating for parents and teachers, who often believe that they must repeatedly redirect

TABLE 4.3. DSM-IV-TR Diagnostic Criteria for Attention-Deficit/Hyperactivity Disorder

A. Either (1) or (2):

(1) six (or more) of the following symptoms of **inattention** have persisted for at least 6 months to a degree that is maladaptive and inconsistent with development level:

Inattention
  (a) often fails to give close attention to details or makes careless mistakes in schoolwork, work, or other activities
  (b) often has difficulty sustaining attention in tasks or play activities
  (c) often does not seem to listen when spoken to directly
  (d) often does not follow through on instructions and fails to finish schoolwork, chores, or duties in the workplace (not due to oppositional behavior or failure to understand instructions)
  (e) often has difficulty organizing tasks and activities
  (f) often avoids, dislikes, or is reluctant to engage in tasks that require sustained mental effort (such as schoolwork or homework)
  (g) often loses things necessary for tasks or activities (e.g., toys, school assignments, pencils, books, or tools)
  (h) is often easily distracted by extraneous stimuli
  (i) is often forgetful in daily activities

(2) six (or more) of the following symptoms of **hyperactivity–impulsivity** have persisted for at least 6 months to a degree that is maladaptive and inconsistent with developmental level:

Hyperactivity
  (a) often fidgets with hands or feet or squirms in seat
  (b) often leaves seat in classroom or in other situations in which remaining seated is expected
  (c) often runs about or climbs excessively in situations in which it is inappropriate (in adolescents or adults, may be limited to subjective feelings of restlessness)
  (d) often has difficulty playing or engaging in leisure activities quietly
  (e) is often "on the go" or often acts as if "driven by a motor"
  (f) often talks excessively

Impulsivity
  (g) often bursts out answers before questions have been completed
  (h) often has difficulty awaiting turn
  (i) often interrupts or intrudes on others (e.g., butts into conversations or games)

B. Some hyperactive–impulsive or inattentive symptoms that caused impairment were present before age 7 years.
C. Some impairment from the symptoms is present in two or more settings (e.g., at school [or work] and at home).
D. There must be clear evidence of clinically significant impairment in social, academic, or occupational functioning.
E. The symptoms do not occur exclusively during the course of a Pervasive Developmental Disorder, Schizophrenia, or other Psychotic Disorder and are not better accounted for by another mental disorder (e.g., Mood Disorder, Anxiety Disorder, Dissociative Disorder, or a Personality Disorder).

Note. From American Psychiatric Association (2000). Copyright 2000 by the American Psychiatric Association. Reprinted by permission.

and remind the child to slow down and think before acting. Risk-taking, which often lasts into adulthood, also seems to arise from impulsivity. For example, studies indicate that adolescents and young adults with ADHD are especially likely to use alcohol, tobacco, and illicit drugs (Molina & Pelham, 2003) and to suffer symptoms of substance dependence (Abrantes, Brown, & Tomlinson, 2003). Adolescents and young adults with ADHD also appear to engage in high rates of vehicular risk-taking, as indexed by self-reports of traffic citations, car accidents, and driver's license suspensions (Barkley, Murphy, DuPaul, & Bush, 2002). Favorably, properly managed pharmacotherapy seems to reduce the risk for later substance abuse (Biederman, 2003; Wilens, 2004) and improves driving performance, at least in a simulator (Cox, Merkel, Penberthy, Kovatchev, & Hankin, 2004).

Compromised interpersonal relations and peer rejection have also been shown to accompany impulsivity and hyperactivity (Abikoff, Hechtman, Klein, Gallagher, et al., 2004; Barkley, 2006; Greene et al., 2001). Poor regulation of affect, overly intense behavioral responses, cognitive distortions, and deficient social skills have been theorized to underlie the rejection children with ADHD often endure (Antshel & Remer, 2003; Pfiffner, Calzada, & McBurnett, 2000). For example, a child with ADHD may be loud, interrupt others, fail to keep his or her hands to self or wait for his or her turn, blurt out rude comments, and overreact when frustrated. It is easy to understand how disregard for social conventions and repeated annoying of peers can foster alienation and negative long-term social outcome (Kupersmidt, Coie, & Dodge, 1990). As reviewed later in this section, improving the social status and interpersonal skills of unpopular children with ADHD is often difficult. Thus, the accumulated research on ADHD-C suggests that, for many children, numerous facets of life, both at school and at home, are affected. For school psychologists, this fact suggests that ADHD-C is likely to affect much more than work completion and classroom productiveness (although work incompletion is the focus of the disorder in this chapter). Accordingly, school psychologists must adopt a broad approach to intervention if they are to maximize their help of the affected student.

Assessment Considerations

The most appropriate method of establishing an ADHD diagnosis is to proceed directly to the DSM-IV-TR criteria and carefully address each. Accordingly, informants (typically parents and teachers) confirm the presence of six or more symptoms of hyperactivity–impulsivity and six symptoms of inattention if ADHD-C is present. Interview of parents, teachers, and child and review of work samples and report cards, plus developmental/medical history, are necessary to identify preliminarily the presence of the requisite symptoms and to decide if supplemental assessment is warranted. To confirm ADHD, these symptoms must be present to a significant degree, cause impairment in multiple settings, and have produced problems before age 7 years. It is also necessary to exclude competing explanations (e.g., autism, anxiety, mental retardation). Of note, another section of this book addresses ADHD-I, which appears to be distinct from ADHD-C in important ways related to etiology, natural history, and optimal method of treatment.

Given their psychometric backgrounds, psychologists may rely on behavioral rating scales to supplement (and sometimes replace) other methods of data collection. Such scales help with the two main questions confronting diagnosticians: Are remarkable levels of hyperactivity–impulsivity and inattention symptoms present? And are other psychiatric conditions (that may be the root problem) absent? Familiar to most school psychologists are broad-band rating scales that assess a variety of symptom clusters and narrow-band rating scales that identify ADHD symptoms primarily or exclusively. A recent review indicates that among narrow-band scales with reasonable reliability and validity are the Attention Deficit Disorder Evaluation Scales (ADDES; McCarney, 1995), ADHD Rating Scales–IV (ADHD-IV; DuPaul, Power, Anastopoulos, & Reid, 1998) and the Conners' Rating Scales—Revised (CRS-R; Conners, 1997; see Demaray, Elting, & Schaefer, 2003). To screen for other psychiatric clusters, we commonly employ broad-band measures like the Achenbach System of Empirically Based Assessment (ASEBA; Achenbach & Rescorla, 2001), which includes the Child Behavior Checklist (CBCL) and Teacher Report Form (TRF), or the BASC-2 (Reynolds & Kamphaus, 2004) Parent Rating Scales and Teacher Rating Scales. Evidence exists that the original versions of the BASC and Achenbach CBCL and TRF all differentiate children with ADHD from children without ADHD reasonably well (Vaughn, Riccio, Hynd, & Hall, 1997). One subsequent study found that the BASC Parent Rating Scales better identified children with ADHD than the Achenbach CBCL (Ostrander, Weinfurt, Yarnold, & August, 1998). Although both rating scales appear appropriate in the assessment of ADHD, we commonly employ the BASC-2. The updated versions of these instruments are likely to be just as effective as their predecessors.

These broad-band instruments provide *T*-scores comparing the referred child with a standardization sample as rated by their parents and teachers on various dimensions, including hyperactivity–impulsivity and inattention. They also afford ratings related to competing diagnoses, such as depression or anxiety. For example, most behavior rating scales, like the BASC-2, report scores in terms of *T*-scores, and a score of 70 often is considered to be in the clinical range, indicating the presence of a notable level of problem behaviors. In the case of a child with ADHD-C, one would expect to find T–scores on the BASC-2 at or near 70 on scales tapping hyperactivity–impulsivity and inattention (Manning & Miller, 2001). Combining parent scales with those from classroom teachers can thus help address the critical challenges of ruling some conditions in and others out.

Unfortunately, rating scales and interviews are silent regarding one challenge confronting the diagnostician considering the performance problems: Does the student actually possess the cognitive, information-processing, and academic skills necessary to succeed at this grade level? Somehow there must be assurance that none of the problems in Chapter 2 (IQ related) or Chapter 3 (narrow information processing) is present, or if they are present, that co-occurrence is documented. Although some data suggest IQ measures (i.e., the Digit Span and Information subtests of the WISC-III in particular) provide reasonable accuracy in identifying the presence of ADHD (Assesmany, McIntosh, Phelps, & Rizza, 2001), we nonetheless caution against the interpretation of these subtests in isolation. There is no evidence of sufficient sensitivity and specificity to use these techniques for clinical purposes; depressed scores on these two scales may result from a wide variety of conditions other than ADHD.

A thorough psychometric evaluation is almost always required when a performance problem such as ADHD-C is at issue. The exception to the must-evaluate dictum is the case of the high-achieving student who has clearly demonstrated that he or she possesses solid academic skills. Consistent with this idea, in clinic settings, we have performed some assessment of ADHD without a comprehensive test battery. This was accomplished by collecting a detailed educational history and screening the student for academic problems. For those without any history of problems acquiring reading, writing, and arithmetic skills and who show average performance in academic domains, the full cognitive and information-processing evaluation may be unnecessary. For these children, confirmation of ADHD symptoms and exclusion of competing psychiatric possibilities then becomes the prime assessment mission.

The use of other psychological tests—such as direct psychometric measures of attention and impulse control or indirect measures of executive function—is subject to debate. On the surface, measuring attention or impulsivity with standard psychometric tests seems quite feasible. Many psychologists are familiar with cancellation tasks or go-no-go tests whose content putatively corresponds to sustained attention and impulse control, respectively. For example, the stop signal task (a computerized test of impulse control commonly used in ADHD research) has been shown to document the impulse control problems of children with ADHD-C (Nigg, Blaskey, Huang-Pollock, & Rappley, 2002). Most straightforward tests of impulse control and executive functioning, however, do not work very well to confirm or disconfirm the presence of ADHD in practical settings. This unfortunate fact is seemingly true of even sophisticated executive function tests designed to tap planning, judgment, efficiency, and impulse control often thought to be associated with frontal lobe brain functioning (Denckla, 1994). Most of these executive tests produce only modest differences between groups of children with ADHD and matched controls. Pennington (2002) pointed out that the effect size associated with executive tests (the departure of the mean of the ADHD group, in standard deviations, from the mean of the control group) is only a modest 0.5 to 1.5, far less than the groups separate themselves on behavioral rating scales. Even more important, almost all of the executive measures fail to predict true cases of ADHD (positive predictive power, PPP) or rule out false cases of ADHD (negative predictive power, NPP; see Barkley & Grodzinsky, 1994).

The exception to this general rule appears to be relatively lengthy, computer-based continuous performance tests (CPT). Examples of CPTs include the Continuous Performance Test—Second Edition (Conners, 2000), the Gordon Diagnostic System (Gordon, 1991), and the Test of Variables of Attention (Greenberg et al., 1997). CPTs typically provide ongoing and fairly rapid stimulus presentation and require the examinee to respond when a target stimulus appears. Most of these tests include an associated requirement to inhibit responding in the presence of non-target stimuli. Thus, most CPTs tax sustained attention and response inhibition but impose few cognitive demands (most CPT tasks are quite simple). Such techniques enjoy wide clinical use and a body of research support (see Ricco, Reynolds, Lowe, & Moore, 2002). For example, the vigilance task from Gordon Diagnostic System presents single-digit numbers at a roughly 1-second rate. The child's task is to await numbers appearing in a specific order (e.g., 4 followed by 7) and to respond with an immediate button press. A computerized system records correct responses, failure to respond to target stimuli, and false alarm hits. In contrast to other executive measures, this test provides strong PPP for ADHD when abnormal scores arise (between 90 and 100%), but only modest NPP when normal scores arise (typically around 50%; Barkley & Grodzinsky, 1994). These were values derived under somewhat artificial circumstances (50–50 split of ADHD and controls was used in the study sample), and the same ability to predict in clinical settings may not exist. Nonetheless, clinicians sometimes supplement parent and teacher interviews, rating scales, and general psychometric batteries with CPTs when ADHD becomes a compelling possibility. In these circumstances, it is generally assumed that normal scores do little to rule ADHD in or out (given weak NPP), but that abnormal scores help to rule in ADHD (given good PPP). Their potential contributory knowledge notwithstanding, these CPTs are not required to confirm the presence of ADHD. Practically, not all child evaluation clinics choose to include CPTs in their standard battery, and it appears that few school psychologists make routine use of CPT techniques. Most psychologists prefer interviews and rating scales.

Other Possibilities

Hyperactivity, impulsivity, and inattention are common to many disorders, not just ADHD. For example, children with mental retardation, ODD/conduct disorder, and other psychiatric disorders listed in DSM-IV-TR that involve psychomotor agitation (e.g., bipolar disorder) may appear overactive and/or impulsive. Thus, consultation with DSM-IV-TR is often needed in order to rule out competing hypotheses or to determine that ADHD is present when another or co-occurring psychiatric disorder is a possibility.

Within this book's framework, IQ-related disorders are the first to be considered (see Figure 5.1). A routine psychometric battery should be sufficient to determine if mental retardation is present. For sake of diagnostic parsimony, if mental retardation is present, we do not advocate for dual diagnoses of mental retardation and ADHD. Rather, it makes more sense to conclude that mental retardation is present and to note that it occurs with hyperactive and inattentive features (i.e., elements of hyperactivity–impulsivity and inattention often accompany low cognitive ability and adaptive delays but are unlikely to be distinct from them or to make up a separate disorder).

After IQ-related disorders have been ruled out, one might question if the disruptive behavior exhibited by a hyperactive–impulsive child is due to an SLD. Because ADHD and learning disabilities often co-occur (Barkley, 2006), a standard psychometric battery is frequently administered and clinical interviews conducted to address the presence of both disorders. When teasing apart the reason for classroom hyperactive, impulsive, or inattentive behavior, it is important to remember that the diagnosis of ADHD requires the presence of some hyperactive–impulsive symptoms before age 7 and that symptoms must occur across two or more settings. In light of these requirements, consultation with teachers and formal classroom observations may be used to confirm symptoms (and accompanying impaired functioning) at school. Alternatively, behavior rating scales, as well as clinical interviews completed with teachers and caregivers at home, are used to demonstrate the presence of problematic behavior that extends across settings.

Behavior rating scales can help in the diagnosis of ADHD and in documenting other psychiatric disorders with clinical features that are similar to or overlap with ADHD. From 54 to 67% of children with ADHD also satisfy diagnostic criteria for ODD, about 25% for an anxiety-related disorder, and between 20 and 30% for a mood disorder (Barkley, 2004). For example, as indicated in DSM-IV-TR, ODD is marked by argumen-tativeness, willful defiance of adults or rules, and both deliberate annoy-ance of and being easily annoyed by others (APA, 2000), these features may be confirmed by parent or teacher ratings. Thus, conduct scales on behavior rating forms (e.g., BASC-2 and Achenbach rating scales), in addi-tion to clinical interviews, help screen for the presence of oppositional or conduct behavior that co-occurs with ADHD and requires treatment.

Using the same techniques, diagnosticians can determine if hyperactivity–impulsivity is part of another psychiatric disorder of which psychomotor agi-tation is a clinical feature. A mood disorder with manic features, like bipo-lar disorder, as well as various psychotic disorders, must be ruled out before ADHD is ruled in. Biederman (1998) argued that pediatric bipolar disorder is commonly mistaken for severe ADHD because the two disor-ders share many symptoms, such as distractibility, motoric overactivity, and excessive talking (Spencer et al., 2001). Although too complex to explain here fully, the methods of subtraction (overlapping symptoms are not considered during diagnosis) and proportion (overlapping symptoms are not considered, and a reduced proportion of symptoms from each crite-ria are required) can help psychologists to differentiate these two condi-tions. In short, elevation on scales tapping anxiety, depression, and atypical behavior, as well as clinical interview, may be used to screen for comorbid disorders or to help form alternative diagnostic hypotheses (see Biederman et al., 1996, for a more thorough explanation). Establishing a clear diagno-sis is important, as the presence of a mood and/or psychotic disorder, instead of ADHD, indicates that different treatment (e.g., psychotherapy, medication) and special education services (e.g., OHI [other health impairment] vs. ED might be required.

Given the overlap of ADHD with other psychiatric disorders, ruling out the presence of competing diagnoses can be a challenge for some school psychologists. In fact, some prefer the ADHD diagnosis be provided by medical professionals. We argue, however, that school psychologists pos-sess the breadth of training necessary reliably to identify the presence of this disorder and to rule out competing explanations for problem behavior. Furthermore, no mental health professional enjoys extended contact with children the way school psychologists do. The ease with which school psy-chologists can repeatedly observe a child at school, across various educa-tional settings, and tap a variety of evaluation sources (e.g., rating scales, psychometric instruments, interview of parents and teachers, observation in the natural setting), places the psychologist in a unique position unavailable to most physicians.

School psychologists' diagnostic advantages aside, collaboration with physicians when diagnosing and treating ADHD remains essential. If the family chooses to access physicians' expertise to explore the presence of

ADHD, school psychologists and other school staff help by providing direct classroom observations (Wodrich & Landau, 1999). In our experience, school personnel are skilled at describing behavior in ways that contribute to accurate diagnosis. With the relentless exposure ADHD receives in the media, awareness is ever-expanding, and families are turning to school-based mental health professionals to help address their concerns and determine if their child has ADHD. In the future, school psychologists will probably both play a more central role in the diagnosis of ADHD and become more involved in medication management, as requested by prescribing physicians (HaileMariam, Bradley-Johnson, & Johnson, 2002). For example, school psychologists can provide prescribing physicians with valuable information that can be used to judge medication effectiveness. Unfortunately, at present, physicians seem more likely to have contact with school staff, including school psychologists, during the initial diagnostic rather than the follow-up treatment phase.

Eligibility Issues

There are two main avenues through which children with ADHD-C receive special services: under Section 504 or IDEA (i.e., OHI or ED). See Table 4.2

TABLE 4.2. Key Elements of Definitions under the Individuals with Disabilities Education Act (Other Health Impairment and Emotional Disturbance) and Section 504

Other health impairment	Emotional disturbance	Section 504
◆ Limited strength, vitality, or alertness ◆ Including heightened alertness to environmental stimuli ◆ Due to chronic or acute health problems ◆ Which affects a pupil's educational performance	◆ Inability to learn that cannot be explained by intellectual, sensory, or health factors ◆ Inability to build and maintain satisfactory relationships with peers and teachers ◆ Inappropriate types of behavior or feelings under normal circumstances ◆ A general pervasive mood of unhappiness or depression ◆ A tendency to develop physical symptoms associated with personal or school problems	◆ Physical or mental impairment ◆ Substantially limits one or more major life activities ◆ Or record of such impairment ◆ Or is regarded as having such an impairment

for a comparison of the key elements of each. If a modified curriculum (e.g., adjustments in grade level) or intensive instruction appears unnecessary, a Section 504 accommodation plan may be considered. Section 504 of the Rehabilitation Act of 1973 mandates accommodations for students with physical or mental impairments that substantially limit one or more major life activities (learning being one) or with a record of such an impairment, or are regarded as having such an impairment (PL 93-112). Regarding ADHD, the challenge of the 504 team is to determine if the disorder substantially limits the child's education. It can be argued that if factors like poor organization and planning, limited time spent on-task, or problems with work completion exist, then a Section 504 plan should be considered. However, some children with ADHD require more than standard and straightforward accommodations in order to succeed. If a student support team believes that a modified curriculum is necessary due to failing performance, or if intensive instruction out of proportion to the spirit of a Section 504 plan seems necessary, special education services probably should be considered. The most common eligibility category is OHI (U.S. Department of Education, 2003). Eligibility in this category requires that a student has

> limited strength, vitality or alertness, including a heightened alertness to environmental stimuli, that results in limited alertness with respect to the educational environment, that—(i) Is due to chronic or acute health problems such as . . . attention deficit disorder or attention deficit hyperactivity disorder . . . and (ii) Adversely affects a child's educational performance. (IDEA, 1997)

Regarding Section 504, ADHD is currently recognized as a chronic health problem that can adversely affect a student. Regarding IDEA, it may be more difficult to determine that ADHD is indeed present than to establish the second criterion that it have a negative impact sufficient to warrant special education designation. It can be argued that failure of a good-faith Section 504 plan implies the necessity for additional, more intensive intervention that may require special education staff and resources (i.e., special education services). Furthermore, the point at which skills deficits become clear (e.g., significantly underdeveloped academic skills compared to peers) beyond mere performance deficits (e.g., poor work completion), the prospect of OHI special education becomes more compelling.

Special education eligibility under the category of ED might also be considered, especially for students with significant behavioral dysregulation or impaired interpersonal function at school. The issues associated with ED eligibility are discussed later in this chapter in relation to the student with CU (see Table 4.5, p. 155). The same decision-making process and special qualifiers also apply when considering eligibility for the child with ADHD-C and ADHD-I (in the book's next section) as apply to CU. The evaluation team will probably consider whether or not the student demonstrates an inability to build or maintain satisfactory interpersonal relationships with peers and teachers and/or expresses inappropriate types of behavior or feelings under normal circumstances (see Table 4.5 for definition of ED). In other words, the key elements of the ED statutory definition must be considered.

If the student with ADHD-C is found to be eligible for special education, regardless of category, related services should also be considered. As GU is commonly seen in children with ADHD, a referral for an occupational therapy evaluation might be in order. Furthermore, consultation with an assistive technology specialist might help to determine if supplementary instructional personnel or devices might be required to assume a "[free] appropriate public education," as required by IDEA. For example, some schools provide graphic organizers to aid in planning and organization, as well as word processing devices to circumvent handwriting deficits. These and other supports are spelled out in the original federal position on special services for students with ADHD (see Davila, 1994).

Treatment Considerations

A consensus about empirically validated treatment for ADHD-C appears to have emerged during the past decade. It is now widely accepted that (1) pharmacotherapy or medication management, (2) parent training, (3) contingency management (behavior therapy), and (4) classroom-based behavior modification are the empirically supported treatments for ADHD-C (American Academy of Pediatrics, 2001a; Barkley, 2004; MTA Cooperative Group, 1999a; Pelham, Wheeler, & Chronis, 1998). Each of these four classes of intervention is considered separately.

The first intervention is pharmacotherapy. It is no surprise to school psychologists that pharmacological interventions have been intensively studied. Although antidepressants, antihypertensives, and norepinephrin reuptake inhibitors are commonly prescribed to treat ADHD (Barkley, 2004), stimulant medications (e.g., methylphenidate, such as Ritalin) are most widely studied and have garnered the most empirical support. Subsequent to an extensive review of treatment outcomes, the American Academy of Pediatrics (2001a) indicated that stimulant medications should be a first-line treatment because they often create significant reduction in core symptoms (inattention, hyperactivity, impulsivity) and have mild side effects. Recent reviews have also looked at the effectiveness of engaging in various psychosocial interventions in addition to stimulant therapy (combined condition) versus stimulant therapy alone. Against intuition and to the surprise of the research group, multimodal psychosocial treatment (Abikoff, Hechtman, Klein, Weiss et al., 2004), social skills training

(Abikoff, Hechtman, Klein, Gallagher et al., 2004), parent training (Hechtman, Abikoff, Klein, Greenfield, et al., 2004), and psychotherapy and academic intervention (Hechtman, Abikoff, Klein, Weiss, et al., 2004) in combination with stimulant therapy did not significantly improve outcome above what was provided by stimulant therapy alone *in stimulant-responsive children*. Thus, there is compelling evidence that stimulant medication is, in fact, an important first-line treatment of ADHD for many children, including those with performance deficits.

Other evidence suggests that psychosocial intervention, in addition to stimulant therapy, is helpful in some instances. Findings from the large-scale MTA Cooperative Group (1999b) indicate that combination therapy (i.e., stimulant medication with psychosocial intervention) is worthwhile in addressing non-core symptoms of ADHD, like aggression/oppositional behavior, internalizing symptoms, social skills problems, parent–child difficulties, and reading achievement deficits. In general, however, stimulant medication was found superior to behavior therapy. These findings might lead one to conclude that the need for supplemental behavioral interventions varies as a function of each child's responsiveness to stimulants. Such general conclusions may not be appropriate. It is important to note that the MTA Cooperative Group study has been criticized for inadequate individualization of treatment groups, insufficient incorporation of cognitive-behavioral treatment strategies, overemphasis of core ADHD symptoms, and treatment sequences in which medication always preceded behavioral treatment in the children who received both medication and behavioral–psychosocial treatments (Anastopoulos, 2000; Hoza, 2001; Root & Resnick, 2003). Additionally, when data from the MTA Group were reanalyzed using a composite score that combined ratings of parents and teachers, the combined treatment group was found to be superior to all other treatment conditions, including medication alone (Conners, Epstein, & March, 2001).

The benefits of medication notwithstanding, it is important to note two facts: (1) approximately 8–25% of children with ADHD fail to respond to stimulant medication to a clinically significant degree, and (2) the behavior of most stimulant-responsive children is not normalized (American Academy of Pediatrics, 2001a; Barkley, 2002). Furthermore, the target behaviors of greatest concern to school psychologists include academic productivity and accuracy, not hyperactivity–impulsivity per se. For example, in a carefully controlled study of medication use, a vast majority of children with ADHD-C responded to carefully adjusted stimulants, but a large subset of positive responders still failed to demonstrate improvement in their rate or accuracy of academic performance (Rapport et al., 1994). Overall, school- and academic-related targets are far less well documented to improve with stimulant use (Hoffman & DuPaul, 2000), or they may be addressed only indirectly by the use of academic rating forms (Wodrich & Kush, 1998). In apparent acknowledgment of some of these facts, the American Academy of Pediatrics (2001a) promotes the use of behavior therapy, parent training, and contingency management at home and school, as well as medication. Likewise, Conners, March, Frances, Wells, and Ross (2001), with the assistance of other experts in the field, developed consensus guidelines regarding the diagnosis and treatment of ADHD that endorse behavioral interventions as first-line under some circumstances (see Table 4.3).

The second intervention involves developing parents' skills. Parent training is well documented to reduce the disruptive behavior of children with ADHD (Barkley, 2002; MTA Cooperative Group, 1999a; Pelham et al., 1998). Among the variety of existing parent training programs, at least one popular program (Barkley, 1997b) is shown to improve the disruptive behavior of children with ADHD in 64% of participant families (Anastopoulos, Shelton, DuPaul, & Guevremont, 1993; Barkley, 2002). This training program is implemented across 10 sessions and provides parents with psychoeducational information regarding ADHD. It explores causes of oppositional behavior, develops positive parent attention skills, provides techniques to increase child compliance, implements a token economy at home, facilitates the use of time-out as a means of discipline, and seeks to manage behavior outside the home and in school through the use of a home–school report card. The program can be implemented with high

---

TABLE 4.3. Consensus Guidelines for the Diagnosis and Treatment of Attention-Deficit/Hyperactivity Disorder: First-Line Treatment Recommendations

Behavioral–psychosocial intervention is indicated as a first-line treatment when any of the following is present:

- Mild symptoms of ADHD
- The focus of treatment is a preschool-age child
- Comorbid internalizing disorders
- Comorbid social skill deficits
- The family prefers psychosocial intervention prior to exploring medication therapy

Medication and psychosocial intervention combined is indicated as a first-line treatment when any of the following is present:

- Severe symptoms of ADHD
- Marked aggression or school problems
- Significant family disruption caused by ADHD-related behavior
- Comorbid externalizing disorders
- Central nervous system dysfunction (e.g., mental retardation, epilepsy)

Note. Data from Conners, March, et al. (2001) and Root and Resnick (2003).

integrity by school psychologists because its material is well organized, sessions are carefully scripted, and extensive handouts for family members are provided. We have implemented this training program and have found that parents generally enjoy it and find its sessions quite helpful. Although valuable, parent training programs are unlikely to alter problems with work completion (unless specifically targeted in a behavior plan) and academic skill development, the concerns addressed in this chapter.

The third intervention is behavior therapy. Contingency management (behavior therapy) is a well-established treatment as well, both at home and school (Barkley, 2004; MTA Cooperative Group, 1999a). Within the realm of behavior therapy, the American Academy of Pediatrics (2001a), based on a review of published studies, promotes the use of positive reinforcement, time-out, response cost, and a token economy for children with ADHD. In a separate review of the psychosocial treatment literature, Barkley (2002) concluded that effective contingency management programs use secondary/tangible reinforcers in addition to attention or other social rewards, as well as a reward system structured through a token economy. Elements in such a system include rewards and response costs (see Table 4.4 for a summary of intervention principles).

Effective classroom management of ADHD behavior may also be undertaken through the use of contingency management procedures (American Academy of Pediatrics, 2001a; Pelham et al., 1998). DuPaul and Eckert (1997) conducted a meta-analysis of 63 outcome studies and concluded that contingency management methods were effective in improving the classroom behavior of children with ADHD. Improving the academic

TABLE 4.4. Summary of Intervention Principles for Attention-Deficit/ Hyperactivity Disorder Suggested by Pfiffner and Barkley

1. Rules and instructions must be clear, brief, and often delivered through highly visible and external modes of presentation.
2. Consequences must be delivered swiftly and immediately.
3. Consequences must be delivered more frequently than for children without ADHD.
4. Rewards must be of sufficient reinforcement value and consequences of sufficient magnitude to provide motivation.
5. A rich schedule of reinforcement for appropriate behavior must be provided before punishment is implemented.
6. Reinforcers must be changed regularly in order to avoid loss of reinforcement value (habituation or satiation).
7. Anticipation of problem behaviors and planning ahead is essential.

Note. Adapted from Pfiffner and Barkley (1998). Copyright 1998 by The Guilford Press. Adapted by permission.

performance of children with ADHD may prove more daunting, as a significant minority of children treated with stimulant medication does not enjoy improved academic work completion and accuracy (Rapport et al., 1994). That is, improvement in core symptoms of hyperactivity–impulsivity or inattention does not automatically equate to improved academics. Of course, applied behavior analysis permits treatment to address precise behaviors of concern (e.g., blurting out answers in class or low rate of worksheet completion) in ways impossible with medication. Contingency management in the classroom appears a logical next step if stimulant medication alone is not successful. The first step is usually performance of a functional behavior analysis (Kazdin, 2001). Some children with ADHD emit hyperactive or disruptive behavior to serve the function of task avoidance and classroom attention, among other considerations (Hoff, Ervin, & Friman, 2005). Understanding the "function" of behavior of students with ADHD, rather than considering their conduct as arising solely from ADHD, permits generation of effective individualized behavior plans. Beyond individualized approaches, Carlson, Mann, and Alexander (2000) studied the broad impact of contingencies. They found that compared to reward, response cost improved the accuracy of completed arithmetic problems, but not completion rate. Accordingly, response cost may be more effective than reward in improving the academic performance of some children with ADHD.

Other data indicate that curriculum modifications may improve the production of children with ADHD. One way to do this is to reduce the amount of work required, recognizing that teachers may argue this modification risks robbing students of the practice necessary to learn concepts (other teachers may be concerned about unfair grading practices). Interspersing relatively simple math problems within assignments has been shown to be a means of increasing on-task classroom behavior via modification of curriculum (Skinner, Wallace & Neddenriep, 2002). McCurdy, Skinner, Grantham, Watson, and Hindman (2001) provided a student referred to the school psychologist for off-task behavior with arithmetic assignments that included simple, brief problems. Interestingly, when these elements were introduced, the student's rate of on-task behavior improved, despite the lengthening of the overall assignment. In addition to interventions like these, peer tutoring (DuPaul & Eckert, 1997; Rabiner et al., 2004), chunking assignments into smaller parts with preestablished time limits for completion, and reducing the amount of production required (Pfiffner & Barkley, 1998) may also prove helpful.

Whereas the preceding interventions have earned general support from empirical research, there are some commonly recommended treatments whose efficacy has not been adequately determined or reported in the peer-reviewed literature. For example, although cognitive-behavioral therapy is the treatment of choice for many internalizing psychiatric disorders (e.g., depression, OCD), this treatment modality has not been shown to be consistently effective for children with ADHD (American Academy of Pediatrics, 2001a; DuPaul & Eckert, 1997; Pelham et al., 1998). Likewise, there is limited empirical evidence for interventions that target remediation of underlying attention processes, such as by providing children with attention-enhancing drills (see Riccio & French, 2004, for a summary of published studies). A program entitled Attention Process Training–II (Sohlberg, Johnson, Paule, Raskin, & Mateer, 1993) does enjoy some tentative support, but social skills training, which is commonly recommended for children with ADHD-C, does not enjoy empirical support (e.g., Antshel & Remer, 2003). Barkley (2004) also cautions that apparent initial positive findings have not been confirmed by subsequent well-controlled experimental replications for vestibular stimulation, oral-motor chewing, EEG/EMG biofeedback, relaxation training, sensory integration training, and dietary treatments (e.g., removal of sugar, additives, coloring; adding vitamins or dietary supplements). For a case example of ADHD-C, see the information on Ryan in Chapter 5.

ATTENTION-DEFICIT/HYPERACTIVITY DISORDER, INATTENTIVE TYPE

Criteria for Attention-Deficit/Hyperactivity Disorder, Predominantly Inattentive Type

1. DSM-IV-TR criteria for ADHD-I.
2. As discussed here, concerns children with academic performance deficits or, more rarely, frank academic skill deficits.

Common Presentation of Attention-Deficit/Hyperactivity Disorder, Inattentive Type

Frequent concern of teacher at time of referral	"Doesn't pay attention; doesn't finish work"
Typical grade of referral	Elementary grades
Gender ratio	Roughly equal boys and girls
Prevalence in referred sample	Common

Note. Estimates from clinic setting.

Manifestations

Some children with ADHD express remarkable problems paying attention even though they are not especially hyperactive or impulsive. They are members of a subgroup referred to as ADHD, predominantly inattentive type (ADHD-I). At the practical level, school psychologists are most likely to hear about such students because they are not paying attention *and* they are not finishing their work. In our experience, there is a lot of tolerance for inattention that does not limit work accuracy or completion. In fact, our system concerns ADHD-I because it clarifies why some children are unable to complete their work despite having acquired reasonable academic skills (i.e., their inattentive nature precludes satisfactory day-to-day academic performance). Thus, as discussed here, this is primarily a performance-related, rather than a skill-related, problem. Children with ADHD-I are particularly susceptible to problems with sustained attention during dull, boring, repetitive tasks, such as schoolwork and chores (Barkley, 2006). DSM-IV-TR, as outlined in the previous section, lists symptoms of inattention that must manifest across settings and cause impairment to reach a threshold for diagnosis (see Table 4.1). Children with ADHD-I as a group struggle to sustain attention and, as a result, often avoid tasks that require concerted and ongoing effort. They also experience a host of related problems that limit work completion: careless mistakes on worksheets or tests, failing to listen when spoken to, not remembering instructions necessary for completing assignments, giving up before tasks are completed, failing to create and follow a plan, and losing things required to accomplish homework.

Some of these problems seem to arise from distractibility, and indeed teachers and parents of children with ADHD-I often complain that these children appear especially vulnerable to environmental distractions. Barkley (2006) argues, however, that although children with ADHD-I may be drawn off-task by extraneous stimuli (e.g., a classmate in the hallway, a conversation in the corner of the classroom), distractibility's role may be more apparent than real. In reality, distractibility may actually represent "diminished persistence of effort or sustained responding to tasks that have little intrinsic appeal or minimal immediate consequences for completion" (p. 57). This proposition may help explain the seeming waxing and waning of inattentive symptoms that can prove perplexing to teachers and parents. For example, a classroom teacher may ask the school psychologist how a child expresses such severe inattention during lectures and when listening to directions, but has no problems at all playing ball with a PE teacher. Similarly, parents may ask why their child is incapable of completing even simple worksheets without repeated prompting but is able to play intricate videogames for hours. The answer may be that when a child is matched with an intrinsically motivating activity or is the benefactor of a rich schedule of reinforcement, then he or she experiences few requirements for self-directed attention; inattentiveness accordingly diminishes or disappears.

Although factor-analytic studies consistently demonstrate that ADHD comprises two factors—hyperactivity–impulsivity and inattention (see Milich, Balentine, & Lynam, 2001, for a review)—it nonetheless appears that the inattention of children with ADHD-C and the inattention of ADHD-I are qualitatively different. For example, the presence of "sluggish cognitive tempo" may be used to distinguish children with ADHD-I from their ADHD-C counterparts (Carlson & Mann, 2000, 2002; McBurnett, Pfiffner, & Frick, 2001; Weiler, Holmes-Bernstein, Bellinger, & Waber, 2000, 2002). Descriptors such as "daydreaming," "drowsy," "apathetic," "amotivation," "underactive," "slow moving," and "lacking in energy" characterize children with ADHD-I but not those with ADHD-C. In fact, recent studies have looked at the processing skills of children with sluggish cognitive tempo. Similarly, Weiler et al. (2002) showed that children with ADHD-I performed more slowly on visual-processing tasks (but not on an auditory-processing task) than children without ADHD (i.e., poor readers). Furthermore, sluggish cognitive tempo was not simply a byproduct of inattention. Thus, the presence of these characteristics may help differentiate children with ADHD-I from those with ADHD-C. Even though qualitative differences may exist in research, teacher and parent ratings of attention for children with ADHD, including and excluding sluggish cognitive tempo, may not actually differ (McBurnett et al., 2001). This suggests that while levels of inattention may be rated as similar for children with ADHD-I and ADHD-C, the substrate may differ.

Based on this research, some have called ADHD-C and ADHD-I "distinct and unrelated disorders" (Milich et al., 2001, p. 463). Others do not share this view, arguing there are no reliable and valid cognitive/neuropsychological profiles to separate the two groups (Hinshaw, 2001). Furthermore, distinguishing the two disorders may actually provide few implications for treatment of the two groups as a whole (Pelham, 2001), although at the individual case level the two groups' characteristics do sometimes matter. Nonetheless, Chhabildas, Pennington, and Willcutt (2001) concluded that attention problems appear to underlie any neuropsychological differences between subtypes, as children with ADHD-C and children with ADHD-I share response inhibition, processing speed, and vigilance impairments, whereas ADHD without attention problems possessed no deficits after subthreshold attention problems were statistically controlled. Still, additional investigations looking at the hallmark symptoms of ADHD-I and compromised domains of functioning are warranted (Barkley, 2001).

In addition to scholastic underachievement and disruption of daily functioning, children with ADHD-I, like children with ADHD-C, often suffer peer rejection. Unlike children with ADHD-C, however, those with ADHD-I typically appear shy and withdrawn to peers. As a result, they are often left out of play activities and neglected by others (Hodgens, Cole, & Boldizar, 2000). These negative social outcomes may be due to a socially passive style and social skills knowledge deficits (Wheeler-Maedgen & Carlson, 2000). On the other hand, children with ADHD-C, who are seen as argumentative, physically aggressive, and emotionally dysregulated, seem to suffer from overt peer rejection (Hodgens et al., 2000; Wheeler-Maedgen & Carlson, 2000). Unfortunately, like children with ADHD-C, the social skills deficits of children with ADHD-I appear difficult to remedy. In general, however, work incompletion, disorganization, and failure to use fully their intellectual and academic skills because of attention problems are the clearest manifestations of ADHD-I likely to be seen by school psychologists.

Assessment Considerations

Like with ADHD-C, the best method of establishing ADHD-I is to examine directly the DSM-IV-TR criteria. In order to diagnose ADHD-I, informants (typically parents and teachers) must confirm the presence of six or more symptoms of inattention that have been present for at least 6 months. The nine-symptom set listed in DSM-IV-TR is included in Table 4.1; it generally includes behaviors related to poor attention span, lack of follow-through, forgetfulness, and distractibility. To satisfy diagnostic criteria, these symptoms must also be present to a significant degree, cause impairment in multiple settings, and have produced problems before age 7 years. As will be discussed in the next section, ruling out competing explanations for the problem behavior is essential. Obviously, it is impossible to meet these criteria unless background information is collected from either parents or existing records (e.g., the student's cumulative folder). In our experience, eliminating alternative explanations for inattention is important because symptoms such as lack of focus and poor concentration are common to a multitude of psychiatric and medical conditions. Some of these conditions are discussed in more detail later.

Many broad-band (those that assess a variety of emotional or behavior problems) and narrow-band rating scales (that assess ADHD symptoms only) may be used to assess the presence of ADHD-I. Among the narrow-band ADHD rating scales that have reasonable reliability and validity are the Attention Deficit Disorder Evaluation Scales (ADDES; McCarney, 1995), ADHD Rating Scales–IV (ADHD-IV; DuPaul et al., 1998) and the Conners' Rating Scales—Revised (CRS-R; Conners; Conners, 1997; see

Demaray, Elting, et al., 2003). Because screening for other psychiatric disturbance is necessary to rule out competing explanations, we commonly employ broad-band measures like the Achenbach behavior rating scales and the BASC-2. At least one study has examined the ability of the parent and teacher forms of these two rating scales to detect the presence of ADHD. The BASC and Achenbach rating scales were both found reasonably to differentiate children with ADHD from children without ADHD. In order to identify ADHD-I, however, data supported the use of the BASC parent and teacher rating scales over Achenbach (Vaughn et al., 1997). In contrast, Ostrander et al. (1998) found the Achenbach parent rating scale (CBCL) superior to the BASC in identifying children with ADHD-I, but did not use teacher rating forms.

As we commonly use the BASC-2, its use is reviewed here. The BASC-2 may be completed by parents and teachers to provide a picture of problem behaviors across settings and to compare the child's behavior with other children of the same age (and sometimes the same sex) on several dimensions. For example, the BASC-2 contains narrow-band scales for depression, anxiety, conduct, hyperactivity–impulsivity, attention problems, and learning problems. If the child demonstrates attention problems in isolation, one would expect to see elevations only on the Attention Problems scale (e.g., "is easily distracted," "has a short attention span," "listens to directions (scored in opposite direction)," "pays attention when being spoken to") and most likely the Learning Problems scale (e.g., "complains that lessons go too fast," "does not complete tests," "gets failing school grades"). Intuitively, this makes sense as most referrals for detailed evaluation in this domain originate with classroom teachers who are concerned that a child perceived as a having an attention problem is not learning up to his or her potential. Other narrow-band scale elevations (e.g., Depression, Anxiety) on parent or teacher rating scales would raise the hypothesis that an alternative emotional or behavioral diagnosis should be considered, or at least that a comorbid psychological disorder might be present.

When rating scales and background data are equivocal, school psychologists might choose to add psychometric measures of attention, executive function, and impulse control. The debate about the value of measures of impulse control or indirect measures of executive function is found in the section on ADHD-C. Briefly, most cancellation tasks or go-no-go tests produce only modest differences between groups of children with ADHD and matched controls (Pennington, 2002), and almost all of the executive measures fail to predict true cases of ADHD or rule out false cases of ADHD (see Barkley & Grodzinsky, 1994). It seems possible that the finding of slow visual-processing tasks (believed to be a manifestation of sluggish cognitive tempo) may be used to aid identification of children with ADHD-I (recalling the findings of Weiler et al., 2002, mentioned earlier) because some psychometric tests include time measures of visual processing. The NEPSY, for example, includes a visual search task (i.e., Visual Attention) that requires sustained attention and quick responses. It will remain unclear if these tests have a direct role in diagnosing ADHD-I until direct research on the possibility is conducted. Therefore, lengthy, computer-based continuous performance tests (CPT) are preferred (see Ricco et al., 2002) as adjuncts to direct interview of parents and teacher or the use of objective rating scales.

Although the same computerized tests of attention (e.g., CPT-II, Gordon Diagnostic System) may be used regardless of subtype of ADHD suspected, one might look to different subtest scales to differentiate the various subtypes of ADHD. For example, if one suspects ADHD-C, commission errors (a measure of impulsive responses) are likely of primary interest. On the other hand, a child with ADHD-I would be expected to underrespond due to inattention and have few commission errors. In this case, omission errors, (not responding when required) are the likely primary index of consideration. Again, performance on computerized tests of attention should be interpreted with caution because normal scores are believed to do little to rule in or out ADHD (i.e., these tests possess only weak NPP).

At present, it appears that few school systems have a detailed system for assessing ADHD. School psychologists regularly employ behavior rating scales, interviews, and behavioral observations as a screening method; however, it appears far less common that computerized tests of attention and executive function are part of the screening battery (Kilpatrick-Demaray, Schaefer, & Delong, 2003). Reasons for the lack of a complex system are likely several: hesitancy to get into the routine activity of diagnosing ADHD, lack of psychometric instruments (i.e., tests of attention and executive function), a potentially unmanageable number of children to screen, and perceived lack of competency on the part of the school psychologist to diagnose ADHD, to list a few (see survey in ADHD-C regarding school psychologists' perceptions of competence and scope of practice by Kilpatrick-Demaray et al., 2003). Still, schools must develop methods for evaluating ADHD as children with this disorder may be entitled to accommodations, or even special education services, given demonstrated educational need.

Other Possibilities

Many conditions besides ADHD-I include difficulty with concentration, poor planning and follow-through, avoidance of activities requiring sustained effort, forgetfulness, and distractibility. DSM-IV-TR warns that PDD, schizophrenia, and various other psychotic disorders may share presenting symptoms with ADHD-I. For example, a child with PDD may not pay attention like her unimpaired classmates, and she may be uninterested in events that readily capture others' attention (e.g., social activities). Of importance for diagnostic purposes, such a child may be especially attentive to objects and activities that are ignored by classmates (e.g., the air-conditioning system of the classroom, bottlecaps, floor tiles). These children have unusual patterns of attention, rather than simple problems with inattention. Likewise, children who are depressed or anxious may be so preoccupied with internal matters that the focus necessary to learn is not present. Clearly, an array of psychiatric disorders needs to be considered before ADHD-I is confirmed.

In the previous section, we suggested that school psychologists use tests of cognitive and information-processing abilities, as well developmental/social–emotional data, to determine if attention problems are better explained by another disorder (e.g., mental retardation). Children who simply cannot understand concepts presented in class or are slow to catch on typically struggle to pay attention. Specific to ADHD-I, it seems especially crucial to rule out a speech and language or hearing impairment. A child who lacks auditory acuity (i.e., has hearing loss) or is unable fully to understand spoken language (i.e., SLI) may appear inattentive. In these instances, targeting the development of language skills or compensatory strategies with respect to hearing, rather than attention, would be the foundation of intervention.

Ruling out the presence of mood disorders or emerging personality disorders, however, can be much more difficult, especially as the child ages and enters adolescence. Teenagers sometimes cease to pay attention, become unconcerned with schoolwork, and grow disorganized and unmotivated because of changing priorities and heightening peer influence that sometimes mimics ADHD-I. Historical data can help establish if this is a longstanding (potentially ADHD-I) versus a new and potentially transient problem (which is not ADHD). Further clouding the diagnostic picture is the comorbidity of ADHD with other mental disorders. Mood disorders such as depression, anxiety (including OCD), and bipolar disorder should be considered as competing hypotheses, especially if the family has consulted a mental health professional outside of the school. These are among the reasons that a full battery of diagnostic instruments and techniques available to school psychologists is often needed to tease apart the presence and/or contributions of all possible disorders. In school settings, a full evaluation is often needed to design a treatment plan after a child has failed to be helped by informal techniques and behavioral consultation alone.

Besides psychiatric and learning problems, there are innumerable medical diseases whose symptoms mimic ADHD-I. Fatigue, weakness, depression, and memory loss are symptoms of a variety of medical illnesses that may result in a child with difficulty attending and concentrating. Some forms of childhood cancer, brain tumor, epilepsy, diabetes mellitus, and hypothyroidism are just a few conditions that share some symptomology with ADHD-I. Therefore, a check of each child's health status is suggested in order to rule out competing medical explanations (see Wodrich & Kaplan, 2005, for situations in which an attention problem warrants an additional medical referral).

Eligibility Issues

Like ADHD-C (see the previous section), there are two main avenues through which children with ADHD-I may receive formal intervention in school settings. If a modified curriculum (e.g., adjustments in grade level) or intensive instruction does not appear necessary and the presence of the disorder is believed to limit substantially the child's education, consideration is given for the construction of a Section 504 accommodation plan. All of the aforementioned behavioral interventions may be considered for inclusion in a Section 504 plan.

Along with the recognition that some children with ADHD-I may require more than standard accommodations in order to demonstrate learning, or even acquire academic skills at all, special education eligibility may become a focus of attention. If the student support team believes that a modified curriculum is required due to below-grade-level performance, or if intensive intervention appears necessary, eligibility for special education under the category of OHI should be considered. It appears that relatively few children with ADHD-I have sufficient problems with conduct or classroom adjustment to warrant ED designation.

Treatment Considerations

Practically speaking, there is a paucity of intervention studies examining the differential effects of treatment between ADHD-C and ADHD-I. In fact, Pelham (2001) commented on the lack of behavioral intervention studies comparing the response of children with ADHD-C versus those with ADHD-I. Thus, to begin with, the reader should refer to the extensive list of interventions for ADHD-C in the preceding section. Briefly, medication management (stimulant medication), parent training, contingency management (behavior therapy), behavior modification in the classroom, and curricular modifications (chunking assignments, interspersing brief problems, peer tutoring, reduction in workload) are empirically supported treatments of ADHD (with attention problems) and should be considered viable treatment options (American Academy of Pediatrics, 2001a; Barkley, 2004; DuPaul & Eckert, 1997; McCurdy et al., 2001; MTA Cooperative Group, 1999a; Pelham et al., 1998; Pfiffner & Barkley, 1998; Rabiner et al., 2004). Additionally, one could infer that, based on ADHD treatment research in general, cognitive-behavioral therapy (American Academy of Pediatrics, 2001a; DuPaul & Eckert, 1997; Pelham et al., 1998), social skills training (Antshel & Remer, 2003), and commonly considered interventions like vestibular stimulation, oral-motor chewing, EEG/EMG biofeedback, relaxation training, sensory integration training, and dietary treatments (Barkley, 2004) would have little to no treatment effect.

The limited research on ADHD-C versus ADHD-I treatment needs notwithstanding, school psychologists can no doubt envision that same approaches may work for some children with ADHD-I that would be ill suited to those with ADHD-C. For example, the slow tempo and "amotivational" description of students with ADHD-I is likely to appear when behavioral interventions are planned. Classroom observation and teacher interview is likely to confirm that there is a substantial problem with work completion or careful attention to detail. Increasing motivation, which entails use of incentives, is accordingly often called for. In fact, much of the role of a school psychologist regarding a student with ADHD-I may be to refine the menu of reinforcers, assure their potency, and modify their rate and timeliness of delivery to guarantee that they possess sufficient reinforcing power to motivate the student. Unlike children with ADHD-C, children with ADHD-I have few conduct problems in class. Thus, use of response cost and behavioral contracts for classroom conduct may be unnecessary for students with ADHD-I. Obviously, each child's presenting problem and unique classroom circumstances, especially behavioral contingencies, must be considered separately. Thus, a functional behavioral analysis is often warranted.

Regarding social skills, school psychologists will also find these students unlike their ADHD-C counterparts. Recalling that these children may be socially isolated and reluctant to initiate interaction, activities that promote contact with peers or behavioral plans that encourage social initiation may be needed. Behavioral techniques such as shaping or modeling of social skills may be required for the individual child. In contrast to children with ADHD-C, few contingencies for maintaining social distance or modulating loud voice tone are typically required for children with ADHD-I. Obviously, these children can be treated via group social skills programs without having to confront issues of behavior management that exist with ADHD-C. Perhaps because issues of impulsive regulation and behavioral control are diminished, these children may be more amenable to social skills training. In fact, at least one aspect of social skills training, assertion training, produced better results for children with ADHD-I than for those with ADHD-C (Antshel & Remer, 2003).

Medication may also need to be managed differently for children with ADHD-I. A classic study, Sprague and Sleator (1977) found that relatively low doses of stimulants were optimal for enhancing cognitive functioning, whereas relatively high doses were most beneficial for behavioral control. Because most children with ADHD-I, in contrast to those with ADHD-C, have problems in the cognitive (close attention to detail, planning ahead, finishing work) rather than the behavioral (self-control, following class rules) domain, relatively low doses of stimulant medication may be needed for many of them. Some research seems to support this idea. Barkley, DuPaul, and McMurray (1991) conducted a commonly cited study that showed children with ADHD-I and children with ADHD-C both respond to stimulant medication. Children with ADHD-I, however, were judged to require a lower dose of methylphenidate reasonably to control their inattentive behavior compared to those with hyperactive–impulsive symptoms, who required a higher dose. Because dosages must be individualized for children with ADHD, school psychologists can provide important monitoring data to prescribing physicians (HaileMariam et al., 2002). For a case example of ADHD-I, see the information on Hannah in Chapter 5.

COMPULSIVE UNDERPRODUCTION

Characteristics of Compulsive Underproduction

1. Presence of obsessive–compulsive disorder (OCD) or OCD-spectrum symptoms.
2. As discussed here, concerns children with academic performance deficits or, more rarely, frank academic skill deficits.

Common Presentation of Compulsive Underproduction

Frequent concern of teacher at time of referral	"Wastes time; doesn't get work done"
Typical grade of referral	Elementary grades
Gender ratio	Roughly equal boys and girls
Prevalence in referred sample	Rare

Note. Estimates from clinic setting.

Manifestations

The pattern seen in this condition is obsessive–compulsive traits that prevent work completion and/or constrain classroom participation. The reduced rate with which the child with compulsive underproduction (CU) completes work is not due to lack of problem-solving abilities or a discrete processing deficit, but rather a perfectionistic manner of approaching tasks, obsessive thoughts, compulsive behaviors, and inflexibility. In theory, if these behaviors are remedied or circumvented, the full complement of academic skills possessed by the student can be expressed. Thus, this condition results in problems of performance, not lack of ability or failure to develop academic skills.

Substantial research exists on childhood OCD. Although it is known that impairments are often present across settings, including school (Piacentini, Bergman, Keller, & McCracken, 2003), relatively little has been published about OCD's direct classroom manifestations. Therefore, children with OCD who additionally fail to complete work may confuse the school-based team. Such a child often appears bright and capable yet remains unable to complete even simple assignments. The same child may be overconcerned with performance but fail to turn in assignments, even when completed. Some children with CU appear anxious and sensitive, unsure of their abilities, seek excessive feedback and reassurance, have trouble initiating responses or erase and rewrite answers, react strongly to negative feedback, and have difficulty transitioning from one activity to the next.

Despite voluminous research on childhood OCD, little appears in the literature about what we call CU. Piacentini and Langley (2004) do present the case of a straight-A, 12-year-old boy with OCD whose impairment extended to the classroom. In addition to other obsessions/compulsions, this child expressed an excessive need for reassurance, rechecking to ensure correctness and avoid perceived negative consequences and "rereading until it felt 'just right.' " The compulsions enacted to reduce anxiety (e.g., rechecking) and to stop intrusive obsessions (e.g., fear of negative consequences) resulted in difficulty concentrating in class and meant that extra time was needed to complete assignments. In this example, classroom achievement was affected by a performance-related disorder rather than any of the disorders of cognition ability or information processing presented in Chapters 2 and 3.

As will be reviewed shortly, the student with CU is often difficult to identify without a complete evaluation, including psychometric data. Students with overt, debilitating anxiety and compulsions may be relatively easily noticed by classroom teachers. Those with CU who merely appear inattentive, require much teacher assistance to start or complete assignments, and may have poor grades are more difficult to spot. Not surprisingly, when referrals concern these symptoms, ADHD is often suspected. A detailed psychoeducational evaluation will be necessary to investigate fully if the root of work incompletion is in fact a disorder of attention, not yet fully appreciated CU tendencies, or some other factor.

Assessment Considerations

In addition to routine background and psychometric data, systematic behavioral observations, clinical interviews, and functional assessments of behavior are vital when conducting an evaluation for suspected CU. Care must be taken to distinguish between problems related to obsessive tendencies and those due to other psychiatric and performance-related disorders (Grados & Riddle, 1999). This is a difficult task as the clinical features of OCD and disorders like ADHD overlap to some degree. Consider the following behaviors: slow to start schoolwork, hard time concentrating with others around, failure to turn in assignments, interruption of teacher, asking for help when it is not needed, and difficulty transitioning. These behaviors are shared by a child with OCD and those with several other performance-limiting disorders, like ADHD. In fact, children with OCD have been disciplined by teachers for being off-task while preoccupied by obsessions (Rapoport, 1989).

With respect to formal observation of behavior, interval recording methods may be helpful in quantifying the amount of off-task time. The BASC-2 Student Observation System (Reynolds & Kamphaus, 2004) and the Behavioral Observation of Students in Schools (BOSS; Shapiro, 2004) are examples of formal observation systems suited to this task. The system of observation we use involves observing the target students, as well as peers of the same sex, in the classroom in alternating 10-second intervals. In addition, off-task occurrences are recorded in terms of motor, verbal, and passive (e.g., staring into space) components. Ironically, the child with CU may obtain the same pattern of off-task behavior as a student with ADHD. However, qualitative aspects of inattention often distinguish the two. For example, a child with CU rarely appears to be merely bored and seldom seems to be just entertaining him- or herself. Rather, a student with CU often appears anxious and typically displays responses suggesting frustration, such as frequent erasure, or facial expressions denoting distress with his or her lack of output. Transitions and ambiguous expectations may be especially likely to involve off-task behavior in a child with CU as compared to students with ADHD, who tend to be off-task when bored (such as when confronted with tedium) or when distractions are present.

The value of observation notwithstanding, a clinical interview is necessary to confirm the presence of CU. Upon interview, children with CU may openly admit perfectionistic tendencies and go on clearly to describe them. Commonly, students report dissatisfaction with their rate and amount of work. They may comment, "It's hard to get started"; "I'm afraid I'll be wrong"; "I can't get my answer to say exactly what I want it to"; "I want my papers to look perfect"; "I'm afraid the teacher can't read my writing and that she'll mark an answer wrong even though it's right because she can't read it." Although perfectionism can appear without the diagnosis of OCD, clinical interviews with teachers, parents, and student may reveal a general pattern consistent with OCD and help explain the array of classroom problems that accompany it.

To this point, we have discussed the evaluation of students suspected of having obsessive qualities. But uncovering these obsessive tendencies at school may not be easy because these children may deny a problem is present, not fully disclose its severity, or rationalize its impact (American Academy of Child and Adolescent Psychiatry, 1998b; Adams, Waas, March, & Smith, 1994). Therefore, it may not be until a formal assessment is finished and observations completed that a student is first suspected of having CU. During testing, the child with CU generally approaches tasks in an apprehensive manner and avoids guessing if unsure. Sometimes the child is even unable to organize him- or herself so as to initiate a response. Considerable finesse and reassurance may be necessary to get the child to respond at all. As a general rule, if the examiner must use copious reassurance and frequent coaxing during testing of a student with a history of performance problems, CU should be considered.

Not surprisingly, formal psychometric testing can help identify the child with CU. Consistent with classroom performance, paper-and-pencil psychometric tasks often evoke these children's perfectionistic tendencies. Unfortunately, slow performance on paper-and-pencil tasks may be misinterpreted as a straightforward information-processing problem. For example, the PSI on the WISC-IV is made up of timed tasks that (1) require the child to write symbols according to numbered code and (2) scrutinize designs for duplications. A low PSI may indeed indicate an information-processing deficit, but careful analysis of how the child executed the tasks should be made. For example, a child with CU may compulsively draw figures on the Coding subtest. She may want to erase to make each figure perfect, even though erasing is prohibited (and a pencil without an eraser is provided). The examiner may find it necessary to cajole the child or reassure her to move forward at the conclusion of one task or the start of another (much like this student's teacher in the classroom); however, even these efforts sometimes fail for children with severe CU.

Visual–motor functioning is another domain of testing that involves paper-and-pencil manipulation and where observation can prove instructive. The NEPSY subtests of Design Copying and Visuomotor Precision can help determine if fine-motor and/or visual–motor deficits are present (see section on GU). Administering these subtests in tandem can also help to identify CU. More often than not, the child with compulsive tendencies is able to copy designs accurately, although slowly. Repeated erasing may be necessary, however, to create a design meeting the child's exacting level. Despite this, a NEPSY Design Copying scaled score within normal limits is usually earned. On the other hand, on the Visuomotor Precision subtest of the NEPSY, children with CU often earn a lower scaled score because of slow but accurate pencil work (see Figure 3.3). Scoring depends on the total time required to traverse a narrow track and the number of times the child's pencil left the track. Separate scaled scores for speed and accuracy are provided. As expected, children with CU commonly earn a substandard scaled score because of slow and deliberate task completion. Although children with true motor deficits may also work slowly, they generally perform inaccurately as well. Accordingly, psychometric data suggesting slow, but accurate, performance should be considered supplemental evidence of CU.

Finally, behavior rating scales, such as the BASC-2 or CBCL, may help document internalizing tendencies associated with CU. The school psychologist will be looking for elevated scores on anxiety-related and internalizing dimensions in order to support the hypothesis of an overly cautious behavioral style as the cause of incomplete schoolwork. Unlike many children who suffer more severe anxiety disorders or frank OCD and have scores in the clinical range, perfectionistic and deliberate students may have only borderline elevations, or none at all. As discussed later, each student's degree of internalizing symptomology may have implications for special education eligibility.

Other Possibilities

Some of the very observations that suggest CU is present—off-task behavior, need for copious prompting and redirection, frequent requests for help—are compatible with any of the learning disorders of Chapters 2 and 3 (e.g., MiMR, SLI). Therefore, psychometric evaluation is helpful to rule out primarily cognitive or information-processing causes. As seen later, use of a flowchart (see Figure 5.1), assures that cognitive and narrow information-processing problems are not a better explanation than CU (or at least a co-occurring one). That being said, obsessive tendencies can coexist with and negatively affect the performance of students with any of this book's other conditions. For example, a child with an SLI may have obsessive or compulsive qualities that stop him from demonstrating the academic skills that he does possess (even if they are somewhat underdeveloped). In this case, verbal skills, reading comprehension, and work completion might all be targets of intervention. Thus, a detailed evaluation is essential for psychologists to assure that all available targets of intervention are identified. Of note, childhood OCD may also coexist with disorders of anxiety and depression, ADHD and disruptive behavior disorders, pervasive developmental disorder, tic disorder, or trichotillomania, as well as other psychiatric, medical, and neuropsychological conditions (American Academy of Child and Adolescent Psychiatry, 1998b; Piacentini & Langley, 2004). Thus, in addition to the conditions covered in this book, school psychologists may need to rule out the presence of various psychiatric disorders or make a subsequent referral so that someone else considers these possibilities.

Eligibility Issues

The overwhelming majority of children with obsessive–compulsive behaviors, in our experience, can be effectively treated in regular classroom settings without special education support. In other words, most children with CU do not require such intensive services or modified curricula that special education eligibility is necessary. That being said, the expertise of school psychologists or behavior intervention specialists may be needed to conduct a functional behavior assessment and to develop an intervention plan. If the child's behavior is not so severe that intensive intervention or a modified curriculum is necessary, eligibility for a Section 504 plan may be considered, although the student would likely need to have a specific diagnosis, such as OCD. A student is 504 eligible if he or she has a "physical or mental impairment that substantially limits one or more major life activities [such as learning], or has a record of such an impairment, or is regarded as having such an impairment" (Public Law 93-112). The option of developing a Section 504 plan may be particularly attractive if the team believes that accommodations, like extended work time or reduced assignment length, will be sufficient to improve performance.

   Some children with CU require more intensive intervention that may be impossible without a special education designation. If the school-based evaluation team believes this to be true, eligibility under the category of ED might be considered (see Table 4.5). Professional judgment must be exercised to establish eligibility under this category considering the vagueness of terms like "long period of time," "marked degree," "adversely affects the child's performance," and "inappropriate types of behavior or feelings under normal circumstances." The school-based team is advised to consider if the presence, frequency, intensity, or duration of the problem behavior is clearly out of the norm for a child of that age. In the case of the child with CU, the school-based evaluation team might find that any of five behavioral descriptors is present, depending on the constellation of behaviors exhibited by each child. Behavioral descriptors extracted from the fed-

TABLE 4.5. Individuals with Disabilities Education Act Definition of Emotional Disturbance

1. The term means a condition exhibiting one or more of the following characteristics over a long period of time and to a marked degree that adversely affects a child's educational performance:
    a. An inability to learn that cannot be explained by intellectual, sensory, or health factors.
    b. An inability to build or maintain satisfactory interpersonal relationships with peers and teachers.
    c. Inappropriate types of behavior or feelings under normal circumstances.
    d. A general pervasive mood of unhappiness or depression.
    e. A tendency to develop physical symptoms or fears associated with personal or school problems.
2. The term includes schizophrenia. The term does not apply to children who are socially maladjusted, unless it is determined that they have an emotional disturbance.

Note. From *Federal Register* (1999).

eral definition of ED in Table 4.5: a (inability to learn), c (inappropriate behavior or feelings) or e (a tendency to develop physical symptoms or fears) are especially apt for children with CU. The adverse educational impact experienced by students with CU sometimes may be manifest in underdeveloped academic skills, but more often in an inability to participate in the classroom setting due to perceived discipline problems or chronic inability to complete work. The application of the adverse educational impact qualification has also been a source of debate, but standards should be applied flexibly for children with emotional problems that prevent school success. For example, rigid adherence to low achievement test scores is inappropriate (Wodrich, Stobo, & Trca, 1998).

The reauthorization of IDEA in December 2004, and specifically the rules for determining eligibility for services under the category of SLD, may also have implications for students with CU. As stated in Chapter 3, the response to intervention (RTI) principle may be applied to establish if an SLD is present; the same notion may be used to justify ED special education placement. Under these circumstances, behavioral consultation will be used to identify targets of intervention, as well as baseline data. Interventions are then designed and progress is monitored to determine if the target behaviors are resistant to intervention. If the team determines that the target behaviors continue at unacceptable levels and that more intensive intervention is necessary, a student may be considered in need of special education services. Thus, the RTI concept may be applicable to ED, even though it currently is not written into regulations for ED.

Treatment Considerations

There are three broad classes of intervention for OCD. Each of these could presumably help students with CU in the classroom, although none yet appears very well supported by classroom-based empirical research: (1) cognitive-behavioral therapy, (2) classroom strategies to disrupt obsessions and compulsions, and (3) medication. Treatment will vary depending on the ways in which each child's problem affects learning and how severe it is. The data gathered during assessment will determine, in part, which interventions are appropriate and guide their implementation.

One treatment with considerable empirical support for anxiety and depression is cognitive-behavioral therapy (Kazdin & Weisz, 2003). Cognitive-behavioral therapy also has been shown effectively to treat OCD (Franklin, Rynn, Foa, & March, 2003; Franklin et al., 1998), and it is now considered a first-line intervention for OCD in children and adolescents (American Academy of Child and Adolescent Psychiatry, 1998b; Barrett, Healy-Farrell, & March, 2004). Cognitive-behavioral therapy is especially attractive because treatment gains are generally well maintained over time (although booster sessions are sometimes necessary), whereas the positive effects of pharmacotherapy tend to decline when medication is discontinued. Of note, insight-oriented therapy has not been shown to reduce OCD symptoms in children and adults (Piacentini & Langley, 2004).

The cognitive-behavioral therapy for OCD typically involves careful assessment of the constellation of problem obsession and compulsions, exposure to identified stress-provoking stimuli, and response prevention (American Academy of Child and Adolescent Psychiatry, 1998b; Barrett et al., 2004; Franklin et al., 1998, 2003; March, 1995). Recent literature suggests that individual and group cognitive-behavioral therapies are equally effective in treating OCD in children (Barrett et al., 2004). Fortunately, detailed cognitive-behavioral therapy manuals have been developed to guide the treatment of children and adolescents with OCD. One such manual that has enjoyed support was constructed by March and Mulle (1998; see Table 4.6 for an outline of sessions and activities). Likewise, Piacentini and Langley (2004) reviewed steps of cognitive-behavioral therapy for children with OCD and presented a case illustration that provides excellent therapist scripts and treatment activities for each stage of intervention (i.e., psychoeducation, construction of a symptom hierarchy, cognitive restructuring, exposure/response prevention, modifying obsessions, and family intervention). The 12-year-old boy with OCD who compulsively rechecked his schoolwork and reread assignments whose case was mentioned earlier (Piacentini & Langley, 2004) was exposed to situations in which he felt the urge to check. He was trained to complete an assignment without rechecking, place it in a folder, and move on to the next assignment. Submitting

TABLE 4.6. Synopsis of a Cognitive-Behavioral Therapy Protocol

Visit number	Goals
Session 1	The psychoeducation phase of treatment includes conceptualizing OCD as a neurobehavioral (medical) condition through the use of medical analogies, analyzing the costs and benefits of treatment, and reviewing the treatment protocol.
Session 2	Cognitive training (CT) teaches the child to engage in constructive self-talk (i.e., bossing back OCD) and to provide self-administered positive reinforcement, and bolsters the child's sense that OCD symptoms can be brought under the individual's control.
Session 3–4	CT advances while a functional analysis of OCD behaviors is conducted (i.e., antecedents, behaviors, consequences, and avoidance behaviors are identified) and the development of treatment metaphors continues. This phase is termed "mapping of OCD."
Weeks 3–18	Exposure and response prevention (E/RP) are introduced and implemented as behavioral treatments of OCD. Both imaginal and *in vivo* E/RP may be undertaken.
Weeks 18–19	Relapse prevention
Sessions 1, 7, and 12	Parent sessions include reviewing the course of treatment, recruiting parent assistance, and defining and maintaining the roles of parents. Of note, parent check-ins are conducted at the start and end of each session.

Note. Adapted from March and Mulle (1998). Copyright 1998 by The Guilford Press. Adapted by permission.

some incomplete assignments was also prescribed to challenge the false belief that devastating consequences would follow submission of incomplete work. Regarding compulsive rereading, the student was coached to cover previously read lines to prevent rereading and to insert intentional miscues, again to challenge the belief that extraordinarily negative consequences would follow imperfection. Once he habituated to working without rechecking and rereading, the child was reinforced by his ability to complete assignments efficiently.

Recognizing that not all children with CU have full-blown OCD, formal cognitive-behavioral therapy may not be necessary. Nonetheless, it remains important for school psychologists to know the theoretical suppositions and related techniques of cognitive-behavioral therapy. Cognitive-behavioral therapy as a school of treatment holds that irrational beliefs lead to maladaptive responses and that behavior therapy, in addition to cognitive restructuring techniques, is needed to correct underlying thoughts and ultimately improve overt behavior (March & Mulle, 1998; Piacentini &

Langley, 2004). When learning is affected by obsessions and compulsions, the child may tremendously underestimate his or her abilities, believe that perfection is absolutely required, or assume that even minor failures will induce catastrophic consequences. As a result, the general goals of cognitive-behavioral therapy are to identify the problem behaviors (though behavioral consultation and formal observation) and the child's cognitive distortions (via clinical interview and formal therapy), reframe those distortions, teach and practice response prevention techniques (if necessary), and reinforce adaptive behavior through a positive behavior plan. No studies to our knowledge have examined the effect of cognitive-behavioral therapy on specific classroom behaviors, like underproduction. It seems logical, however, that addressing the irrational beliefs and worries that accompany obsessive–compulsive behaviors while reinforcing work completion would lead to positive outcomes. This is so because cognitive-behavioral therapy is effective for many problems related to OCD (e.g., anxiety and depression).

Even though overt problem behaviors (e.g., poor work completion or crying) may be easily identified via behavioral consultation, discovering underlying cognitive distortions may be more difficult. Children with CU may hold a variety of false beliefs, and reporting them may be limited by developmental status and expressive language skills. Children are better able to share the basis of their fears and behaviors as they mature, but some may not fully understand what false beliefs trouble them. In the absence of a disclosing child, the psychologist might consider common distortions of students with obsessive–compulsive tendencies. Among recurring themes appear to be an intrinsic need to be perfect, intense fear of failure, possible catastrophic consequences that may result from imperfection, and unfounded worry (e.g., obsessive worry about the safety of loved ones, natural disasters, fire). Likewise, researchers have compiled a list of common childhood intrusive thoughts: fear of germs/contamination, concern about harm befalling self and others, exorbitant moralization, and the feeling that something might be just "not right" (Piacentini & Langley, 2004).

The subset of students with obsessive–compulsive tendencies who can be especially difficult to treat are those unable to stop thinking about possibilities, especially unpleasant ones. Again, examples include a litany of dangerous prospects and potential harm befalling loved ones. Once treatment begins, it may be hard, and in some instances inappropriate, to tell a child that the most dreaded outcome will never happen. For example, unfounded concern about the safety of parents can be a recurring theme and, obviously, no one can absolutely guarantee the safety of any individual. Nonetheless, many worried children enjoy great relief when reassured by an adult that their worries simply will not come true. In cases of extreme worry, cognitive therapy (i.e., addressing false beliefs) in isolation can be unsuccessful. Consequently, behavior modification consisting of reinforcement of behavior incompatible with obsessions/compulsions is necessary (i.e., differential reinforcement of other behavior). With respect to children who are failing to complete classwork, a behavior program that rewards work completion, in conjunction with supportive counseling, in our experience has the greatest chance of success.

A second broad category of intervention, exposure/response prevention (E/RP) techniques, is key in the treatment of CU. In fact, there is some evidence that E/RP techniques are equally as or more effective than medication management for children with frank OCD (Benazon, Ager, & Rosenberg, 2002; Piacentini, Bergman, Jacobs, McCracken, & Kretchman, 2002). The purpose of these techniques is to teach the child to work through anxiety-provoking times while demonstrating that the distortions he or she holds are irrational or, at best, extremely implausible. Children may be responsible for implementing some techniques, whereas other strategies may be carried out by teachers and parents. An important first step is to teach children to identify when they are engaging in compulsive behaviors. Some children possess enough insight into their own behavior to realize when they will engage in such acts, whereas other children do not. Given this reality, school psychologists and teachers need to intervene sensitively and discreetly when it appears the child cannot recognize the signs of his or her harmful obsessions and compulsions (e.g., visible frustration, expressed worry). For example, a child whose work production is derailed by thoughts of her parents' safety may recognize, sometimes to her dismay, that the class is relentlessly moving forward while she stares, filled with concern and nervously twisting her hair. Some children may lack awareness of their look of concern and indicators of stress (in this case, hair twirling and underproduction). In the latter case, a teacher may gently put a hand on the child's shoulder when she begins to twist her hair. If the child does not realize when she is ruminating, it will be difficult to teach her to identify when to start response prevention techniques. Commonly implemented response prevention techniques include thought stopping, guided imagery, and relaxation exercises. The purposes of these techniques are to break the pattern of obsessive worrying and to replace the maladaptive thoughts with non-anxiety-provoking thoughts and images (see March & Mulle, 1998).

At other times, children may be too immature to implement response prevention strategies independently; therefore, adults' assistance is needed. Consultation with teachers can introduce cognitive-behavioral techniques and allow their effective implementation in the classroom. A teacher may have to cue a child that he is engaging in compulsive behaviors and lead him through response prevention techniques, gently challenge distortions (if appropriate), or just provide reassurance. Other times, a teacher may have to disrupt the problem behavior physically in a firm but sensitive manner. For example, a teacher may literally have to collect a child's assignment while he is compulsively erasing or impose time limits for assignments while reinforcing the student's effort. When implementing techniques that interrupt or physically disrupt counterproductive habits, confirming that the child understands the plan before it is started can be wise.

A positive behavior plan can be important for children with anxiety disorders, and especially OCD-spectrum problems. Children with OCD often possess a heightened sense of fairness and therefore overreact to perceived injustices. This may appear as oppositional behavior and may predate the appearance of obviously OCD characteristics (American Academy of Child and Adolescent Psychiatry, 1998b). Thus, techniques like response costs may cause the child to dwell on the fairness of the punishment (thereby shifting the focus of obsession) and promote obstinacy in the face of redirection. For this reason, rewarding students for work completion and issuing frequent reminders that perfection is not expected may be much more successful. One way this may be done is by praising effort, not accuracy, because lauding accuracy may inadvertently reinforce a belief that work must be done perfectly. Likewise, a token economy whereby a child earns points or stickers exchangeable for a back-up reinforcer (valued object or privilege) might also be tried to improve work completion (which is a response that may be incompatible with obsessions and compulsions).

Yet another positive behavior technique is to circumvent situations that provoke compulsive behavior and slow work completion. Take a student whose written work must be completed with perfect penmanship but who seldom turns in work on time. Oral presentations and audiotaped responses can be used to bypass problem behavior (Adams & Burke, 1999). If time is of the essence, the child may be asked to provide verbal responses at the teacher's desk or use computerized dictation software while classmates are writing. These alternative methods of work completion can then be assessed for their effectiveness in promoting timely accomplishment of tasks for each student.

Modeling effective coping strategies may also be used. Specifically, parents and teachers may be taught how to display effective management of frustration when they make mistakes in the presence of the child (Parker & Stewart, 1994). For example, after a mistake a teacher may follow a script like: "I made a mistake, but it is all right. Everyone makes mistakes." The extent to which such interventions have been studied empirically is unknown.

Medication may be necessary for students with severe problems or those who fail to respond to behavioral interventions. If medication is tried, the school psychologist and school-based team can play an important role in evaluating its effectiveness. In our experience, most prescribing physicians value the observations of trained professionals at school because they are unable to observe the child outside the office. Behavioral observations, as well as rating scale data, may be provided to the prescribing physician as feedback from which to make treatment decisions. When academic productivity is at issue, the Academic Performance Rating Scale can be an effective monitoring tool (DuPaul, Rapport, & Perriello, 1991).

Selective serotonin reuptake inhibitors (SSRIs) have been identified as first-line medications. These may be preferred to avoid negative side effects related to other pharmacological options, like clomipramine (Grados & Riddle, 2001). A recent meta-analysis confirmed that SSRIs, such as paroxetine, fluoxetine, fluvoxamine, and sertraline, reduce OCD symptoms in children and adolescents (Geller et al., 2003). It is important for those practicing in schools, however, to realize that symptom improvement may not be immediate. For example, fluoxetine (Prozac) has been shown to improve pediatric OCD symptoms (Geller et al., 2001). Up to 8 weeks may be necessary for full effects to manifest (Liebowitz et al., 2002), but it may appreciably reduce core OCD symptoms. For example, Riddle et al. (1992) found that obsessive–compulsive symptoms were reduced by 44% after 8 weeks of pharmacotherapy in a sample of children ages 8–15 years. Similarly, Geller, Biederman, Reed, Spencer, and Wilens (1995) confirmed a 74% reduction of childhood OCD symptoms at follow-up over 19 months. That being said, these studies looked at symptom reduction in children with diagnosed OCD on a recognized instrument designed to detect core symptoms of OCD. The extent to which pharmacotherapy reduces compulsive behavior in the classroom or promotes work completion in children with CU is unclear. For a case example of CU, see the information on Alicia in Chapter 5.

CHAPTER 5

♦ ♦ ♦

How to Use the System through Case Examples

♦

Diagnosticians need two things to be able to use this system. The first is a list of potential conditions (patterns) and their potential treatments. The second is information on how to determine which, if any, of the patterns is present—that is, a guide for decision making. This chapter contains such a guide. We begin with a step-by-step schema for evaluating students. A flowchart (Figure 5.1) is provided to guide you through the system. It reveals a system of analysis that follows a structured set of questions. In some ways, this affords a means of hypothesis testing similar to that used by both medical and educational decision makers (Bartolo, Dockrell, & Lunt, 2001). We conclude with 12 case examples, in which each condition is depicted, along with background information, observations, analysis of results, and recommended interventions. To illustrate the system's use, we show how available psychometric and case information is used at each decision point in the flowchart. Following the decision-making process as individual cases are discussed should prepare school psychologists to use the system independently. We have intentionally made the case examples uncomplicated by the coexistence of a second condition. Of course, in the real world, more than one of these conditions may be present in the same case (see Box 1.1 in Chapter 1).

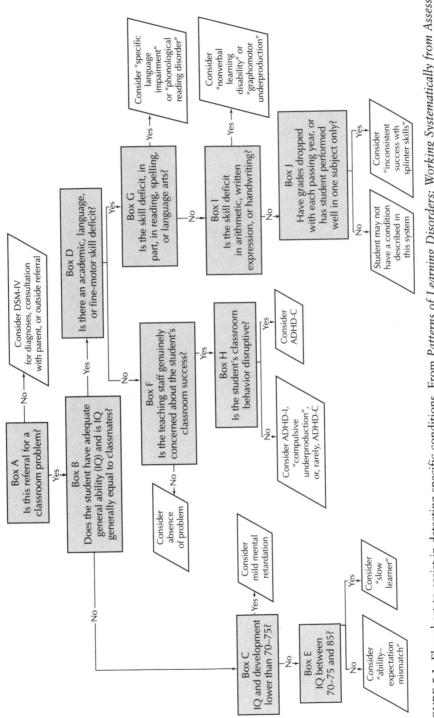

FIGURE 5.1. Flowchart to assist in detecting specific conditions. From *Patterns of Learning Disorders: Working Systematically from Assessment to Intervention* by David L. Wodrich and Ara J. Schmitt. Copyright 2006 by The Guilford Press. Permission to photocopy this figure is granted to purchasers of this book for personal use only (see copyright page for details).

CASE 1: DANIEL

Background Information

Daniel is a 7-year-old biracial boy (white father, black mother) who was referred by his teacher because of concern about his inability to read.

Daniel is a healthy child who has passed hearing and vision screenings. He was born at 40 weeks of gestational age (weighing 8 pounds, 13 ounces) after an uneventful pregnancy and delivery. His first independent steps and first words were at 12 and 14 months, respectively. He was toilet trained at 27 months. He was noted to have minor speech articulation problems as a preschooler. His older brother, age 13 years, sometimes interpreted Daniel's words for listeners.

Daniel attended preschool at his local church beginning at age 3 years. He was viewed as social and popular. He was always eager to attend. Preschool teachers, who indicated that their program emphasized socialization and religious instruction over academics, had few complaints. Beginning handwriting was described as excellent. Records provided by his parents revealed that he mastered names of only about half of the letters and 80% of colors by the conclusion of his preschool program at 5 years old, even though these skills were practiced repeatedly.

Daniel then enrolled in a public school kindergarten. By midyear, his teacher expressed concern that he was failing to read. Problems persisted even though his parents began to work with him nightly on pre-primer-level books sent home by his teacher. His reading was described as extremely slow paced, few words were recognized immediately even if they had been repeatedly practiced, and letter sounds were only inconsistently retained; sometimes even initial consonant sounds were missed when an unknown word was encountered. Daniel spelled a bit better than this, although by midyear his kindergarten teacher had drastically reduced the length of his weekly spelling list. He was able to write little interpretable narrative material in his journal. His teacher indicated, as reflected in his report card, that he sometimes had trouble paying attention and that a lot of his schoolwork was left uncompleted. He remained, however, a popular and ostensibly happy child who was eager to attend school. He was ultimately promoted to first grade, although his parents hired a private tutor (a former elementary school teacher) to instruct him in reading twice a week during the summer between kindergarten and first grade.

During an interview, his first-grade teacher described him as far below peers in reading and spelling but at grade level in arithmetic. In fact, Daniel's teacher was able to provide curriculum-based data from a schoolwide screening that indicated his oral reading fluency fell at the 10th percentile compared to local norms, while his first-grade math computation skills fell at the 70th percentile. His handwriting was described as good. His teacher said that he had not yet "broken the code" in reading. She stated that Daniel was either the poorest reader or the next to poorest reader in the lowest reading group. Simplified spelling lists and adjusted reading assignments were provided. None of this seemed to help, and he was eventually referred for a formal evaluation.

The parents' social and developmental history questionnaire failed to illuminate the reason for school problems. Boxes were checked suggesting that Daniel was a pleasant, cooperative child at home. His health history appeared to be unrelated to school problems. He was treated for eczema twice as a preschooler and once had an emergency room visit for a dog bite, but he had no chronic health problems. He reportedly slept and ate well. Daniel rarely missed school.

Daniel's mother accompanied him to the evaluation and provided the following additional information. The family was concerned about his indistinct speech earlier but had been counseled by his pediatrician that he would likely outgrow the problem. Indeed, his speech is now generally understandable and he did not appear frustrated when communicating. His mother viewed her son as focused, well regulated, and cooperative. He was described as compliant at home and had no obvious problems with mood, temper, or anxiety. She believed he is a fairly bright child, although he does not especially enjoy board games, television, or listening to her read stories.

Family history was described as negative for psychiatric problems and genetic/developmental syndromes. Daniel's mother said that his father always found school hard and that he continues to struggle when reading technical material and in spelling. He works in air-conditioning sales, but his wife often must assist him because of limited literacy. One of his two brothers (Daniel's paternal uncles) and his father (Daniel's grandfather) also were reported to be poor readers, and all three dropped out of school prior to graduation. Parents have been married for 15 years, and there are no significant conflicts or sources of stress in the home.

Assessment Procedures

Wechsler Intelligence Scale for Children–IV; Woodcock–Johnson III Tests of Achievement; Gray Oral Reading Test: 4; A Developmental Neuropsychological Assessment (NEPSY) (Design Copying, Visuomotor Precision, Memory for Faces, Memory for Names, Narrative Memory, Phonological Processing) subtests; Behavior Assessment System for Children–2 (Teacher Report Form, Parent Report Form); informal assessment with curriculum material, parent interview, child interview. Scores on standardized instruments for Daniel are listed in Table 5.1.

TABLE 5.1. Summary of Assessment Scores for Daniel

Name	Age	Sex	Dominant hand	Grade
Daniel	7 years	Male	Right	1

Wechsler Intelligence Scale for Children–IV

Verbal Comprehension		Perceptual Reasoning		Working Memory		Processing Speed	
Similarities	10	Block Design	11	Digit Span	7	Coding	10
Vocabulary	9	Picture Concepts	12	Letter–Number Sequence	9	Symbol Search	11
Comprehension	10	Matrix Reasoning	11	(Arithmetic)		(Cancellation)	

Scale	Composite score		Percentile rank
Verbal Comprehension	98 (91–105)	VCI	45th
Perceptual Reasoning	108 (100–115)	PRI	70th
Working Memory	88 (81–97)	WMI	21st
Processing Speed	103 (94–112)	PSI	58th
Full Scale	100 (95–105)	FSIQ	50th
General Ability Index	103 (97–109)	GAI	58th

Woodcock–Johnson III Tests of Achievement

WJ III subtests	Scaled score
Letter–Word Identification	70
Passage Comprehension	75
Reading Fluency	76
Calculations	102
Math Fluency	99
Spelling	79
Writing Samples	82
Writing Fluency	83
Word Attack	60

A Developmental Neuropsychological Assessment (NEPSY)

Phonological Processing	4
Visuomotor Precision	10
Design Copying	11
Memory for Faces	10
Memory for Names	5
Narrative Memory	9

Gray Oral Reading Test–4

Scale	Score
Fluency	5
Comprehension	4
Oral Reading Quotient	67

(continued)

TABLE 5.1. *(continued)*

Behavior Assessment System for Children–2 (Parent Report)

Scale	Level
F	Acceptable
Response Pattern	Acceptable
Consistency	Acceptable
Hyperactivity	55
Aggression	50
Conduct Problems	53
Anxiety	47
Depression	53
Somatization	48
Atypicality	52
Withdrawal	51
Attention Problems	56
Adaptability	51
Social Skills	52
Leadership	57
Activities of Daily Living	49
Functional Communication	51

Behavior Assessment System for Children–2 (Teacher Report)

Scale	Level
F	Acceptable
Response Pattern	Acceptable
Consistency	Acceptable
Hyperactivity	50
Aggression	52
Conduct Problems	46
Anxiety	50
Depression	50
Somatization	54
Atypicality	53
Withdrawal	50
Attention Problems	56
Adaptability	57
Social Skills	51
Leadership	52
Learning Problems	56
Study Skills	53
Functional Communication	50

Observations

Daniel presented as a handsome, well-groomed 7-year-old who appeared physically mature. He was, however, initially reticent. After warming up, he talked comfortably about school and friends, with only occasional articulation errors. Nonetheless, his speech was almost always able to be fully understood. He engaged in turn-taking conversations. Daniel's behavior was well controlled, his attention was unremarkable, and he easily worked through the examination during a single morning, with several breaks.

Daniel was observed in his class on three occasions. He did not appear to experience general problems with attention to detail, distractibility, task persistence, impulse control, or motor restlessness. However, when reading and spelling worksheets were presented, Daniel was indeed more off-task than classmates, at least some of the time. Twice he actually put his head on his desk and stopped working until prompted by his teacher. Subsequent review of these work samples indicated very low accuracy and substantial material left incomplete. In contrast, he was far more focused on arithmetic and art activities. Overall, Daniel's difficulty paying attention appeared to arise from the nature of assigned work (i.e., reading and spelling) rather than cross-situational problems that might reflect ADHD.

Analysis of Results

The first question concerns whether Daniel was referred for a classroom problem. It is clear that both teacher and parents are alarmed about lack of progress in reading. He continues to make little progress despite informal assistance. The answer to Box A is "yes," and the subsequent use of this system is appropriate.

Box B poses a question about general cognitive development. All sources of information should be considered. Daniel's developmental milestones were generally on time (only speech articulation was of concern), his parents view him as capable, he has acquired same-age playmates, and he has had success in some cognitively related academic domains (i.e., arithmetic). Nonpsychometric material suggests a pervasive problem with ability is unlikely. So do psychometric data. The WISC-IV index scores most indicative of general cognitive ability are both solidly average (VCI = 98; PRI = 108), and the composite of these two was average (GAI = 103). He also scored in the average range on speeded WISC-IV tasks requiring visual attention and pencil usage (PSI = 103). He was in the low average range on WMI (88), the relatively lower score here due almost entirely to limited success repeating digits forward and backward. His Full Scale score (100) substantiates that general cognitive problems are absent. The answer to Box B is "yes."

The task in Box D is to confirm academic skill deficits. In Daniel's case, there is abundant relevant information. Records document his difficulty in reading and spelling compared to peers, and so do standardized measures. Daniel was administered simple tests of word recognition and silent reading (for meaning) using a cloze procedure and foundered on both (WJ III Letter–Word Identification and Passage Comprehension subtests = 70 and 75, respectively). When required to read passages aloud for speed, accuracy, and comprehension, he had equal difficulty (Gray Oral Reading Test: 4 [GORT-4] Fluency score = 5; Oral Reading Quotient = 67). He was unable to answer questions about what he had just attempted to read (GORT-4 Comprehension score = 4). An informal procedure was then used (testing the limits); when GORT-4 passages were read orally to Ryan he answered comprehension questions with surprising accuracy, up to approximately a third-grade level. Word attack was extremely poor when he was confronted with pseudowords (WJ III Word Attack subtest = 60). In fact, even when presented with nonwords with patterns nearly identical to real words, Daniel made only a single correct response on the entire subtest. Daniel's spelling was equally undeveloped, which constrained his writing scores.

Finally, Daniel brought a book from a first-grade literature series that he had been practicing at home for the past several evenings. His rate and accuracy were low even in this familiar material (WPM = 17; accuracy rate = 74%). He did no better with spelling words already encountered in the first-grade curriculum. Of 10 words on which he had been tested during a recent weekly exam, he had only two correct responses. The answer to Box D is "yes."

Turning to Box G, we address the question of which type of academic deficits are present. As the above suggests, language arts (especially reading) are poorly developed. The answer to Box G is "yes."

The flowchart indicates that SLI and PRD are possibilities. Substantial data have already been provided to help in considering each of these possibilities, and we have additional psychometric data that has yet to be analyzed. Daniel's academic pattern implies that his greatest problem is word identification or an inability to decode words as he reads. Furthermore, word identification seems to be hindered because he fails to produce sounds (phonemes) in the presence of symbols in a predictable manner so they can be blended to produce whole words. Failure of sound–symbol associations is a hallmark of PRD. Consistent with the primary emerging phonological deficit hypothesis is his intact understanding of material (recall that listening comprehension was not a problem) but meager ability to read nonwords (a task with extreme phonological demands).

Does the rest of Daniel's information agree with the PRD hypothesis? Might he be equally limited because of inadequately developed general language competence (e.g., suffer an SLI)? Daniel's supplemental scores are relatively low in some dimensions and high in others. Phonological Processing on the NEPSY, which required segmentation and reconstitution of sounds, was among his lowest scores (scaled score = 4). Recalling names, a task with some phonological demands, was also poor (NEPSY Memory for Names = 5).

In contrast, although Daniel has fairly modest general language skills, these are not impaired, and they are unlikely to explain his classroom learning problems. Recall that his VCI was in the average range, his score on a subtest requiring him to recall a passage was average (NEPSY Narrative Memory = 9), and no problems understanding directions or explaining himself were observed during testing, reported by his teacher, or was mentioned by his parents. He clearly possesses conversational skills. SLI is an unlikely explanation.

Lastly, Daniel's family and personal history may be illuminating. PRD (and variations thereof) appears to be heritable, it is especially common in males, and phonological deficits themselves appear to be the most heritable component. Recall that Daniel's father, uncles, and grandfather all experienced problems reading. His father, perhaps like Daniel himself, presumably enjoys well-developed expressive and receptive language, and he possesses a good vocabulary (he is a salesman). Also recall that Daniel suffered articulation problems earlier, which have mostly resolved, and that he earlier had poor memory for rote linguistic material (letter and color names). All of these facts point toward PRD.

Intervention Plan

The following are suggested for Daniel:

1. An intensive oral reading program combining oral reading, phonics instruction, and phonemic awareness is recommended. A structured program such as the Lindamood Phoneme Sequencing Program for Reading, Spelling, and Speech is proposed to develop sound–symbol relationships so that he can rapidly identify words. Abandoning simple work with basal reading series in lieu of a clinical approach is suggested. Moreover, to help Daniel close the gap, intensive services for several hours per week are suggested. Daniel may need to receive SLD designation to assure that such services are provided and to increase the prospect of working with a teacher who possesses specific training in reading problems.

2. A parallel program to teach spelling is also suggested. To back up direct instruction, Daniel's written work should be checked and errors corrected by applying the same algorithms to teach sound–symbol pairing applied during reading instruction.

3. Daniel should be promoted to second grade. However, classroom accommodations may be needed to assure that he can read instructions and has sufficient support to complete writing tasks that classmates may execute independently. A peer tutor, an arrangement to seek assistance from an aide, or other procedural steps to assure success are recommended as supplements to direct instruction.

4. Computerized assistive technology that reads aloud to Daniel may be used to circumvent his inability to read in content areas.

5. A speech–language evaluation is suggested. The purpose of this evaluation, (explicit referral questions should accompany all interdisciplinary referrals), is to determine Daniel's candidacy for speech therapy and to determine whether accommodations are necessary regarding speech articulation.

6. Daniel risks discouragement. Teachers and parents should acknowledge his successes (e.g., in arithmetic) as an antidote to discouragement and potentially declining academic self-confidence.

CASE 2: CARMEN

Background Information

Carmen is a 6-year-old kindergarten student who lives with her mother and stepfather. She was referred by the preschool special needs program for a routine evaluation before starting kindergarten. She has participated in a special needs preschool program under the designation of mild/moderate developmental delay since age 3 years.

Carmen is a white female. She was born after a full-term pregnancy with no record of birth-related difficulty. Her mother said that she was under an obstetrician's care throughout her pregnancy. Carmen came home from the hospital on time and encountered no obvious difficulty until age 3 years. At that point, her pediatrician became concerned that her language was "immature." Simultaneous review of her history indicated that motor milestones were also slightly delayed. Her pediatrician requested an evaluation to determine her candidacy for preschool services. An evaluation by a team consisting of professionals from occupational and physical therapy, speech, and social work established that she was more than 1.5 standard deviations behind age-mates on motor, linguistic, and social dimensions. This information was sufficient to enroll her in a half-day program designed to promote development in each of these areas, principally through direct instruction that targeted the next developmental task as outlined in documents that describe standard toddler and child development.

Carmen's preschool teacher characterized her as a pleasant, somewhat quiet child who socialized with just one or two other children in the heterogeneous setting where she attended class (i.e., the class was composed of children with special needs and those with unimpaired development). Favorably, her teacher had seen steady progress. For example, Carmen had advanced from reticence, using extremely simple phrases and incomplete sentences only, to frequent spontaneous utterances, sometimes involving full sentences, and with generally good intelligibility. Regarding self-care, she had grown from being dependent on others for toileting to complete independence. Her teacher believed that she acquired about half the readiness skills desired for beginning kindergartners by her local school, a substantial improvement during the course of 2 years.

Carmen's pediatrician indicated that she was healthy. She documented that Carmen has normal hearing and vision. There was no evidence of physical stigmata that might signal a genetic syndrome. Carmen's immunizations were reported up-to-date.

Carmen's mother stated that she, herself, had been a special education student, participating in what she called "a classroom for students who were slow." She did graduate from high school (with special education participation throughout her school years) but had never been employed outside the home. She stated that most of the decisions in her home are made by her husband, who is 11 years her senior and regularly employed as a janitor. Carmen's mother said that most of her siblings dropped out of school before graduation. Carmen has a 4-year-old half-sister who attends the same special needs preschool. The home is described as stable, although her mother said that money is often tight.

Assessment Procedures

Wechsler Intelligence Scale for Children–IV; Woodcock–Johnson III Tests of Achievement; NEPSY (Design Copying, Visuomotor Precision, Memory for Faces, Memory for Names, Phonological Processing); Grooved Pegboard Test; Peabody Picture Vocabulary Test—Third Edition; Vineland Adaptive Behavior Scales–2: Interview Edition; Behavior Assessment System for Children–2 (Teacher Report Form, Parent Report Form); parent interview. Scores on standardized instruments for Carmen are listed in Table 5.2.

Observations

Carmen is an age-appropriate-appearing 6-year-old. She was a bit tentative at the outset of the evaluation. Her mother sat in on administration of the first test (PPVT-III) and then departed with no protest or signs of apprehension from her daughter. Carmen's attention span did seem to be relatively brief, and at times she clearly struggled to understand what was expected of her. This meant that the examining psychologist sometimes had to elaborate on directions or demonstrate exactly what was expected. Carmen's effort, however, was excellent during the entire evaluation (two sittings). She was obviously eager to please; she reveled in compliments and always responded enthusiastically to encouragement. Because Carmen was assessed during the summer preceding kindergarten, no classroom observation was conducted.

TABLE 5.2. Summary of Assessment Scores for Carmen

Name	Age	Sex	Dominant hand	Grade
Carmen	6 years, 4 months	Female	Right	Kindergarten

Wechsler Intelligence Scale for Children–IV

Verbal Comprehension		Perceptual Reasoning		Working Memory		Processing speed	
Similarities	5	Block Design	6	Digit Span	4	Coding	6
Vocabulary	6	Picture Concepts	6	Letter–Number Sequence	5	Symbol Search	5
Comprehension	4	Matrix Reasoning	5	(Arithmetic)		(Cancellation)	

Scale	Composite score		Percentile rank
Verbal Comprehension	71 (66–80)	VCI	3rd
Perceptual Reasoning	73 (68–83)	PRI	4th
Working Memory	68 (64–77)	WMI	2nd
Processing Speed	75 (70–86)	PSI	5th
Full Scale	66 (62–72)	FSIQ	1st
General Ability Index	69 (65–76)	GAI	2nd

Woodcock–Johnson III Tests of Achievement

WJ III subtests	Scaled score
Letter–Word Identification	73
Story Recall	52
Calculations	71
Spelling	65

A Developmental Neuropsychological Assessment (NEPSY)

Phonological Processing	5
Visuomotor Precision	4
Design Copying	3
Memory for Faces	7
Memory for Names	5

Motor Exam

Pegboard

Dominant hand (right): 69 sec
Nondominant hand (left): Unable to perform

Peabody Picture Vocabulary Test—Third Edition

Receptive Vocabulary Index = 73

(continued)

TABLE 5.2. *(continued)*

Vineland Adaptive Behavior Scales–2: Interview Edition, Survey Form (Parent)

Scale	Standard score
Communication Domain	69
Daily Living Skills	66
Socialization Domain	68
Motor Skills	70
Adaptive Behavior Composite	66

Behavior Assessment System for Children–2 (Parent Report)

Scale	Level
F	Acceptable
Response Pattern	Acceptable
Consistency	Acceptable
Hyperactivity	61
Aggression	56
Conduct Problems	56
Anxiety	46
Depression	56
Somatization	51
Atypicality	66
Withdrawal	61
Attention Problems	62
Adaptability	40
Social Skills	39
Leadership	36
Activities of Daily Living	36
Functional Communication	31

Behavior Assessment System for Children–2 (Teacher Report)

Scale	Level
F	Acceptable
Response Pattern	Acceptable
Consistency	Acceptable
Hyperactivity	62
Aggression	59
Conduct Problems	59
Anxiety	54
Depression	59
Somatization	57
Attention Problems	70
Learning Problems	63
Atypicality	63
Withdrawal	40
Adaptability	39
Social Skills	40
Leadership	38
Study Skills	35
Functional Communication	32

Analysis of Results

Regarding the first question (in Box A), Carmen is in a different situation than most other children. She has participated in preschool only. Nonetheless, her teacher identifies significant limitations in her skills when they are compared to those of others beginning kindergarten. Work samples provided by her mother documented extremely immature handwriting (little legible writing), limited grasp of numerical concepts, and scant evidence of appreciation of sound–symbol associations on prereading tasks. Given this information and her history, the answer to Box A was concluded to be "yes." An affirmative answer to this question means that it is appropriate to use the rest of the flowchart.

Box B concerns general cognitive ability; it is a pathway for considering whether IQ-related problems may explain Carmen's school difficulty. In considering the answer to Box B's question, her history needs to be taken into account. She was slow to develop based on judgments by her pediatrician, and several professionals' developmental evaluations confirmed language, social, and motor delays. IQ and other psychometric scores are now essential to establish her ability level objectively.

Carmen's WISC-IV scores point to clear and pervasive delays. She has relatively little difference among VCI, PRI, WMI, and PSI indices, and the differences that do appear fail to reach statistical significance. Accordingly, her Full Scale IQ of 66 represents the best psychometric indicator of her current global ability. Accordingly, the preponderance of evidence indicates that the answer to Box B is "no."

Box C addresses whether significant cognitive delay exists when Carmen's current status is compared to national standards. The quantifiable aspect of this question makes standardized tests, especially IQ tests, essential. Referring to the WISC-IV scores just considered, Carmen's scores are clearly more than two standard deviations (IQ < 70) below the mean. Furthermore, the bulk of her psychometric data reveal scores in the same range. This is determined by looking at the rest of her scores on the NEPSY, PPVT-III, Grooved Pegboard, and Woodcock–Johnson III Tests of Achievement. That is, all domains—visual–motor, linguistic, declarative memory, academic-related, and readiness—converge around a standard score of 65. The answer to Box C is "yes."

Thus, a formal designation of mental retardation should be considered. To do so, the three criteria for mental retardation must be considered. Regarding the first criterion, Carmen has general cognitive delays, evidenced by IQ scores and other developmental data, below the cut-off value. Regarding the second criterion, she also suffers adaptive delays. To some extent, these are reflected in the comments made by her teacher and mother. However, formal corroboration of adaptive delays (i.e., using quantifiable adaptive behavior scales) is routine if parents' and teachers' reports contain any ambiguity or if the child's development is close to the cut-off level. In this instance, a face-to-face interview was conducted with Carmen's mother during which the Vineland Adaptive Behavior Scales–2: Interview Edition was administered. Carmen's mother was extremely cooperative, but her responses to several questions were hard to interpret and, accordingly, challenging to score. Nonetheless, the composite score (Adaptive Behavior Composite) of 66 agrees with the remainder of the available information on Carmen. Thus, the second mental retardation criterion was satisfied. A final formal requirement is that delayed development appears before age 18 years. This stipulation is clearly met in Carmen's case.

Intervention Plan

The following are recommended:

1. Carmen requires direct instruction in language, motor, and social development by participation in special education programs. She will require direct instruction from a resource teacher. Children at this level seem to benefit from multisensory methods and use of peer tutoring. Later, she may require use of technology (e.g., calculators). Clearly identified instructional goals that use close monitoring and frequent feedback are also suggested.

2. Integrated with the above activities, she needs to work on readiness (and subsequently actual academic skills) in reading, spelling, and arithmetic.

3. Because Carmen currently expresses mild mental retardation, the goal of teaching academic skills should not be abandoned. She shares many "normal" interests and characteristics with her unimpaired classmates. In contrast, she possesses cognitive and social strengths above children with moderate, severe, and profound mental retardation. Special services programming that would group her with children in the moderate, severe, or profound range risk unnecessary stigma and may lead to reduced expectations. Such instructional grouping should be avoided, even if placement with lower-functioning students seems convenient or economically advantageous to her school.

4. Information needs to be shared with parents, and an integrated plan that encourages parents to provide stimulation and services consistent with those in points 1 and 2 above should be considered.

5. Carmen's information needs to be considered by a school-based multidisciplinary team. She appears to be eligible for services under the category of MiMR, but the team needs to make a formal judgment of this label's appropriateness.

6. Despite this designation, Carmen is not recommended for placement in a self-contained classroom where her interactions would be confined to other students with similar delays. For the sake of cognitive stimulation and development of social skills, she should be placed in a regular kindergarten classroom and supplemental services (as indicated above) provided on a pull-out basis.

CASE 3: RYAN

Background Information

Ryan is a 9-and-a-half-year-old white male who is healthy, free of hearing and vision problems, and lives with his biological parents. He attends the fourth grade at a public school. Ryan was born following a term pregnancy without perinatal complications. He mastered developmental milestones at expected ages. No motor or linguistic problems, including subtle auditory-processing problems that might predict subsequent reading difficulties, were noted in his preschool history. Ryan sleeps adequately, although he sometimes resists going to bed unless his parents become insistent. He eats adequately but with strongly expressed food preferences. He is sometimes restless at the table, reportedly getting up and down more often than his three older brothers.

Ryan represents a moderate behavior problem at home. He is sometimes noncompliant with requests, especially those made by his mother. He resists chores, tends toward impatience, dislikes tedious activities (such as board games), and complains of boredom on car trips or visits to restaurants. He demonstrates an adequate attention span at home on self-selected tasks only (e.g., videogames). If his parents ask him to do something that he finds uninteresting (e.g., cleaning his room), he has a remarkably hard time paying attention. Rather than working consistently, he is apt to find excuses to get up and move around during homework. He can often be described as restless and impatient. For example, he has left his seat in class to talk with friends several times even though warned not to do so. He tends to race through schoolwork or volunteer an answer before it is his turn. Regarding cooperation, he is apt to resist requests from adults, especially if much effort is required, unless requests are repeated or backed up with imminent consequences. Despite his parents' good efforts, he still forgets routine activities, such as grooming, unless reminded and encouraged.

Ryan has some social problems, although he is overtly friendly. His play is said to be loud and animated, both at home and school. Favorably, he does well in sports, where he is seen as coordinated and assertive. Nonetheless, he seems to lose focus (e.g., requires reminders and redirection during tennis practice) and sometimes disrupts activities by roughhousing, loud talk, and interrupting the instructor. Apparently because of the intensity level of his play and social intrusion, he fails to keep friends, although other boys like him a great deal at first.

Ryan has three older brothers who have always done well in school. His mother was a high achiever, and his father reportedly did adequately. There are two uncles who have been diagnosed with ADHD-C, but no other family history of learning, developmental, or psychiatric disorders.

Ryan is a fourth grader in a middle-class, rural school district. Both his parents and his current teacher express concern about his classroom status. Work quality fluctuates from acceptable to poor. Writing work samples, which were provided by his teacher, ranged from approximately 10% to nearly 100% correct. On untimed arithmetic worksheets involving multiplication and division, he ranged from 50–85% correct. Extremely inconsistent penmanship was noted; all work was done in manuscript, and much of it was hard to read. Ryan's mother stated that he has consistently found all subjects (including reading) harder than his classmates, perhaps because he resists work and is disorganized. Concern from parents and teacher notwithstanding, he made C's in all subjects on his last report card. Group achievement test scores have also fluctuated, but generally have fallen in the 25th–60th percentile (national norms). His group achievement test scores do not demonstrate obvious strengths or weaknesses.

The pre-referral team at Ryan's school reviewed his case three times. On the first occasion, the team's brainstorming process led to conclusions that he was easily bored. Accordingly, his teacher attempted to engage him in frequent discussions and, consistent with suggestions from fellow teachers, used a more animated speaking style. Two weeks later, with no reported improvement, a second meeting was held that resulted in a change of seating to a location closer to the teacher. Again, the team felt that little progress was made. The school's psychologist, a consultant to the team, was then asked to contribute. She devised a daily report card targeting work completion and in-class compliance. Also fearing that poor phonological awareness may underlie Ryan's reading difficulties, she suggested he participate in a remedial reading program with a phonetic emphasis. RTI was measured by the administration of oral fluency curriculum-based measurement (CBM) probes and monitoring of work completion. After administration of reading CBM probes to determine a baseline from which to judge progress, it became obvious that Ryan's word reading skills were commensurate with peers, and the reading intervention with related response monitoring was discontinued. Despite a slight improvement in compliance and minor gains in work completion, both Ryan's teacher and his parents requested a comprehensive evaluation better to understand the causes of his marginal school status. Because of an anticipated 2-month wait for an evaluation at school, Ryan's parents took him to a local, independent-practice psychologist.

Observations

As this was a clinic-based evaluation, no classroom observation was made. Ryan was observed in the clinic to be a handsome, well-groomed boy who was somewhat large for his age. He was cooperative but quick to complain about being expected to work. He frequently stated that the work was "boring" and asked how long he would be expected to work. He appeared to give up quickly, although he was quite responsive to encouragement. He was slightly restless but not especially impulsive or interpersonally intrusive. He made good eye contact, conversed easily, and appeared comfortable. The evaluation was planned for a single morning session, but a second morning session was needed because of concern about flagging effort.

Assessment Procedures

Wechsler Intelligence Scale for Children–IV; NEPSY (Design Copying, Visuomotor Precision, Memory for Faces, Memory for Names, Narrative Memory); Grooved Pegboard Test; Gordon Diagnostic System (Vigilance Task and Delay Task); Wechsler Individual Achievement Test–II; Behavior Assessment System for Children–2 (Teacher Report Form, Parent Report Form), parent interview, child interview, review of school documents. Scores on standardized instruments for Ryan are listed in Table 5.3.

Analysis of Results

In order to use our system, we first had to determine whether Ryan was referred because of concern about school performance or academic success, as queried in Box A. Review of his mother's comments and those of his teacher confirmed that this was the case. Consequently, the rest of the flowchart could be followed. Box A was answered "yes." A positive answer to this preliminary question meant that we could use the current system (i.e., one designed to understand learning problems, not psychiatric or genetic syndromes).

The next question is whether Ryan's development level, or current level of cognitive functioning, is at issue. Put another way, is it safe to assume that general cognitive ability is not the principal explanation for Ryan's presenting problems? To address this question, we wanted to consider all pertinent information, not just test scores. In Ryan's case, the following are relevant: developmental history (normal), mother's comments about development (seems to be roughly average, but not as bright as older

TABLE 5.3. Summary of Assessment Scores for Ryan

Name	Age	Sex	Dominant hand	Grade
Ryan	9 years, 6 months	Male	Right	4

Wechsler Intelligence Scale for Children–IV

Verbal Comprehension		Perceptual Reasoning		Working Memory		Processing Speed	
Similarities	9	Block Design	10	Digit Span	7	Coding	10
Vocabulary	11	Picture Concepts	7	(Arithmetic)	14	Symbol Search	5
Comprehension	11	Matrix Reasoning	7				

Scale	Composite score		Percentile rank
Verbal Comprehension	100 (93–107)	VCI	50th
Perceptual Reasoning	88 (81–97)	PRI	21st
Working Memory	102 (94–109)	WMI	55th
Processing Speed	85 (78–96)	PSI	16th
Full Scale	92 (88–98)	FSIQ	30th
General Ability Index	95 (90–101)	GAI	37th

A Developmental Neuropsychological Assessment (NEPSY)

Visuomotor Precision	7
Design Copying	8
Memory	
Memory for Faces	7
Memory for Names	9
Narrative Memory	7
Domain Score	83

Motor Exam

Pegboard
Dominant Hand (Right): 95 sec
Nondominant hand (left): 94 sec

Gordon Diagnostic System

Delay task	Score	Normal Borderline/Abnormal
Efficiency ratio	70%	Borderline
Total correct	49	Average
Vigilance task		
Total commissions	79	Abnormal
Total correct	30	Abnormal

Wechsler Individual Achievement Test–II

WIAT-II subtests	Scaled score
Word Reading	111
Reading Comprehension	100
Numerical Operations	93

(continued)

TABLE 5.3. *(continued)*

WIAT-II subtests	Scaled score
Spelling	103
Written Expression	92

Behavior Assessment System for Children–2 (Parent Report)

Scale	Level
F	Acceptable
Response Pattern	Acceptable
Consistency	Acceptable
Hyperactivity	69
Aggression	40
Conduct Problems	46
Anxiety	40
Depression	37
Somatization	50
Atypicality	41
Withdrawal	65
Attention Problems	72
Adaptability	44
Social Skills	56
Leadership	53
Activities of Daily Living	39
Functional Communication	52

Behavior Assessment System for Children–2 (Teacher Report)

Scale	Level
F	Acceptable
Response Pattern	Acceptable
Consistency	Acceptable
Hyperactivity	69
Aggression	48
Conduct Problems	57
Anxiety	48
Depression	42
Somatization	50
Attention Problems	68
Learning Problems	58
Atypicality	46
Withdrawal	39
Adaptability	35
Social Skills	34
Leadership	44
Study Skills	42
Functional Communication	48

brothers), progress in school (borderline to adequate), and standardized cognitive ability scores (WISC-IV IQ).

Similarly, we needed to examine all of Ryan's scores on the WISC-IV. The two most important index scores in this case are an FSIQ of 92 (30th percentile, average range) and VCI score of 100 (50th percentile, average range). The first score is a bit concerning. Recalling that Ryan attends an average school, he may be slightly less cognitively able than some of his classmates, at least if scores are taken at face value. This is an important point because we want to be certain that Ryan's problems do not derive from the simple fact that he is less cognitively mature and capable than his classmates (e.g., has SL status or AEM) before entertaining other possibilities. However, his VCI of 100 (comprising language conceptual ability, work knowledge, and vocabulary) is solidly average. These skills measured by Vocabulary, Similarities, and Comprehension subtests are highly related to school success; they are also good measures of g. Moreover, Ryan's response style may have contributed to his relatively low scores and, accordingly, diminished the degree to which his FSIQ reflects overall ability. For example, on the Picture Concepts subtest, which requires repeated examination and hypothesis testing, he sometimes responded quickly and carelessly; on Symbol Search, his pace slowed noticeably after 1 minute. Lack of effort and persistence, rather than limited general cognitive ability, probably caused his scaled score to fall to 5. Reflecting on standard error of measurement, it may be that Ryan's FSIQ would be close to the upper bound of his range (which extends from 88 to 98). Thus, although Ryan may not find school easy based on his current level of cognitive ability, the expectations at his local school are unlikely to be so high that a student of average or even low-average ability could not succeed. This consideration, coupled with other background facts, would lead us to conclude that Box B is answered "yes."

The next question (Box D) concerns the prospect of genuine deficits in academic skills. That is, are any of Ryan's skills (i.e., academic, language, fine-motor) appreciably lower than average for someone of his age and school experience? It is again important to consider all sources of information, not just test scores. Pertinent available information included report card marks (generally average), teacher ratings of academic level (generally average, except for penmanship), group achievement test scores (generally average), progress through the curriculum (Ryan had been promoted each year in school), and individually administered achievement test (WIAT-II) scores. On the WIAT-II, Ryan's scores were average to high-average on language-related tasks (Word Reading = 111; Reading Comprehension = 100; Spelling = 103; Written Expression = 92). Ryan showed a fairly well-developed sight vocabulary (automatically pronounceable words); he also demonstrated reasonable word attack skills on words that were not immediately recognized. Overall, he seemed to use fairly well-developed appreciation of phonics rules, based on an analysis of his reading responses to single words and spelling. Ryan's handwriting, executed in manuscript form, was marginal, and he wrote relatively short sentences. He did seem to struggle slightly with pencil control, although he demonstrated a mature pencil grip. He wrote very quickly and apparently with little concern about legibility. His NEPSY Visuomotor Precision score, which might speak to true graphomotor problems, is only slightly low, as is his NEPSY Design Copying score. He scored in the average range on mechanical arithmetic (Numerical Operations = 93). His errors here occurred on both simple and complex tasks, the former apparently due to carelessness and failure to attend closely to details. Although the data here are a bit equivocal, it was concluded that academics and/or fine-motor control was not clearly deficit. The answer to Box D is "no."

The next question concerns the extent to which the teacher(s) are convinced that a classroom problem actually exists. The question should be thought of in broad terms, and several sources of information merit consideration. Those include input from current instructional teachers, aides, tutors, and even parents, if they have routinely been involved in the student's homework routine (as was the case with Ryan's father). His teacher brought his case to the pre-referral team and attempted various interventions. It was apparent that Ryan's parents were concerned. They sometimes spend 3 hours at home helping him complete assignments he failed to finish in class. Both parents and teachers, including his second-grade teacher, noted drastically fluctuating performance, much work left undone, and some low grades. At least occasionally, Ryan's handwriting was judged to be below standard. The answer to Box F, therefore, was "yes."

By now, the decisions that we have made imply a performance, rather than a skill development, problem. That is, we have established that Ryan's apparent school difficulties are unlikely due to either lack of ability or failure of actual academic skills. The next question (Box H) helps us determine which, if any, performance-related problem is actually present. This question concerns whether Ryan's behavior is seen as disruptive; in other words, do his actions require behavior management techniques, and is he prone to disturb other students? This question is primarily about classroom behavior, but information from home and social settings is also relevant. In reviewing comments from teachers, the following were noted: out of seat, talkative, occasionally blurts out answers, and interactions with classmates that can be intrusive and rough on the playground. His behavior at home speaks more directly to the question. His mother confirmed noncompliance, argumentativeness, and impulsiveness so that she often finds herself reminding, threatening, physically redirecting, or using time-out. Furthermore, Ryan's conduct during testing was such that finesse, limit-setting, and use of contingencies were required. The decision Box H is also answered "yes." This affirmative answer suggests that ADHD, especially combined type, needs to be considered.

In attempting to confirm that ADHD is Ryan's primary condition, all sources of information once again merit consideration. We turn first to the DSM-IV-TR criteria for ADHD. The history provided by Ryan's parents confirms the following DSM-IV-TR symptoms of ADHD: often does not follow through on instructions and fails to finish schoolwork, chores, or duties; often does not seem to listen when spoken to directly; and often fails to give close attention to detail or makes careless mistakes in schoolwork and other work. His teacher's classroom reports appear to substantiate the following DSM-IV-TR symptoms: often leaves seat when remaining seated is expected; often talks excessively; often blurts out answers; often interrupts or intrudes on others (peers). Furthermore, his parents' reports indicate that symptoms appeared before age 7 years, cause clinically significant impairment in several settings, and do not appear to be attributable to other factors, such as chronic illness. Each of these points must be addressed if confirmation of ADHD by DSM-IV-TR criteria is sought (see Chapter 4).

We next consider objective rating scales completed by his classroom teacher and his parents. The BASC-2 shows borderline clinical elevations on the two applicable scales (Hyperactivity T score = 69; Attention Problems T score = 68). Only the Learning Problems scale (T score = 58) among other BASC-2 scales was even slightly elevated. This scale's slight elevation probably reflects his teacher's uneasiness about Ryan's lack of work completion and its threat to long-term academic skill development. His parents also completed the BASC-2 and the resulting profile fits with his teacher's BASC-2 scores. Both the Hyperactivity and Attention Problems scales were elevated (T scores of 69 and 72, respectively). In our clinic setting, one additional source of information was available to address the prospect of ADHD. Ryan was administered a computerized continuous performance test, the Gordon Diagnostic System. Despite limitations, this test is sometimes useful when questions of ADHD are on the table (see Chapter 4). On the Delay task, Ryan worked persistently and earned a total correct value that was in the average range. However, his responses tended to be impulsive and reflected impatience. His percentage of correct responses (called the "efficiency ratio") was 70%, a borderline abnormal score for 9-year-olds. On the Vigilance task, Ryan had extremely poor scores. The number of inappropriate button presses (called "commission errors") was many times the average value for 9-year-olds. Furthermore, he missed (or committed "omission errors" on) 15 of the 45 target combinations, far beyond the average range cut-off. When these poor scores are combined with his history, objective rating scales, and psychometric scores, the aggregate information is sufficient to establish the conclusion of ADHD-C. Additionally, an interview with Ryan (and available BASC-2 scores) failed to suggest another social–emotional problem that might better explain his presenting behavior and history (i.e., he did not appear to be demonstrating an anxiety or mood problem).

Although arriving at a decision about Ryan's core problem is helpful, the process should not stop here. In Ryan's case, we had collected additional psychometric information, and his history also required consideration. As Ryan had a significant VCI/PRI discrepancy on the WISC-IV, one might consider the possibility of a coexisting NLD. Some information supports this hypothesis: his drawings (NEPSY Design Copying) were of slightly poor quality (scaled score = 8), his WIAT-II computational arithmetic subtest score was lower than his scores in reading, and he tended to play with children younger than himself, raising the possibility of social skills deficits. All of these seem somewhat compatible with an NLD. Alternatively, many facts are incompatible with an NLD designation: Ryan was quite socially adept and appeared accomplished in recognizing social cues during the evaluation, he reportedly excelled at gross-motor tasks and in tennis, he was viewed by his parents as attuned to feedback and generally adaptive in new situations, there was no speed–dexterity asymmetry between his performance with right and left hand on the Grooved Pegboard Test. Thus, it was deemed unlikely that Ryan had a predominant (or even coexisting) NLD. Nonetheless, Ryan's pattern does suggest relative strengths on verbal tasks and corresponding weaknesses on nonverbal, visual–spatial, and graphomotor tasks (he appears, likewise, to be below the threshold for designation with GU). The most parsimonious explanation is that Ryan's facts match ADHD-C and that most other problems derive from core problems with hyperactivity–impulsivity and inattention. All of the information, not just the fact that ADHD-C has been established, should be considered in making recommendations.

Intervention Plan

Ryan's most pressing need is to enhance work completion and to see that work is done consistently. This is entirely compatible with our conceptualization of a performance, rather than a skill development, deficit. For that reason, we suggested that the following be considered.

1. An incentive plan to encourage work completion should be individually tailored to Ryan and his classroom and, ideally, would follow a functional behavior analysis completed by a school psychologist or behaviorally trained educator. This plan might encompass, for example, a daily report card, with or without incentives. Although rudimentary at-

tempts were already made to use a daily report card, a similar intervention overseen by a psychologist who remained available to suggest revisions in workload, frequency, and method of report of daily performance to Ryan's parents and to schedule an array of reinforcers may be needed. Furthermore, ongoing involvement by a psychologist to monitor progress and assure treatment integrity is often needed.

2. The pattern of work completion should be investigated to determine if either written assignments or those that were particularly slow-paced or tedious were associated with poorer performance. This decision might be reached by discussion of a problem-solving team or as a result of the functional behavior analysis mentioned above. If written or slow-paced assignments were consistently associated with failure to complete work, then substituting oral or fast-paced assignments would be suggested.

3. Ryan might benefit from learning to keyboard in lieu of writing. He might also benefit from a structured handwriting program that could make writing easier for him to execute and more legible for his readers.

4. Ryan appears to be acquiring academic skills well, even if he is not always completing work at school. It may be helpful, therefore, to emphasize skill acquisition, rather than productivity, when assigning grades. That is to say, low report marks attributable to incomplete assignments may be unduly pessimistic, and they may discourage rather than motivate him.

5. An in-class plan to discourage disruptive or impulsive responding may be in order. Again, a functional behavior analysis might help to specify the plan's exact elements.

6. Ryan's teacher may benefit from learning more about the classroom manifestations of ADHD. Assigned reading may be in order.

7. To address points 1–7, and to assure that reasonable adjustments are made, Ryan should be considered for a Section 504 accommodation plan or, perhaps, special education services under the OHI category for ADHD.

8. If a recent physical examination has not been conducted, then one is suggested to rule out any health problems that might mimic ADHD (see American Academy of Pediatrics guidelines for evaluation of ADHD, 2000). Generally, a final conclusion about the presence of ADHD would await this evaluation, although a physician's documentation is not deemed necessary to conclude that ADHD is present (U.S. Department of Education, 2003).

9. Related to #8, psychopharmacology may have a role in Ryan's performance in class and his behavior at home. Information from this evaluation should be shared with his primary care physician, and his parents are encouraged to discuss the potential role of medicine in his management.

Regarding this topic, many parents benefit from learning factual information, such as from books for parents by Barkley (2000), Hallowell and Ratney (1994), and Wodrich (2000).

10. If Ryan's mother and father are interested, a 10-session training sequence for parents, as scripted by Barkley (1997b), might be considered.

CASE 4: TODD

Background Information

Todd is an 8-year-and-1-month-old white male whose only language is English. He is a first grader in a middle-class, urban school district. The request for an evaluation was initiated by his teacher and parents. The chief concern was trouble learning all, or nearly all, school subjects. Todd is said by his teacher to be substantially behind classmates in each academic area, and he is becoming increasingly frustrated.

Todd is a healthy youngster. He has passed hearing and vision screenings. He was born following a term pregnancy without complications. He came home from the nursery on time and mastered developmental milestones at what his parents describe as "a little slower than other children." They indicated that, even now, he sometimes seems immature. He had a history of thumb sucking (evident at bedtime only) that resolved at about age 5 years, but the habit reappeared this year. His parents attribute this occurrence to mounting stress associated with school failure. Todd reportedly sleeps and eats well, although he often complains of being tired in the morning. His parents often find it tough to get him out of bed on school days.

Todd attended preschool programs for 3- and 4-year-olds without behavioral or social problems. Similarly, no teachers in these settings reported concern about his development. He began a half-day kindergarten at age 5, but soon encountered trouble in all subject areas. He repeated kindergarten in a whole-day program and reportedly did well the second time through the same material. However, in his first-grade year, his teacher stated that he was behind classmates in reading (seemed to lack any sight words and only inconsistently sounded out unknown words), spelling (demonstrated little appreciation of letter–sound associations and had poorly formed letters), and math (struggled to grasp concepts and appeared confused over simple facts). Todd's teacher was concerned that he sometimes failed to speak clearly; thus, he was referred to the school's speech–language pathologist for an evaluation. That evaluation rated his articulation as "within acceptable limits" for his age while designating him with mild receptive and expressive language delays. As a result of the evaluation and after his parents agreed to services under the category of speech–language impairment, he received school-based language services in a group with four other students for 20 minutes three times weekly.

Reading has been a special concern of Todd's mother and his maternal grandmother, who worked many years as an instructional aide and was well aware of various approaches to reading instruction. Todd complained that he did not like the way in which his teacher taught reading and stated that he was introduced to new material too quickly. Besides direct instruction, worksheets were frequently used, even though Todd complained that he seldom understood what he was supposed to do with these. Favorably, Todd was well behaved in class. He sometimes isolated himself from classmates and played alone at recess. By the same token, his parents saw him as hesitant in sports and painfully short of confidence. He reportedly seldom socialized with classmates outside of school.

Todd lives with his biological parents. His father reportedly had a hard time in school and "hated it." He ultimately finished high school by taking vocational courses, but now does well as a skilled laborer. One of Todd's older brothers had school trouble, including retention in second grade. His marks are reportedly marginal now that he is a fifth grader. Family history is otherwise negative for learning, developmental, or psychiatric problems. An older sister is said to find school "easy."

Observations

Todd was slightly anxious when his parents brought him to be evaluated, but he soon warmed up when he stated that the examiner reminded him of his karate coach. His effort was excellent, although he appeared slightly inattentive and restless. He tended to forget directions and required repeated explanations to grasp what was expected of him. Despite interpersonal comfort, he seemed to need more reassurance and encouragement than most first graders. The evaluation was easily completed in a single morning with several rest/snack breaks that he spent with his parents.

Assessment Procedures

Wechsler Intelligence Scale for Children–IV; Wechsler Individual Achievement Test–II; NEPSY (Design Copying, Visuomotor Precision, Memory for Faces, Memory for Names, Narrative Memory, Phonological Processing); Behavior Assessment System for Children–2 (Teacher Report Form, Parent Report Form); informal assessment of curriculum material, parent interview, child interview. Scores on standardized instruments for Todd are listed in Table 5.4.

TABLE 5.4. Summary of Assessment Scores for Todd

Name	Age	Sex	Dominant hand	Grade
Todd	8 years, 1 month	Male	Left	1

Wechsler Intelligence Scale for Children–IV

Verbal Comprehension		*Perceptual Reasoning*		*Working Memory*		*Processing speed*	
Similarities	6	Block Design	7	Digit Span	8	Coding	8
Vocabulary	5	Picture Concepts	6	Letter–Number Sequence	6	Symbol Search	7
Comprehension	7	Matrix Reasoning	7				

Scale	*Composite score*		*Percentile rank*
Verbal Comprehension	77 (72–85)	VCI	6th
Perceptual Reasoning	79 (73–88)	PRI	8th
Working Memory	83 (77–92)	WMI	13th
Processing Speed	85 (78–96)	PSI	16th
Full Scale	75 (71–81)	FSIQ	5th
General Ability Index	77 (72–84)	GAI	6th

Wechsler Individual Achievement Test–II

WIAT-II subtests	*Scaled score*
Word Reading	75
Reading Comprehension	70
Pseudoword Decoding	72
Numerical Operations	86
Math Reasoning	81
Spelling	88
Written Expression	81

A Developmental Neuropsychological Assessment (NEPSY)

Phonological Processing	8
Visuomotor Precision	6
Design Copying	6
Memory for Faces	9
Memory for Names	4
Narrative Memory	7

Behavior Assessment System for Children–2 (Parent Report)

Scale	*Level*
F	Acceptable
Response Pattern	Acceptable
Consistency	Acceptable
Hyperactivity	41
Aggression	37

(continued)

TABLE 5.4. *(continued)*

Scale	Level
Conduct Problems	37
Anxiety	55
Depression	57
Somatization	36
Atypicality	41
Withdrawal	44
Attention Problems	67
Adaptability	37
Social Skills	39
Leadership	36
Activities of Daily Living	34
Functional Communication	37

Behavior Assessment System for Children–2 (Teacher Report)

Scale	Level
F	Acceptable
Response Pattern	Acceptable
Consistency	Acceptable
Hyperactivity	41
Aggression	43
Conduct Problems	42
Anxiety	55
Depression	55
Somatization	43
Attention Problems	68
Learning Problems	72
Atypicality	43
Withdrawal	44
Adaptability	37
Social Skills	40
Leadership	37
Study Skills	36
Functional Communication	34

Analysis of Results

The first step in using our system is to verify that this referral is for truly academic concerns. This was easily accomplished by noting that both Todd's parents and his teacher expressed unequivocal concern about his academic progress. Furthermore, he encountered so much trouble learning in kindergarten that he was actually retained. Box A is answered "yes." The rest of the flowchart is then usable.

The next step is to decide whether Todd's level of general development might be part of the explanation for his classroom learning problems. That is, we needed to rule out lack of general cognitive ability before considering other possibilities. Several sources of information require consideration. These were: (1) his developmental history (grossly normal), (2) his parents' comment about their son's development level (seems to be a little less mature than some children his age), (3) progress in school (below average in every subject area), (4) subjective appraisal of his ability during testing (slow to catch on), and (5) standardized ability scores (i.e., WISC-IV IQ). In this case, his WISC-IV required special scrutiny. The two index scores that most accurately reflect cognitive ability, VCI and PRI, were in the borderline range, (VCI = 77, 6th percentile; PRI = 79, 8th percentile). His FSIQ of 75, at the 5th percentile, is also in the borderline range, even though he enjoyed a bit more success on tasks tapping working memory and speed. These scores are quite suggestive of a child whose overall cognitive abilities are less developed than his age peers. At the subtest level, too, Todd's scores suggested that reasoning, problem solving, and conceptual sophistication were below average. This appeared to be true regardless of the type of cognitive task presented. Besides actual test scores, the quality of Todd's responses implied the same conclusion. Regarding verbal tasks, Todd's responses appeared to contain immature ideas when describing relations among words and concepts (Similarities), his vocabulary looked small and he provided only simple, unelaborated explanations for the words that he knew (Vocabulary); he also provided simplistic and unelaborated responses when confronted with practical problems (Comprehension). Similarly, regarding nonverbal tasks, Todd used trial-and-error in construction (Block Design), and he had limited success in recognizing similarities among objects (Picture Concepts) and patterns among visual arrays (Matrix Reasoning). None of the six subtests with the highest cognitive loading was in the average range (all VCI and PRI subtest scores were 7 or lower). Even considering scores within the 95% confidence interval, neither of the two cognitive index scores reached the average range. On the rest of the WISC-IV—Working Memory (83, 13rd percentile) and Processing Speed (85, 16th percentile) indexes—Todd scored better. However, neither of these indexes is a strong measure of cognitive ability. Todd's FSIQ of 75, thus, probably represents a fairly accurate estimate of his current cognitive ability.

Other indicators of general ability also warranted review. The reports of his parents that Todd seems "immature" correspond to his objective ability scores, although the description of milestones as acquired on time may not. His school history is probably more pertinent because he encountered such consistent trouble keeping up with classmates. The fact that he performed adequately when kindergarten was repeated matches the notion that he possesses ability to master material with repetition. It also suggests that he does better when he is older than classmates (a 1-year age advantage can be important among young children but diminishes with passing

years). Todd's pattern in academics is also pertinent. He had uniform difficulty; reading, spelling, handwriting, and arithmetic skills are underdeveloped compared to most of his peers. One might interpret the findings from
a speech–language evaluation in the same light. Reports of "receptive and
expressive" language delays may simply reflect lack of general ability. That
is, even though receptive and expressive language might be identified as
separable skills, they both reflect general development. The most parsimonious explanation for Todd's limited school success is general (albeit mild)
delay in all cognitively related dimensions, rather than delayed
development on several unrelated dimensions.

The flowchart does not require that the rest of his scores be examined,
but most diagnosticians choose to review all scores before resolving questions of general cognitive delay. That is to say, if Todd truly has general
cognitive immaturity, then many of his other special ability and academic
achievement scores should appear to be about equally delayed. This is to be
expected because almost all psychometric tasks, despite their varied titles
and intention to measure narrow skills, unavoidably measure g to some
extent. In Todd's case, the expected pattern on supplemental tests appears.
Each of his memory, graphomotor, and academic subject matter scores fall
in the below-average range. Thus, when the accumulated evidence is
brought to bear on Box B, an answer of "no" results. In other words, Todd
lacks general ability compared to classmates.

The next questions address the magnitude of general cognitive problems. Specifically, they concern whether Todd's deficits are so great that he
might warrant consideration for mental retardation designation (Box C). If
this were the case, then additional adaptive behavior data would need to be
collected, and the evaluation might ultimately result in provision of formal
special education services in the MiMR category. Fortunately, the information already collected is sufficient to answer these questions. Although
Todd's overall ability appears to be sufficiently low to cause academic failure, it is not below the 70–75 IQ, the recognized threshold for MiMR.
Accordingly, the answer to Box C is "no." The question posed in Box E is
similarly answered with the existing data set. After weighing the information, Todd's general ability does appear to fall between the 75 and 85 IQ
level. Thus, the answer to Box E is "yes." The flowchart hence points to the
conclusion that Todd's problems are those of a student with SL status.

To tie up loose ends, it is appropriate to look at other information that
has yet to be reviewed. Todd's BASC-2 scores are especially noteworthy.
Both his parents and his classroom teacher rate him as below average
regarding adaptive functioning, and both rate him as having learning and
attention problems (viz., the scales related to Adaptability and those
labeled Attention Problems and Learning Problems). This is not surprising
given the content of these scales and what we have now concluded about

this youngster's overall status. Cumulatively, these BASC-2 scales tap attention, organization, efficiency, and actual mastery of school subject matter—all dimensions that generally prove difficult for someone with low-average or borderline cognitive ability. It is perhaps more concerning to notice that his internalizing scales of Anxiety and Depression are in the at-risk range, according to forms completed by both parents and teacher. Scores like these match his parents' initial comments that their son is experiencing mounting frustration with school, discouragement regarding the prospect of success, and perhaps even frank apprehension about entering school each morning. This is a common pattern: repeated failure often produces frustration, fear of losing face, negative self-image, and avoidance of tasks. Thus, it was not surprising that during an interview Todd appeared somber as he talked about school. His fondest wishes also fit with the idea of a discouraged youngster: "already be grown up," "to be a baseball player," and "to never have any more school." Thus, in addition to determining the presence of ability consistent with SL status, the evaluation concluded that demoralization and anxiety are problems that could reach clinical significance unless interventions are made. Accordingly, these factors should be considered in any comprehensive intervention plan.

Finally, work samples brought by parents were reviewed, as was Todd's performance when working with curriculum material provided by his classroom teacher. Todd presented a basal reading book that he had been using in a reading group. His parents indicated that they believed he had attained "pretty good" mastery of the material, and they were certain that he had been reading in the same book for several weeks. When presented a text passage, however, Todd's oral responses consisted almost entirely of paraphrasing the story and showed almost no correspondence with the literal text. Suspicious that he was unable to recognize the story's words, we isolated several of them and showed them to him individually. Todd had about a 20% rate of recognizing these words in isolation. Likewise, a recently completed math worksheet was brought to the evaluation. His accuracy on it was about 55%. When a set of problems of equivalent difficulty was generated and Todd tried them, he had only about 60% accuracy. This information suggested that Todd may be placed in material beyond his current instructional level. This situation is common among children with delayed general ability; most will find grade-level material too difficult for them unless modifications are made. Obviously, this situation would also require attention in his intervention plan.

Intervention Plan

Todd does not have a diagnosable disorder or a formal handicap, at least as those terms are typically currently used. Rather, he expresses general cognitive development that is less than ideal for the demands of most elementary classrooms. This is a recognizable pattern known to be associated with school problems (i.e., SL) even if it is not a formal disorder with obvious special education entitlement. This fact seems to have caused him to struggle in each academic area, contributed to misplacement in the curriculum, and led to discouragement and psychological distress. Although he is not likely to be eligible for any type of special services, recognizing the core of his problem is helpful in creating a coherent plan and informing his parents and teachers why he is struggling. The following were recommended.

1. The first recommendation is for Todd to be properly placed in material so that he stands a reasonable chance of success. Formal CBA or informal procedures can be used to assure that this is accomplished in each academic area. In fact, given his current situation, he may need to be placed temporarily where success is guaranteed. That is, rather than placing him in material where most students enjoy optimum academic growth (90–95% success), Todd may now need tasks of sufficient simplicity (and with enough support) to guarantee success approximating 100%. After a period of enriched success, and with concurrent monitoring of his sense of self-efficacy, slightly more demanding material could be introduced, but with frequent feedback.

2. A related, second, recommendation is to provide classroom support. This might be accomplished by a peer tutor, supplemental explanations and encouragement by his teacher or an aide (to provide concrete descriptions of abstract concepts), or pre-instructional exposure to some curriculum material that could be sent as homework (i.e., permitting parents to explain what is expected in each day's upcoming schoolwork).

3. Explanations may need to be simplified and the necessary steps to complete school assignments demonstrated. Despite Todd's contention that his teacher talks too fast, his difficulty with understanding probably arises from lack of insight and deficits in background ideas, rather than a receptive language problem or problems with auditory working memory. Problems like this are common among students with ability in the SL range. Consequently, cognitive supports, rather than circumventions related to language, are often the key to success.

4. Likewise, as Todd moves into more complex material in later school years, he may require background explanations and discussion of concepts before they are presented in class. This provision for ideational scaffolding may be particularly beneficial in areas such as social studies or science. In these areas specifically, he may lack prerequisite ideas that might be acquired ultimately with support and simplified explanation.

5. In the long term, mentoring in problem solving (perhaps through peer tutoring) may be used so that he can learn systematic ap-

proaches for tackling unknown or confusing situations and class material (e.g., learning metacognitive strategies), including self-management strategies. Also, sensitizing Todd to background ideas and concepts via regular discussion with his parents may help expand his base of background ideas, vocabulary, and knowledge of current events.

6. Given his current situation, Todd's anxiety level and sense of discouragement should be monitored. He may need direct treatment in these dimensions if problems do not abate. He will almost certainly require treatment if problems intensify.

7. A behavior plan to eliminate thumb sucking may be needed. As this behavior is typically done privately, there may seem be little reason to intervene. Nonetheless, Todd has complained that this habit makes him feel like a baby. Self-efficacy may be enhanced by helping him overcome this self-identified problem. In addition, he may feel more comfortable in social situations (e.g., sleepovers) if he is confident that this potentially embarrassing habit will not appear.

8. As long-term academic success will be influenced by cognitive growth and as such growth depends in part on exposure to appropriate models, all means of promoting social contact with age peers (or those older than Todd) should be encouraged. In other words, isolation may have negative impact on ultimate cognitive development.

CASE 5: BRODY

Background Information

Brody is a 10-year-old white, English-speaking male who attends fourth grade in a suburban school district. He was referred by his classroom teacher, who expressed concern about poor reading and spelling. His grades have fallen to the point where retention in fourth grade is being considered. Beginning in the fall, his parents instituted supplemental reading practice at home each evening. After this failed to produce improvement, a private tutor worked with Brody twice a week in his basal reading series and with his assigned spelling list. His teacher has also tried peer tutoring and a charting system to encourage accuracy by providing him with explicit feedback of his success in a graph. None of these interventions has worked.

Brody is a healthy child who has always passed hearing and vision screenings. He takes over-the-counter allergy medication during spring, but allergies do not appear to interfere with school attendance or ability to focus on academic tasks. He reportedly sleeps and eats well. He has always had regular school attendance and has been enrolled in his current school throughout his entire career. He was born following a term pregnancy without perinatal complications. He came home from the nursery at 2 days and established regular biological rhythms. Developmental milestones were reported by his parents to be "about average," although his mother stated that Brody always seemed to be quieter than his sister, who is 3 years older. His father added that Brody has never been good at explaining things. For example, his attempt to describe a recent classroom visit by a zoo outreach program left his parents confused. Brody's account of events was so unclear that his parents at first believed that a fellow student was attacked by a bird on the playground.

Brody lives with his biological mother and stepfather. His parents were divorced when he was 2 years old. He and his sister spend weekends and Wednesday evening with their father, which both children reportedly enjoy. His biological father is a bricklayer who makes a good living. His biological mother is an office worker, and his stepfather is a salesman. There are no obvious stresses or conflicts in his living arrangement. Family history is negative for psychiatric disorders, but two paternal uncles reportedly struggled in school and never graduated from high school. No one in the family has ever had a formal special education label or been diagnosed with a developmental or genetic disorder.

Brody's teacher describes him as a pleasant and cooperative student who appears to try hard. However, she is concerned that he appears slow to catch on and immature. His work is intermittently incomplete. His handwriting is reportedly satisfactory, but reading is apparently a major concern. Brody has been instructed in a whole-language approach. He reads slowly, with poor inflection, and often forgets words that he has seemingly already mastered. Spelling is also a problem, although with practice he appears to master weekly spelling lists. Spelling accuracy, however, declines in his journal and the overall quality of his journal entries is said to be poor compared to classmates.

Observations

Brody is a short-stature, well-groomed lad who appears a bit younger than his age. Although generally reticent, he made good eye contact and had a pleasant smile. He appeared confused by directions several times. For example, he initially seemed bewildered by the rules of the WISC-IV Symbol Search subtest but caught on with demonstration and clarification. He provided extensive information about his favorite baseball team, including naming players and their positions and identifying some of their unique skills. However, he failed to remember the name of last year's Little League team, his current coach's name, or the names of any recent opponents. He could not describe where he lives or the route his school bus takes to school. The evaluation was completed during a single morning session with several breaks. His effort was excellent.

Assessment Procedures

Wechsler Intelligence Scale for Children–IV; Woodcock–Johnson III, Tests of Achievement; Gray Oral Reading Test: 4; NEPSY (Design Copying, Visuomotor Precision, Memory for Faces, Memory for Names, Narrative Memory, Phonological Processing), Peabody Picture Vocabulary Test—Third Edition; Behavior Assessment System for Children–2 (Teacher Report Form, Parent Report Form); informal assessment of curriculum material, parent interview, child interview. Scores on standardized instruments for Brody are listed in Table 5.5.

Analysis of Results

The first step in our system requires that Brody's referral reasons are confirmed to be related to academic problems. This is clearly the case. The primary concern is reading, and there is no apprehension about his conduct, personal adjustment, or social acceptance. Consequently, the answer to Box A is "yes." The flowchart is appropriate to use for subsequent decision making.

The next task is to rule out general cognitive limitations as a cause of Brody's problems. Once again, all available information should be considered. Developmental history, school history (which includes several years of success and continuing competence in computational math), and Brody's family's summary opinion suggest that lack of general ability is unlikely. Then again, Brody's teacher expresses doubt that he catches on as fast as peers, and he has encountered intensifying trouble with advancing curricular demands. Formal IQ scores are obviously needed. Brody's scores are extremely informative. He earned a FSIQ score of 97, which places him well in the average range. However, he expresses an extremely large difference among WISC-IV index scores. Strengths are evident on PRI (standard score = 112) and PSI (standard score = 121) compared to VCI (standard score = 77), a domain where he encounters clear-cut deficits. His WMI is average (standard score = 91) but, like his VCI, is meaningfully lower than PRI and PSI (and somewhat higher than VCI). As always, psychologists need to adhere to standard procedures for determining when WISC-IV index score differences are large enough to be considered significant. Such information is available in the WISC-IV manual and in scoring software available from the publisher. Regarding our crucial question, Brody has more than adequate overall cognitive ability to compete with classmates. The answer to Box B is "yes." Importantly, not only do IQ scores document adequate ability to learn, they refute a potentially troublesome hypothesis held by Brody's teacher that he is not especially bright. His PRI scores suggest just the opposite.

TABLE 5.5. Summary of Assessment Scores for Brody

Name	Age	Sex	Grade
Brody	10 years	Male	4

Wechsler Intelligence Scale for Children–IV

Verbal Comprehension		Perceptual Reasoning		Working Memory		Processing Speed	
Similarities	6	Block Design	14	Digit Span	9	Coding	12
Vocabulary	7	Picture Concepts	11	Letter–Number Sequence	8	Symbol Search	15
Comprehension	5	Matrix Reasoning	11	(Arithmetic)		(Cancellation)	

Scale	Composite score		Percentile rank
Verbal Comprehension	77 (72–85)	VCI	6th
Perceptual Reasoning	112 (103–119)	PRI	79th
Working Memory	91 (84–99)	WMI	27th
Processing Speed	121 (110–127)	PSI	92nd
Full Scale	97 (92–102)	FSIQ	45th
General Ability Index	94 (89–100)	GAI	34th

Woodcock–Johnson III Tests of Achievement

WJ III subtests	Scaled score
Letter–Word Identification	96
Passage Comprehension	74
Reading Fluency	86
Calculations	102
Math Fluency	100
Spelling	90
Applied Problems	80
Writing Samples	80
Writing Fluency	84
Word Attack	89

A Developmental Neuropsychological Assessment (NEPSY)

Phonological Processing	10
Visuomotor Precision	8
Design Copying	11
Memory for Faces	9
Memory for Names	10
Narrative Memory	4

Gray Oral Reading Test-4

Scale	Score
Fluency	8

(continued)

TABLE 5.5. *(continued)*

Scale	Score
Comprehension	3
Oral Reading Quotient	73

Peabody Picture Vocabulary Test—Third Edition

Standard Score = 78

Behavior Assessment System for Children–2 (Parent Report)

Scale	Level
F	Acceptable
Response Pattern	Acceptable
Consistency	Acceptable
Hyperactivity	50
Aggression	48
Conduct Problems	48
Anxiety	50
Depression	55
Somatization	42
Atypicality	41
Withdrawal	47
Attention Problems	43
Adaptability	60
Social Skills	65
Leadership	68
Activities of Daily Living	50
Functional Communication	52

Behavior Assessment System for Children–2 (Teacher Report)

Scale	Level
F	Acceptable
Response Pattern	Acceptable
Consistency	Acceptable
Hyperactivity	53
Aggression	43
Conduct Problems	45
Anxiety	52
Depression	53
Somatization	47
Attention Problems	51
Learning Problems	62
Atypicality	50
Withdrawal	52
Adaptability	56
Social Skills	67
Leadership	66
Study Skills	51
Functional Communication	41

The next question is whether genuine deficits exist in Brody's array of academic skills and related skills (i.e., language or fine-motor). Again, all information should be considered. Brody's teacher rated him as far below peers in basic reading, reading comprehension, spelling, and written expression when completing a brief screening form. She indicated fairly well-developed arithmetic skills. When questioned, she clarified that Brody does excellently in arithmetic, which has focused primarily on facts and computation this year, but he sometimes struggles on story problems. Because her class uses small-group instruction, however, potential problems in the latter have not been obvious. Students are encouraged to consult with one another to determine what is required on story problems and to help set up the calculations, support which Brody apparently consistently uses. At any rate, Brody's teacher is certain that he is below grade level in these areas. Group achievement test scores suggest the same.

Individual achievement testing was used to confirm suspected academic problems and establish their severity. As is seen in Table 5.5, Brody indeed suffers extreme skill deficits, but their precise configuration is somewhat surprising. Brody actually demonstrated word-identification skills within the normal range (WJ III Letter–Word Identification = 96). Furthermore, he was able to read passages out loud only at a slightly below-average level (GORT-4 Fluency scaled score = 8). In confronting passages, however, he sometimes produced all necessary phonemes in the correct sequence but failed to identify the precise target word (e.g., produced the sounds *mi'l it er i* but failed to say the word *military*). This raises the possibility that he was attempting to sound out words that were not in his speaking vocabulary. Furthermore, he tended to read in a mechanical manner, with little inflection, and provided guesses for unknown words with little appreciation of context. In other words, his responses were reminiscent of a student able to identify words but unable to process their meaning when they are combined into sentences and passages. This supposition is borne out by the rest of his achievement test scores. Reading comprehension scores were dramatically poorer than oral reading scores. This was true both when he was asked to read orally and answer comprehension questions (GORT-4 Comprehension scaled score = 3) and when required to read silently and provide missing words as evidence of understanding (WJ III Passage Comprehension standard score = 74). Also comporting with the emerging hypothesis that comprehension skills are inferior to word reading skills was that Brody demonstrated reasonably well-developed phonics skills on the WJ III Word Attack subtest (standard score = 89). Thus, a pervasive reading problem does not appear to be present. Instead there looks to be one that is dominated by limited understanding of text rather than inability to identify words or read passages aloud.

Brody's problems are not confined to reading comprehension, and it is important to document their full scope. Although able to spell reasonably well (WJ III Spelling standard score = 90), he revealed little ability to write a passage (WJ III Writing Samples standard score = 80). His efforts here contained immature language, little organization, and poor punctuation and capitalization. Interestingly, he does not appear to be free of mathematics problems. Despite his teacher's perceptions that he possesses adequate development in math, Brody was unable to solve math problems that involved quantitative concepts and terms and required solution of verbally formatted problems (Applied Problems standard score = 80). The answer to Box D is "yes."

Turning to Box G, the nature of Brody's academic problems provide powerful clues to the underlying information-processing and cognitive deficits. For Brody, reading and written expression problems dominate. Furthermore, the rest of his academic profile fits parsimoniously into a description of deficits in language arts. Accordingly, the answer to Box G is "yes."

Our flowchart suggests two possibilities, SLI and PRD. Establishing if either condition contributes to (or causes) Brody's problem is important. Brody's history is relevant. He had less trouble learning to identify words and sound out unknown words, a crucial task during grades K–2, than in understanding the meaning of what he read. His history has no suggestion of articulation problems or failures of memory for sounds (i.e., compatible with PRD). Alternatively, he has encountered intensifying problems in recent years as reading comprehension replaces simple word identification as the central reading challenge. Furthermore, Brody's history includes difficulty understanding math concepts, following directions, and catching on (presumably when things are explained to him in words). Problems with vocabulary, language concepts, verbal comprehension, and word-related general knowledge are compatible with these facts; problems at the sound (phonological) level are insufficient to explain these manifest problems. In other words, a PRD would not explain the myriad academic problems he has encountered nor would that condition fit all of the facts of his case.

Formal test results appear to fit with our emerging hypothesis of an SLI. Brody shows striking deficits in verbal skills, and these are most clearly indicated by his WISC-IV VCI score of 77, which documents lexical/vocabulary and conceptual deficiencies. To be certain that Brody did not suffer from mere reticence or a more isolated problem related to an inability to express himself verbally, he was administered the PPVT-III, which taps word knowledge without a need to verbalize. Children simply point to one of four pictures matching a vocabulary word that is provided orally. The fact that Brody did no better here, when expressive requirements were eliminated, substantiates the prospect of a pervasive general language problem or SLI.

Simply put, Brody lacks concepts and terms needed to succeed in class.

When he reads, he appears to identify words and to move through passages orally, but this helps him little because he fails the final crucial task; he does not derive meaning from what he reads. Writing success, which depends upon conveying meaning with words and phrases, is similarly limited. Not surprisingly, he shows little ability to recount a story after hearing it (note that NEPSY describes this ability as Narrative Memory, emphasizing a recall component, even though Brody's poor score likely reflects limitations of vocabulary and initial comprehension). Brody's scaled score here was 4. Because listening comprehension generally sets an upper limit on reading comprehension, Brody's weak reading comprehension scores are quite predictable. So, too, is limited success on math tasks that presuppose the ability to read and understand passages. Also hard have been those tasks that depend on mastery of underlying concepts related to time, money, measurement, and geometry. It is easy to see why Brody struggles with each of these school tasks. Although the manifestations cross several academic domains and may be more or less obvious depending on task demands, a common language core is identifiable.

Unlike many children with SLI, Brody appears to enjoy intact phonological processing (NEPSY Phonological Processing scaled score = 10). Favorably, he scores well on measures of phonological processing and word attack, including reading pseudowords (WJ III Word Attack standard score = 89). He can identify unknown words and retain spelling patterns, especially if they are phonetically regular. These intact phonological abilities and word attack skills represent assets that may be used during instruction.

Intervention Plan

The following may help Brody:

1. Because he is struggling in reading, writing, and math reasoning, he requires ongoing and consistent instruction in each area. Small group or individual instruction to supplement regular classwork is suggested.

2. Notwithstanding the above recommendation, Brody's assistance in each academic skill area needs to be individualized either to circumvent language limitations or to provide immediate, targeted language assistance before or during each lesson. Regarding the former, self-selecting "level books" on topics of his own interest may help him get around limitations of vocabulary and background knowledge that might otherwise constrain comprehension. For example, choosing from an array of books at his oral reading level that match his interest in baseball may foster understanding. Similarly, promoting writing on topics that correspond to his interest or permitting Brody to pick freely among writing topics may encourage more

and better written production. In arithmetic, story problems with familiar content may accomplish the desired end (i.e., application of computational skills to real-world situations). Regarding the second approach, prereading review of vocabulary and concepts may boost comprehension. For example, before reading a passage on a Civil War hero, Brody may need to be told the meaning of the terms "military," "musket," and "heroism." By the same token, in arithmetic, clarification of "deposit" and "withdrawal" may ameliorate problems performing a set of addition and subtraction problems related to a savings account. Providing Brody with supporting vocabulary words and simply and concretely teaching their meanings could ease the challenge of writing assignments. For example, giving Brody four words whose meanings have been made clear may help him tackle a writing assignment about which he possesses limited vocabulary and few ideas.

3. Long-term plans to build vocabulary size, increase store of general knowledge, and enhance conceptual sophistication may promote subsequent academic success in reading, written expression, and math reasoning. Well-developed language skills also are essential when instruction in the content areas (e.g., science, social studies) receives greater emphasis, especially in the fourth grade and after. To accomplish this, exposure to oral language models, current events, and discussion is suggested. Examples are parents reading to their children and then discussing the content of what was read, selected viewing of current events on television, reading high-interest, low-vocabulary books, and group language stimulation provided by a special educator or speech–language pathologist. Activities to build vocabulary with a resource teacher might include mnemonic strategies, cognitive strategy instruction, the constant delay technique, concept mapping, and activity-based methods. Dictionary drills that involve writing are not suggested, although Internet access that allows children to find definitions and hear synthetic voice pronunciation may work. To effect change, these types of activities must be regular, of sufficient duration, and well matched to the child's current understanding level.

4. Children with SLI often become frustrated and discouraged. Finding obvious areas of success and making these patent may help. In Brody's case, emphasizing his computational arithmetic strengths may be one such avenue.

5. Fostering positive expectations is also suggested. Children with SLI are often thought to be cognitively limited. Conveying his outstanding nonverbal abilities to his teacher, as well as tapping these (e.g., in art, designing posters or visual aids for the class) may help. It should be made clear to all that linguistic competence is one expression of cognitive ability and that Brody possesses other abilities, which may be less obvious but are at least as advanced as those of most of his peers.

6. He should be monitored for social problems and considered for structured play activities or social skills training, if needed.

7. Regarding special services, Brody is probably eligible for SLD designation with reading comprehension, written expression, and math reasoning as the areas in which achievement problems manifest. If evidence of poor RTI is needed, Brody would probably require a focused, nonspecial education instructional program and simultaneous monitoring before he is deemed eligible for special services.

CASE 6: JAMES WILSON (J.W.)

Background Information

James Wilson (who is called J.W. by his family) was referred by his parents to an outpatient clinic. His family has long-held concern about his school status; they sought the evaluation to determine what was wrong with him.

J.W. is a 15-year-old high school sophomore. He is the youngest of three children. His father is a surgeon, and his mother is an art dealer. His mother suffers from an anxiety disorder and has had panic attacks. Family history is otherwise negative for learning, developmental, or psychiatric disorders. Parents describe their relationship as good and that there are no meaningful sources of stress in the home. Mother confirmed that she misses J.W.'s older sister, who attends a private college in Massachusetts, and his brother, who attends college in California. Both parents were reportedly superior students.

J.W. is reportedly a healthy youngster, free of hearing problems. He wears contact lenses. He had been taken to a developmental optometrist who suspected problems with visual tracking. As a result of this evaluation, he was prescribed a 6-month course of visual exercises with the hope that improving his ability to track objects and to shift his gaze quickly from far to near point would make school easier. For the past several months, J.W. has reported trouble falling asleep, occasionally remaining awake until 2:00 or 3:00 A.M. Even if he remains awake until quite late, he denies that he is fatigued or drowsy at school the next morning. J.W. has taken prescription medication for acne, but is currently healthy and using no medication.

No problems with cooperation or conduct were present at home. He has always been seen as "a good kid," although he has complained recently that his parents pick on him about his diet, sleeping routine, taste in music, and study habits. Always a popular child, he has maintained friendships with several neighborhood friends who attend the same upper-middle-class, competitive high school. He has dated a little, but does not have a girlfriend. Parents believe that he has experimented with alcohol while with friends but never used drugs.

J.W. has been a puzzle to his parents, and accordingly a source of anxiety for them, since kindergarten. Although he acquired developmental milestones on time, he in no way experienced the school successes that seemed to come easily to his brother and sister. Even though he learned to read by mid-first grade, he was never especially proficient in reading (e.g., he sometimes seemed a bit halting on passages), and he rarely expressed interest in independent or leisure reading. J.W. was generally more successful in math and spelling than reading throughout his elementary years. Review of his cumulative folder reveals that his report card and group achievement test scores have always been at or near average, with no obvious pattern of subject-to-subject strength or weakness. None of his report cards contained indications of work habit, citizenship, or interpersonal problems.

Beginning in junior high, his parents became increasingly worried because J.W. had failed to snap out of his "learning malaise." They sent their son to a commercial learning center where he received individual instruction. Here he was taught strategies (3QSR), but most time was spent in individual tutoring to support homework completion and to prepare him for upcoming tests. Nonetheless, by high school, this assistance proved insufficient to prevent trouble. His first-quarter sophomore report card included D's in geometry, English/creative writing and French II. Frustrated, his parents withdrew him from tutoring and sought an evaluation from a psychiatrist, suspecting that an undetected problem with attention or depression might explain his lack of success. The psychiatric evaluation, which consisted of an interview with J.W. and his parents, resulted in the conclusion that he had normal attention and impulse control for a teenage boy, but that he was experiencing intensifying feelings of sadness and discouragement now approaching clinical significance. Family therapy and monitoring of his mood state, but no medication, was suggested. Despite the insight gained from the psychiatric evaluation, J.W.'s parents remained concerned that there was something wrong with him that had eluded detection. Hence, he was referred for a comprehensive psychoeducational evaluation.

Assessment Procedures

Wechsler Intelligence Scale for Children–IV; Woodcock–Johnson III, Tests of Achievement; Wide Range Assessment of Memory and Learning–2 (screening subtests only); Grooved Pegboard Test; Gordon Diagnostic System; Behavior Assessment System for Children–2 (Teacher Rating Form, Parent Rating Form); parent interview, child interview. Scores on standardized instruments for J.W. are listed in Table 5.6.

Observations

J.W. presented as a mature, well-groomed, and pleasant 15-year-old. He was cooperative, well focused, and hard working during the entire evaluation, which was conducted in a single morning session. There were no limitations in understanding tasks, following directions, or regulating actions or impulses. He spoke well, using full sentences, with grammar, syntax, and prosody that seemed age-appropriate. It was a bit unusual to hear a student express expectations for the assessment; however, J.W. indicated that he hoped the evaluation would discover why school had long been so hard for him.

No in-class observation was conducted. Nonetheless, on a rating form, his first-hour (American history) teacher described J.W. as a slightly below-average student who tried hard, completed work, and sought to please. He was viewed as fairly popular with classmates. His teacher doubted that he was a "druggie" or that he ever came to class under the influence of alcohol or illegal substances. Furthermore, his teacher remarked that he had none of the attitude of disinterest or financial/cultural superiority that sometimes characterized the well-off students attending his high school.

Analysis of Results

The first question to consider is whether our system is applicable. In Box A, the question concerns if this is a classroom problem. Reviewing background information, we note that the evaluation was requested by parents, not teachers. Nonetheless, J.W.'s school status has made his parents anxious for a long time. Furthermore, some of his grades are now clearly below average. Finally, J.W. was obviously referred for issues other than emotional or adjustment problems (viz., concern about school). Considering all of this information, the tentative answer to Box A is "yes." Accordingly, the system is an appropriate vehicle to use in attempting to understand J.W.'s apparently limited learning success.

Box B requires determination of whether J.W.'s situation is explainable by his general cognitive status. In other words, might he experience an IQ-related problem? Background information rules out frank developmental delay (e.g., MiMR); his school grades, group achievement test scores, and social presentation contraindicate that possibility. The same is almost certainly true regarding SL status. Recalling that his social milieu and school environment comprise average to above-average performers, it is entirely plausible that J.W.'s level of development may be lower than the majority of his classmates. Unquestionably, he has never experienced the academic successes of his siblings (and perhaps of his parents).

Psychometric data, especially indicators of general cognitive ability,

TABLE 5.6. Summary of Assessment Scores for J.W.

Name	Age	Sex	Dominant hand	Grade
J.W.	15 years	Male	Right	10

Wechsler Intelligence Scale for Children–IV

Verbal Comprehension		*Perceptual Reasoning*		*Working Memory*		*Processing Speed*	
Similarities	8	Block Design	11	Digit Span	10	Coding	8
Vocabulary	10	Picture Concepts	9	Letter–Number Sequence	10	Symbol Search	11
Comprehension	9	Matrix Reasoning	10				

Scale	*Composite score*		*Percentile rank*
Verbal Comprehension	95 (89–102)	VCI	37th
Perceptual Reasoning	100 (92–108)	PRI	50th
Working Memory	99 (91–107)	WMI	47th
Processing Speed	97 (88–106)	PSI	42nd
Full Scale	97 (92–102)	FSIQ	42nd
General Ability Index	97 (91–103)	GAI	42nd

Woodcock–Johnson III, Tests of Achievement

WJ III subtests	*Scaled score*
Letter–Word Identification	102
Passage Comprehension	95
Reading Fluency	100
Calculations	102
Math Fluency	104
Spelling	96
Writing Samples	97
Writing Fluency	96

Motor Exam

Pegboard

Dominant hand (right): 61 sec   (within normal limits)
Nondominant hand (left): 62 sec   (within normal limits)

Wide Range Assessment of Memory and Learning–2

Subtest	*Scaled Score*
Picture Memory	10
Design Memory	9
Verbal Learning	10
Story Memory	11

(continued)

TABLE 5.6. *(continued)*

Gordon Diagnostic System

Vigilance task	Score	Normal Borderline/Abnormal
Total Correct	44	Normal
Omission Errors	1	Normal

Behavior Assessment System for Children–2 (Parent Report)

Scale	Level
F	Acceptable
Response Pattern	Acceptable
Consistency	Acceptable
Hyperactivity	50
Aggression	48
Conduct Problems	48
Anxiety	54
Depression	58
Somatization	57
Atypicality	56
Withdrawal	44
Attention Problems	50
Adaptability	52
Social Skills	50
Leadership	49
Activities of Daily Living	53
Functional Communication	50

Behavior Assessment System for Children–2 (Teacher Report)

Scale	Level
F	Acceptable
Response Pattern	Acceptable
Consistency	Acceptable
Hyperactivity	51
Aggression	46
Conduct Problems	46
Anxiety	49
Depression	51
Somatization	52
Attention Problems	54
Learning Problems	56
Atypicality	48
Withdrawal	44
Adaptability	52
Social Skills	54
Leadership	54
Study Skills	49
Functional Communication	49

are thus invaluable in addressing the emerging central question posed in Box B. Reviewing Table 5.6, a clear and easy to interpret pattern is seen. J.W. earned nearly identical index scores on the WISC-IV. His FSIQ score of 97 places him in the average range compared to national standards. Equally important, there is nothing in his profile to suggest ability much above this score. In fact, the two most crucial indices, VCI (index score = 95) and PRI (index score = 100), fall quite close to his FSIQ. Moreover, the bulk of his psychometric data agree with ability in the range depicted by his FSIQ. For example, declarative memory, language, motor speed, fine-motor speed and all academic domain scores fall in the average range.

These facts thus set the stage for the crucial inference. Is J.W.'s IQ generally equal to classmates? Local knowledge suggests that J.W.'s high school is among the most competitive in the state. It is certainly plausible that the mean IQ among classmates is 115 or even 120. Perhaps unfortunately, no universally administered IQ tests (e.g., group tests) are available to provide a basis for comparison. On the other hand, group achievement tests are. Each year, the state releases median scores on the Stanford Achievement Test–9 for each school, and these are subsequently published. The percentile ranks for J.W.'s high school were: Total Reading: 87th; Language: 88th; Total Mathematics: 81st. If these percentile values were converted to standard scores, they would fall between 113 and 118. Although IQ and achievement are not synonymous, J.W.'s cognitive ability probably is 15 to 20 points lower than many classmates. Similarly, comparing his individual achievement test scores (and historical group scores) with these Stanford Achievement Test–9 values, he would be many percentile ranks below a typical classmate. Considering all this information, it is hardly surprising that his history teacher describes him as slightly below average.

Turning back to the flowchart, the answer to Box B is "no." This answer reflects the conclusion that J.W.'s IQ is not commensurate with many of his classmates. Box C is easily answered. J.W. clearly possesses ability higher than the 70–75 IQ range associated with MiMR. Box E is equally straightforward. J.W.'s overall ability surpasses the SL range. The facts of the case support a conclusion of an AEM.

This finding helps place J.W.'s school history and, indeed, his present standing in a new light. He does not suffer a disorder or condition in the traditional sense, but he certainly has a recognizable pattern of psychometric scores, disappointment at school, and high parental expectations. Although his parents may be discouraged by findings on the one hand, they can abandon their search for a cause (and hope for a ready fix) on the other hand. In that sense, J.W.'s case is like others with AEM—his parents' repeated efforts to find the underlying cause of his nonexistent problem have prevented intelligent planning. Such efforts to find the elusive cause often leave parents frustrated, and they can result in perplexed and discouraged students. In J.W.'s case, the search for understanding has included stops at the offices of optometrists, tutors, and psychiatrists. His psychiatrist may have been correct in concluding the presence of feelings of demoralization and dissatisfaction. Without a full evaluation to reveal the source of J.W.'s distress, however, psychotherapy is likely to be only partially helpful. A comprehensive psychoeducational evaluation permitted his family to reach closure and to develop a plan matching J.W.'s particular skills and circumstances.

Intervention Plan

The following are suggested:

1. Parents need a detailed explanation of their son's psychometric scores and the relationship of those scores to his presenting problem. Accordingly, the chief task is to convince them that their son is cognitively average and does not suffer a diagnosable learning problem.

2. Parents and school personnel are advised against supplemental evaluations that may divert effort away from helping improve J.W.'s current situation. In other words, trips to music therapists, biofeedback specialists, or movement therapists (each of whom might offer a seemingly plausible explanation for his "problem") should be avoided.

3. J.W. is not recommended for special services. He does not have an SLD or an ED. Placing him in an SLD program because he has apparently failed to respond to interventions (e.g., tutoring) violates the intent of IDEA (viz., to educate children with *disabilities*) and the letter of the SLD definition (see Table 3.3; note that J.W. suffers no disorder of "basic psychological processes").

4. Guidance counseling and careful selection of school courses is suggested. He may need to be advised to avoid some extremely competitive college preparatory courses or to spread them out (e.g., take some during summer sessions).

5. Concomitantly, careful selection of a college, including in-depth investigation of less competitive settings, is in order.

6. Parents are encouraged to seek areas of success and highlight them. This is particularly important because comparing J.W.'s academic success with that of his siblings may leave him feeling discouraged.

7. Parents and J.W. need an explanation of the importance and limitation of IQ scores and especially the fact that scores may change over time.

8. A follow-up conference in 6 months is suggested. Parents risk reverting to old habits of seeking explanation and stepping up expectations without these findings periodically being reviewed and reemphasized.

CASE 7: HANNAH

Background Information

Hannah is an 8-year-old girl of mixed Asian (Filipino) and Caucasian heritage who was referred by her third-grade teacher. The reason was failure to keep up with classmates.

Hannah attends a middle-class school in a suburban area that is designated as a "basic skills" school. Traditional academics are emphasized, and art, music, and creative writing are deemphasized. Hannah has had trouble since transferring to this school at the beginning of first grade. She reportedly was performing about average in a typical kindergarten setting. Hannah's teacher has worked to revise her teaching approach since the second week of school by moving Hannah closer to the front of class, providing her a study carrel when she feels troubled by distractions, and encouraging her to "make a plan and then stick with it." Nonetheless, Hannah has remained the most unproductive student in class, often requiring twice as long as classmates to complete tasks. She has also needed much more of her teacher's time to remind her what to do and to encourage her to stick with her goals. She seems confused about assigned tasks, unable to find assignment-related materials, easily diverted by others' actions, and frequently out of her seat to sharpen her pencil or visit the restroom. As a result, Hannah has earned below-average marks in each academic area and now is being considered for retention in third grade. The rationale for retention is that even greater demands for independence, task persistence, and organization exist in fourth grade.

Hannah's teacher describes her as friendly and generally cooperative but immature and spacey. She lacks a group of steady playmates and sometimes wanders from one group to the next during recess without ever staying anywhere for long. She reportedly has reasonable spelling and math skills, although she loses points in math because of disregard for addition and subtraction signs, failure to remember directions, and a hurried, chaotic pace. She demonstrates well-developed sound–symbol associations when spelling, but only sometimes in reading. On passages, for example, she seems to lose her place, guesses based on initial sounds only, and utters words that bear no correspondence to the passage's context. Reading worksheets are sent home nightly, but they are apt to be forgotten (causing further loss of points).

Her parents told the school psychologist that their daughter was without significant health or developmental problems. She was born after an uneventful pregnancy, with continuous prenatal care, at full term with Apgar scores of 9/9. She crawled at 6 months, walked at 12 months, said her first words at 15 months and two-word combinations at 18 months, and was potty trained at 24 months. She had a good memory for rote linguistic facts (home address, telephone number, names of colors) at the start of kindergarten. She also had memorized letter names readily by the start of kindergarten. Her speech has always been clear, free of articulation problems, and without dysfluency.

She has never enjoyed board games, even though her two older sisters love to play them with parents. Hannah forgets activities of daily living (grooming, dressing) unless prompted by parents, who view her as "slow, disorganized, and in her own world."

English is the only language spoken at home. There have been financial stressors related to her father's unemployment, but these have now been resolved. Her parents reportedly agree on discipline, although her father is less patient than his wife with Hannah's need to be reminded. Both parents express concern about grade retention. Older sisters have been solid students, and the family places great value on formal learning, although neither parent completed post-high school instruction.

Group achievement test scores were reviewed. Hannah's pattern was extremely uneven. For example, one year she scored at the 22nd percentile in math, but the next year at the 72nd in the same subject. Likewise, she scored at the 51st and 17th percentiles in reading in back-to-back years.

Assessment Procedures

Wechsler Intelligence Scale for Children–IV; Wechsler Individual Achievement Tests–II; NEPSY (Design Copying, Visuomotor Precision, Memory for Faces, Memory for Names, Narrative Memory, Phonological Processing); Gordon Diagnostic System; Behavior Assessment System for Children–2 (Parent Report Form, Teacher Report Form); Academic Performance Rating Scale (Teacher); informal assessment of curriculum material, parent interview, child interview. Scores on standardized instruments for Hannah are listed in Table 5.7.

Observations

Hannah was observed during three class sessions, two in the morning and one in the afternoon. The Behavioral Observation of Students in Schools was used. Hannah had nearly twice as many intervals of off-task behavior as the composite of her classmates; virtually all such intervals were characterized as "passive" rather than "verbal" or "motoric." No conspicuous antecedents or consequences of off-task were noted. Hannah was about as apt to be off-task during math as reading. There was no difference between the morning and afternoon. Likewise, no obvious contingencies supporting off-task behavior were detected. When Hannah was off-task, she was not especially likely to elicit teacher or peer attention or support and assignments were not reduced, although she may have experienced covert rein-

TABLE 5.7. Summary of Assessment Scores for Hannah

Name	Age	Sex	Grade
Hannah	8 years	Female	3

Wechsler Intelligence Scale for Children–IV

Verbal Comprehension		Perceptual Reasoning		Working Memory		Processing Speed	
Similarities	8	Block Design	11	Digit Span	8	Coding	12
Vocabulary	13	Picture Concepts	12	Letter–Number Sequence	11	Symbol Search	12
Comprehension	12	Matrix Reasoning	11				

Scale	Composite score		Percentile rank
Verbal Comprehension	102 (95–109)	VCI	55th
Perceptual Reasoning	108 (100–115)	PRI	70th
Working Memory	97 (90–105)	WMI	42nd
Processing Speed	112 (102–120)	PSI	79th
Full Scale	107 (102–112)	FSIQ	68th
General Ability Index	107 (101–112)	GAI	68th

Wechsler Individual Achievement Test–II

WIAT-II subtests	Scaled score
Word Reading	99
Reading Comprehension	95
Pseudoword Decoding	105
Numerical Operations	102
Math Reasoning	99
Spelling	107
Written Expression	98

Gordon Diagnostic System

Vigilance Task	Score	Range
Total correct	41	Normal
Commission Errors	4	Normal

A Developmental Neuropsychological Assessment (NEPSY)

Phonological Processing	10
Visuomotor Precision	8
Design Copying	9
Memory for Faces	10
Memory for Names	11

Behavior Assessment System for Children–2 (Parent Report)

Scale	Level
F	Acceptable
Response Pattern	Acceptable

(continued)

TABLE 5.7. *(continued)*

Scale	Level
Consistency	Acceptable
Hyperactivity	41
Aggression	46
Conduct Problems	43
Anxiety	52
Depression	47
Somatization	50
Atypicality	57
Withdrawal	56
Attention Problems	74
Adaptability	53
Social Skills	42
Leadership	44
Activities of Daily Living	42
Functional Communication	45

Behavior Assessment System for Children–2 (Teacher Report)

Scale	Level
F	Acceptable
Response Pattern	Acceptable
Consistency	Acceptable
Hyperactivity	46
Aggression	46
Conduct Problems	45
Anxiety	42
Depression	42
Somatization	47
Attention Problems	70
Learning Problems	68
Atypicality	46
Withdrawal	39
Adaptability	50
Social Skills	42
Leadership	44
Study Skills	43
Functional Communication	46

forcement via reduction in the prospect of facing tedious worksheets (self-reinforced for task avoidance).

Hannah presented during testing as a somewhat shy and tentative 8-year-old. She worked persistently, although she sometimes forgot expectations (e.g., on the Similarities subtest she lapsed into giving differences between words; on WISC-IV Digit Span Backwards, she reverted to giving numbers forward). She disregarded signs on arithmetic problems and several times required repeated directions, apparently due to inattention.

Analysis of Results

Hannah's information is analyzed by following the flowchart (Figure 5.1), even though diagnosticians may detect symptoms that remind them of a particular disorder even before they start the process. The first step is to consider whether Hannah's teacher launched a referral because of classroom problems (Box A). Clearly, Hannah's teacher feels doubt about her preparedness to move onto the fourth grade, and she has assigned Hannah low grades. Parents also harbor concern about their daughter's school status. The answer to Box A is "yes." The bulk of the flowchart is thus applicable in our attempt to understand Hannah's problem.

Box B requires consideration of Hannah's overall cognitive ability as the source of classroom problems. We once again must consider all sources of information. Recall that Hannah's behavior has been described as immature (a description sometimes denoting general cognitive delay). She also encountered some problems during second grade, and she has not developed enduring friendships, a developmental task associated with the elementary years. On the other hand, developmental milestones were attained on time. Also, some of Hannah's group achievement test scores seem too high for a child with significant general cognitive delay. Obviously, IQ scores are important in addressing this question.

Hannah's WISC-IV scores answer the question unequivocally. Her FSIQ of 107 is far above the cut-off for either MiMR or SL status. There is insufficient scatter among index scores (and among subtests) to suggest that the FSIQ score cannot be trusted as an indication of general cognitive ability. Furthermore, Hannah's school- and home-based comparison groups appear to be quite representative; it is unlikely that Hannah's average complement of reasoning and problem-solving skills place her at a disadvantage compared to classmates. The answer to Box B is "yes." Hannah does benefit from ample general ability.

Box D exists to determine if Hannah's problems involve genuine skill deficits. This is quite important in Hannah's case because her teacher's comments are unclear. At this stage her teacher was requested to complete the Academic Performance Rating Scale for 2 weeks. Crucially, her teacher rated her academic productivity (amount of work finished) as low but her academic accuracy (amount of material correct) as average. Regarding the same point, we checked Hannah's complement of academic skills compared to others her same age. It was found that, indeed, she possessed an adequate array of reading, spelling, arithmetic, and writing skills. Her scores on the WIAT-II were all equal to or above 95. Crucially, Hannah generated these scores when tested in a one-to-one situation where prospective problems with attention, effort, and understanding of directions could be mitigated. Use of curriculum-based material also verified that she was correctly placed in reading and math curricula. Furthermore, there were no problems evident in her work samples or psychometric testing suggesting that fine-motor or language problems (e.g., WISC-IV VCI and NEPSY Visuomotor Precision) would constrain classroom performance. The answer to Box D is "no." The pattern of adequate cognitive and academic skills in a child with classroom concerns points toward a performance problem. We turn to Box F for further clarification.

Box F again substantiates that her teacher is genuinely concerned. The answer to Box F is "yes." Box H asks if Hannah's presentation includes disruptive behavior. Her background information is devoid of references to conduct or oppositional behavior. None of her teachers or parents has described the need to resort to behavior management techniques. No such issues were evident during testing. Nonetheless, objective rating scales completed by parents and teachers are helpful. Both BASC-2 scales show Aggression, Conduct Problems, and Hyperactivity scores in the average range. The answer to Box H is "no." We finally consider whether ADHD-I or CU might be present, according to the flowchart.

ADHD-I symptoms are numerous and obvious. Hannah appears to meet the following DSM-IV-TR symptoms: fails to give close attention to detail or makes careless mistakes; difficulty sustaining attention; does not follow through on instructions and fails to finish schoolwork; difficulty organizing tasks and activities; avoids tasks that require sustained mental effort; loses things necessary for tasks or activities; forgetful of activities of daily living. Furthermore, her symptoms have been evident for at least 6 months, cause impairment in home and social situations, and are not attributable to another psychiatric disorder. In this sense, and complying with our overall approach's requirement to work consistently, we need to consider Hannah's entire database. To complete the task, the prospects of CU and ADHD-C need to be eliminated.

Regarding CU, none of the cardinal characteristics is present. Hannah has a disorganized, inattentive, and spacey approach, but her history contains no indication of obsessions or compulsions. In fact, her mother lamented that "we can't get Hannah to be concerned about anything." When interviewed, Hannah disavowed obsessive thoughts, worry, anxiety, and other indicators of internalizing psychopathology.

Regarding ADHD-C, there were no elevations on the BASC-2 Hyperactivity scale as completed by parent and teacher. Finally, the Gordon Diagnostic System was used and its results should be considered. Hannah had normal-range values for errors of commission and errors of omission on the Vigilance task. Commission errors suggest hyperactivity–impulsivity symptoms, whereas omission errors suggest inattention. The fact that neither score was elevated means that the evaluation was silent on the prospect of either type of problem. Although abnormal scores on the Gordon Diagnostic System are helpful, normal-range scores are not as valuable (see Chapter 4). ADHD-I was ultimately concluded to be present.

Intervention Plan

The following were suggested:

1. Before a final determination is made, health problems may need to be considered. A physical exam should be conducted if one has not occurred recently.

2. An escalating set of procedures to increase work productivity or work habits is suggested. These would begin by establishing a baseline of work completed and percentage correct. The first step is objective monitoring and use of conspicuous charting. The second step is a daily report card that is sent home providing the same information. The third step is an incentive plan with reinforcers dispensed at home. The fourth step is the same plan with reinforcers dispensed at school. The time between work and reinforcement, the richness of the reinforcement schedule, and the amount of work required for reinforcement can be modified. The intervention begins with the least intrusive procedures and is stepped up only when targets for behavior change have not been reached.

3. Although increasing productivity is worthwhile (as in point #2), the primary goal of education is to assure the acquisition of academic skills. Hannah actually is proceeding well in that regard. Accordingly, her teacher may wish to reduce the emphasis on work completion and correspondingly increase the emphasis on tangible skills acquired when assigning grades. Grading practice may need to change and failing grades or consideration of grade retention be abandoned if Hannah shows mastery of core academic skills. Obviously, emphasis on mastery requires repeated probes and explicit tracking of her skill development against clear standards.

4. A Section 504 accommodation plan or OHI designation may be needed to assure that these services are in place and monitored. Such services can be accessed with a diagnosis of ADHD.

5. Social interaction targets, such as peer contact during recess, should be sought. Social skills training, which might involve teaching play and social conversation skills, is similarly suggested. A school counselor or school psychologist should oversee this element of the intervention.

6. Hannah may be a candidate for medication to treat ADHD. The evaluation results and recommendations can be sent to her pediatrician. Like any treatment with targeted outcomes, use of medication to improve academic proficiency requires ongoing monitoring. The American Academy of Pediatrics (AAP) guidelines specify that medication for the treatment of ADHD should be used with input from school personnel (AAP, 2001a).

7. Parents should be provided basic information about ADHD-I and offered support, either through school or a mental health agency,

health care provider (e.g., pediatrician), or parent group (e.g., Children and Adults with Attention-Deficit/Hyperactivity Disorder [ChADD]).

CASE 8: ALICIA

Background Information

Alicia is a 12-year-old sixth grader of Hispanic background. She was referred because of dramatically fluctuating classroom performance, especially on written assignments. Her grades have dropped to near-failing levels in social studies and English, and there is concern about an underlying problem that has escaped previous detection.

Alicia lives with her biological parents and three younger brothers (ages 10, 8, and 7). Her father is from Mexico and speaks both Spanish and English with his coworkers and friends; her mother is of Hispanic background but speaks only English. Alicia also speaks English only, as her parents have insisted that their children develop maximum English proficiency and believed that hearing Spanish at home might not be helpful. Her father works as a skilled craftsman, and her mother has an in-home secretarial business. Parents disagree on the presence of stressors in the home; her father indicates that the family is well off, but her mother is reportedly "constantly worried about finances." Her mother's side of the family is described as high achievers, and the mother herself did extremely well in school. She now prefers to work alone at home to avoid what she describes as "work-associated stress." She has two sisters (Alicia's aunts) currently treated with Paxil (an antidepressant/anti-anxiety agent in the SSRI category) for work-related anxiety. The father's family is negative for learning, developmental, or psychiatric disorders.

Alicia was reportedly born after an uneventful, planned pregnancy and easy delivery. She came home from the hospital at 2 days and enjoyed typical acquisition of developmental milestones, although her temperamental style was described as shy. She suffered intermittent bouts of otitis media as a preschooler and had pressure equalizing (PE) tubes inserted twice. She has passed all hearing and vision screenings conducted since she started school. Due to her recently declining school grades, she underwent a complete physical examination by her pediatrician, who deemed her to be in excellent health.

Alicia has attended the same rural school district, described as diverse with a range of achievement levels, since kindergarten. Review of her report cards reveals a fairly high-achieving student with above-average marks from kindergarten through third grade. No obvious pattern of strengths and weaknesses was apparent across subjects until fourth grade, when occasional low marks first appeared in English and social studies.

Indications in Alicia's record of slow work pace, incomplete assignments, and poor use of time first appeared during the fourth grade and continue to the present.

Now, as a sixth grader, her report card includes D's in English and social studies. She currently has several outstanding writing projects and, under questioning, is unable to tell her parents and teacher why she failed to submit the completed papers. Favorably, Alicia has continued to do well on tests, including those in English and social studies. Nonetheless, she has made repeated comments about fear of failing, being embarrassed for providing wrong answers, and believing that she is not as smart as her classmates. Her parents also notice that she seems noticeably preoccupied at times. Under questioning, she revealed foreboding feelings about the health of her paternal grandfather, who resides in Mexico. Her parents report diminishing contact with classmates. Review of work samples also is interesting. Responses to open-ended writing questions are exceptionally sparse, whereas responses to convergent probes, such as answering post-reading social studies questions, are universally full and complete. When questioned, Alicia says that she has trouble deciding what to write. Furthermore, Alicia's written work has an odd quality. Manuscript letters appear to be overworked, and they are frequently erased—her papers' overall appearance is messy, smudged, and wrinkled. Attempts to help her by peer tutoring and cooperative drills with a popular and academically able classmate produced no noticeable improvement. Alicia complained that her study partner worked too fast and always had to do things her own way, which Alicia frequently believed to be wrong.

Observations

Alicia presents as an extremely well-groomed, pleasant, age-appropriate-appearing 12-year-old. She was slightly apprehensive at the start of the formal evaluation, but she remained poised, well focused, and cooperative. Her effort was excellent throughout the evaluation. She was reluctant to take breaks, as she obviously wanted to do her best and impress the examiner. Alicia routinely sought reassurance that she was doing well, even though it was made clear at the start of the evaluation that feedback was not permitted and that everyone should expect to encounter some items beyond their ability.

Assessment Procedures

Wechsler Intelligence Scale for Children–IV; Woodcock–Johnson III, Tests of Achievement; NEPSY (Design Copying, Visuomotor Precision, Memory for Faces, Memory for Names, Narrative Memory, Phonological Processing); Behavior Assessment System for Children–2 (Teacher Report Form, Parent Report Form); informal assessment with curriculum material, parent interview, child interview. Scores on standardized instruments for Alicia are listed in Table 5.8.

Analysis of Results

The question contained in Box A, regarding whether the presenting problem is classroom in nature, is answered without difficulty. Alicia's low marks and declining school status mean that this question can be met with a "yes." The remainder of the flowchart is accordingly suitable for use.

Regarding Box B, which concerns eliminating general cognitive influences as explanations for Alicia's apparent problems, abundant information is available. Review of her history alone strongly suggests that she is a reasonably bright child who possesses considerable facility to master conceptually demanding school subject matter (e.g., she learned well until the fourth grade and continues to do adequately in some subjects). Examination of her current psychometric test scores, however, is more definitive. Her WISC-IV VCI of 108 and PRI of 110 suggest that she possesses general cognitive ability at least commensurate with classmates. It is interesting that her other WISC-IV index scores separate, with speed tasks (PSI = 118) better than working memory (WMI = 94). Data permit an unequivocal "yes" answer to Box B, that Alicia has plenty of cognitive ability to achieve in her current grade placement.

Box D is then addressed, namely whether Alicia suffers genuine skill deficits. Several sources of information are pertinent. First, she demonstrates numerous solidly developed academic skills in class. On a rating scale, her teacher estimated her as average or above in reading, spelling, and arithmetic but expressed concern about Alicia's writing skills. During a direct interview, however, her teacher indicated that Alicia often seems on the verge of writing but then hesitates to do so. This supposition seems to agree with the previously reviewed work sample: success on convergent writing tasks coexisting with reluctance, and perhaps insufficient skills, on divergent writing projects. In this situation, standardized individual achievement tests can be invaluable. With assurance that Alicia's full cooperation was secured, and with the added advantage of watching her approach, it was possible to estimate whether legitimate academic deficits exist. Review of Alicia's WJ III scores is instructive. She shows herself to be a skillful reader (all WJ III reading scores ≥ 110) with solid math skills (Calculations standard score = 105). Likewise, spelling proved no problem (standard score = 101). She had mixed results in writing: generating sentences to a prompt was well within normal limits, as was a timed task calling for generation of novel response by combining words into sentences. Notably, Alicia appeared more anxious and required repeated encourage-

TABLE 5.8. Summary of Assessment Scores for Alicia

Name	Age	Sex	Grade
Alicia	12 years	Female	6

Wechsler Intelligence Scale for Children–IV

Verbal Comprehension		*Perceptual Reasoning*		*Working Memory*		*Processing Speed*	
Similarities	11	Block Design	12	Digit Span	8	Coding	14
Vocabulary	13	Picture Concepts	13	Letter–Number Sequence	10	Symbol Search	12
Comprehension	11	Matrix Reasoning	10				

Scale	*Composite score*		*Percentile rank*
Verbal Comprehension	108 (101–114)	VCI	70th
Perceptual Reasoning	110 (102–117)	PRI	75th
Working Memory	94 (87–102)	WMI	34th
Processing Speed	118 (107–125)	PSI	88th
Full Scale	110 (103–113)	FSIQ	75th
General Ability Index	111 (105–116)	GAI	77th

Woodcock–Johnson III, Tests of Achievement

WJ III subtests	*Scaled score*
Letter–Word Identification	110
Passage Comprehension	112
Reading Fluency	115
Calculations	105
Math Fluency	99
Spelling	101
Writing Samples	95
Writing Fluency	93

A Developmental Neuropsychological Assessment (NEPSY)

Phonological Processing	10
Visuomotor Precision	8
Design Copying	11
Memory for Faces	9
Memory for Names	10
Narrative Memory	11

Behavior Assessment System for Children–2 (Parent Report)

Scale	*Level*
F	Acceptable
Response Pattern	Acceptable
Consistency	Acceptable

(continued)

TABLE 5.8. *(continued)*

Scale	Level
Hyperactivity	44
Aggression	40
Conduct Problems	44
Anxiety	68
Depression	52
Somatization	55
Atypicality	44
Withdrawal	57
Attention Problems	58
Adaptability	33
Social Skills	35
Leadership	32
Activities of Daily Living	40
Functional Communication	35

Behavior Assessment System for Children–2 (Teacher Report)

Scale	Level
F	Acceptable
Response Pattern	Acceptable
Consistency	Acceptable
Hyperactivity	42
Aggression	44
Conduct Problems	43
Anxiety	66
Depression	53
Somatization	55
Attention Problems	60
Learning Problems	55
Atypicality	44
Withdrawal	49
Adaptability	35
Social Skills	34
Leadership	34
Study Skills	31
Functional Communication	40

ment during this second task. Although both writing tests are relatively open-ended, the latter is more so, and thus may have engendered more intense anxiety. Nonetheless, Alicia accomplished both tasks reasonably well, with scores in the average range. The final writing challenge, which required preparation of a narrative, appeared to elicit marked anxiety. After complaints of lacking ideas and inability to select a topic, Alicia was ultimately told simply to try her best. With this support, she eventually produced a reasonably written story that was scored as within normal limits. Thus, it is likely that Alicia does not experience authentic academic skill deficits, including those of written expression, even though her performance in class often is lacking. Moreover, there are no language or fine-motor problems present. In other words, Alicia appears to express a performance problem rather than one of skill deficits. The answer to Box D is consequently "no." Even though Alicia appears to lack a true skill deficit, her teacher and parents nonetheless are deeply concerned about her classroom status. Her marks are unacceptably low, and everyone wants to know the nature of Alicia's problem and what to do about it. Box F is answered "yes," there is genuine concern among the teaching staff.

At this point, important (perhaps compelling) information has been collected about Alicia's potential core problem. Turning to Box H, it is easy to discern that she represents no management problem in class (and her presentation is not remotely compatible with an externalizing condition, such as ADHD-C). The "no" answer suggests that either an ADHD-I or a CU problem should be especially considered, although ADHD-C is still a possibility. Recalling that CU is often related to obsessive and compulsive symptoms, the possibility of this condition should be considered especially carefully. Alicia's history and her classroom presentation correspond to numerous symptoms of obsession and compulsion: reluctance in the face of even mild uncertainty, apparent preoccupation, recurring worry about events beyond control (e.g., grandfather's health), repeated erasures and overwriting, withholding of assignments (perhaps for fear of being wrong), and reduced social contact. As CU is a classroom-based category, rather than a psychiatric diagnosis, we sought to confirm school-related manifestations. In an interview, Alicia confirmed presence of each of the following during an interview.

- Tries very hard to have a neat paper.
- May do a paper over to make sure that it is perfect.
- Is careful not to mess up in school.
- Spends a lot of time erasing.
- Is slow to start work (if at all unsure about chances of success).
- Avoids turning in papers that might contain mistakes.
- Writes darkly and writes numbers over so they will look "just right."

We also reviewed her BASC-2, as completed by parent and teacher. Both suggest near-clinical levels of anxiety, a finding that sometimes exists with CU.

The assessment process was concluded with interview of Alicia's parents. During questions about her daughter's tendency to worry, Alicia's mother disclosed her own anxiety, for which she was currently considering treatment. Furthermore, an extensive family history of worry, social avoidance, and panic attacks was revealed. Such information buttressed the emerging conclusion that Alicia's problems were generally related to anxiety and obsessions and compulsions. Her particular manifestation was to take a deliberate and guarded approach to school that sometimes precluded submitting completed work and at other times led her to proceed so cautiously, and only after compulsive repetition, that little work was ever finished.

Following the steps in the flowchart to their conclusion, we note that ADHD-I remains a possibility. Here, history, observations, and rating scales are helpful. None of Alicia's teachers had previously complained about inattention, nor had her parents ever thought of her as disorganized, distractible, forgetful, or spacey (the hallmarks of ADHD-I). During extensive testing, she remained focused and persistent, and there were no indications of careless errors or lapses of concentration. Similarly, both parent- and teacher-completed BASC-2 forms are incompatible with inattention as the most plausible pattern. Alicia's parents place her near the at-risk range, whereas her teacher places her just into the at-risk range on the Attention Problems scale. More significantly, each of these scales' elevations is dwarfed by Anxiety scale elevations. Some inattention is expected among anxious children, and the mild elevations reflecting inattention are most parsimoniously explained as part of her anxious presentation. CU, however, is the salient classroom-based condition in this case.

Intervention Plan

Alicia obviously has unique needs, and understanding them is the only reasonable way to help her. As such, she illustrates very well the notion that interventions must be targeted to be effective. Using standard nostrums, such as increasing engaged academic time, would be misdirected for her (even though they may be wonderful for many struggling students). Below are the suggestions to help Alicia:

1. In class, reassurance probably needs to be repeatedly, clearly, and assertively provided. Specifically, Alicia may need to be told that her work quality is satisfactory and that her overall progress is acceptable. This intervention addresses Alicia's apparent underlying false assumption that her work must approach perfection and that mistakes are catastrophic. Phrases such as these may be appropriate: "You are responsible for your best work only"; "No one is perfect and we don't expect you to be"; "I'm interested in what you have written, not if it is perfect, so be sure to turn it in"; "Your handwriting is easy to read, and you don't need to make it darker or perfect." These strategies are designed to diminish false beliefs

and change covert negative thought sequences (e.g., are cognitive-behavioral modification techniques applied in a classroom setting).

2. Alicia may also benefit from learning to address false attributions during regularly scheduled sessions with a psychologist or counselor. This is a straightforward cognitive-behavioral therapy approach designed to support her teacher's efforts along the same lines. Overall adjustment and personal happiness, besides enhanced school status, may result.

3. Classroom behavioral strategies are also suggested to address the target behavior of excessive erasures, procrastination when starting writing assignments, and hoarding of completed work. A response cost system, given Alicia's likely aversion to negative feedback, may be necessary. Straightforward disruption of compulsive slowness may also work (e.g., teacher statements indicating that x amount of work must be completed within y minutes can capitalize on Alicia's compulsive need to avoid failure).

4. Assignment modifications may also help. Reducing written work and concomitantly increasing opportunities to respond orally may help. Likewise, emphasizing convergent over open-ended writing assignments may prevent problems. Accommodations of this type try to alleviate the problem by changing situational factors and task demands, rather than changing the child. Obviously, adjusting expectations may be easier than changing long-standing habits and strong constitutional (biologically based) tendencies. In behavioral terms, both of these interventions are changes in antecedent variables.

5. Alicia's family should be informed that pharmacotherapy may be valuable. For this particular family, the role of medication in the treatment of anxiety-related symptoms probably is known already. Nonetheless, an obligation to share such important information and to contextualize Alicia's classroom problems as akin to the anxiety disorders already known to the family is required if the school team is to do a thorough job.

Although Alicia may not qualify for SLD services because her problems are performance, rather than skill-related (and she lacks underlying processing problems), potential services eligibility should still be considered. If services outlined in #1-5 are impossible without an IEP, then consideration of ED designation is suggested. Regarding the ED definition, Alicia demonstrates: (1) a tendency to develop physical symptoms or fears associated with personal or school problems, (2) behaviors that have been present for a long period of time and to a marked extent, and (3) that adversely affect educational performance (see Table 4.5). Prospective services probably would be best delivered in Alicia's regular classroom, perhaps with a resource teacher determining expectations and orchestrating instructional modifications. Individual sessions emphasizing cognitive-behavioral therapy with a school psychologist, counselor, or social worker might be provided as a special education related service.

CASE 9: CARLOS

Background Information

Carlos is a 12-year-old sixth grader of Hispanic background, although he speaks little Spanish. He was referred because his parents are worried that he is losing skills.

Carlos was always among the best students in his class from kindergarten through third grade. He routinely completed his work quickly, demonstrated superior penmanship, and listened well. His primary-grade teachers thought of him as more mature than some of his classmates. Beginning in fourth grade, however, his status in class seemed less stellar; this was particularly the case in English/writing and in social studies. Now, as a sixth grader, he has begun to earn C's, which prompted his mother and father to seek an evaluation. He was taken to a private clinic for assessment.

Carlos's parents brought work samples, group achievement test scores, and report cards dating from kindergarten. These were meticulously organized. Indeed, his grades showed a gradual decline, with the exception of math, where he continued to earn A's. However, his teacher failed to express alarm; her comments were that Carlos was an excellent worker who was making adequate progress in most subjects, but who was above average in math.

Carlos's personal and family history failed to enlighten. He was born by cesarean section after an uneventful pregnancy. He came home from the hospital at 3 days, thrived physically, and made normal attachments to parents. He walked at 10 months and spoke single words at 13 months and two-word combinations at 16 months. He was easily toilet trained at 24 months and rode a two-wheeler at 5 years. He had clear articulation and good rote auditory memory as a preschooler.

Carlos's mother was born in the United States, and her primary language is English. His father came to the United States from Nicaragua at age 11; Spanish is his preferred language, although he insists on speaking English only at home. The family owns a small landscape business and is self-described as successful. Family history is negative for learning, developmental, and psychiatric problems.

At home, Carlos is described as always busy, although his parents insist that he is not impulsive or motorically chaotic, simply always engaged in something. When there is nothing to do, he can spend hours finding hidden words in workbooks. He is scrupulous about starting homework as soon as he comes home from school. He has never had a missing assignment and has been absent only 1 day of school in nearly 7 years of public school attendance. He has relatively few friends, indicating that their interests and his do not match.

Carlos is described by his parents as healthy. There is no history of vision or hearing problems. He sleeps and eats well. He had a noteworthy blow to the head in a bicycle accident at age 6, but he never lost consciousness, and his pediatrician described this as a subclinical concussion.

Assessment Procedures

Wechsler Intelligence Scale for Children–IV; Woodcock–Johnson III, Tests of Achievement; NEPSY (Design Copying, Visuomotor Precision, Memory for Faces, Memory for Names, Narrative Memory, Phonological Processing); Behavior Assessment System for Children–2 (Parent Report Form, Teacher Report Form); informal assessment of curriculum material, parent interview, child interview. Scores on standardized instruments for Carlos are listed in Table 5.9.

Observations

Carlos is a thin, tall 12-year-old Hispanic male who was well groomed. He is free of obvious physical stigmata and dysmorphic signs. His attention, effort, and cooperation were excellent throughout the evaluation, which was conducted during a single morning session.

Carlos was not observed in class. An interview with his teacher, however, suggests that he is a hard worker who is extremely compliant and organized. He is sometimes isolated on the playground and a bit reluctant to open up on team projects. He reportedly reads well orally but sometimes fails to understand what he has read.

Analysis of Results

Beginning with Box A in the flowchart, the question is about the nature of Carlos's prospective problem and specifically whether it has a classroom component. As always, all sources of information should be examined. Carlos's parents are quite concerned about his progressively declining grades, which are documented by report cards. Thus, legitimate concern exists about his academic status, taking the long view, even if his teacher expresses little immediate concern (taking the short view). Accordingly, the answer to Box A is "yes." Use of the flowchart to analyze the rest of Carlos's data is appropriate.

Regarding Box B, pertaining to the question about adequate general

TABLE 5.9. Summary of Assessment Scores for Carlos

Name	Age	Sex	Grade
Carlos	12 years	Male	6

Wechsler Intelligence Scale for Children–IV

Verbal Comprehension		*Perceptual Reasoning*		*Working Memory*		*Processing Speed*	
Similarities	7	Block Design	10	Digit Span	14	Coding	11
Vocabulary	9	Picture Concepts	7	Letter–Number Sequence	13	Symbol Search	13
Comprehension	7	Matrix Reasoning	7	(Arithmetic)		(Cancellation)	

Scale	*Composite score*		*Percentile rank*
Verbal Comprehension	87 (81–95)	VCI	19th
Perceptual Reasoning	88 (81–97)	PRI	21st
Working Memory	120 (111–126)	WMI	91st
Processing Speed	112 (102–120)	PSI	79th
Full Scale	99 (94–104)	FSIQ	47th
General Ability Index	87 (82–93)	GAI	19th

Woodcock–Johnson III, Tests of Achievement

WJ III subtests	*Scaled score*
Letter–word Identification	110
Passage Comprehension	88
Reading Fluency	115
Calculations	90
Math Fluency	117
Spelling	104
Writing Samples	86
Writing Fluency	87

A Developmental Neuropsychological Assessment (NEPSY)

Phonological Processing	10
Visuomotor Precision	12
Design Copying	11
Memory for Faces	14
Memory for Names	12
Narrative Memory	8

Behavior Assessment System for Children–2 (Parent Report)

Scale	*Level*
F	Acceptable
Response Pattern	Acceptable
Consistency	Acceptable

(continued)

TABLE 5.9. *(continued)*

Scale	Level
Hyperactivity	50
Aggression	47
Conduct Problems	48
Anxiety	53
Depression	56
Somatization	49
Atypicality	57
Withdrawal	57
Attention Problems	53
Adaptability	46
Social Skills	43
Leadership	44
Activities of Daily Living	45
Functional Communication	43

Behavior Assessment System for Children–2 (Teacher Report)

Scale	Level
F	Acceptable
Response Pattern	Acceptable
Consistency	Acceptable
Hyperactivity	52
Aggression	50
Conduct Problems	45
Anxiety	53
Depression	53
Somatization	51
Attention Problems	49
Learning Problems	57
Atypicality	58
Withdrawal	55
Adaptability	45
Social Skills	47
Leadership	44
Study Skills	44
Functional Communication	46

ability, the data are mixed. Based on history, Carlos is thought to be extremely bright. This supposition arises from his outstanding classroom performance during the primary grades and his contemporary solid arithmetic performance. Furthermore, Carlos acquired milestones somewhat ahead of expectations. Also, he earned a WISC-IV FSIQ of 99, which places him in the average range. This score is surprisingly low given elements of his school history, which sounds terrific. It is noteworthy that Carlos has extreme scatter among his WISC-IV index scores, as well among other non-IQ measures. These discrepancies warrant attention (which they will receive later). At this point in the flowchart, there is sufficient evidence to suggest that Carlos's difficulties do not derive primarily from simple general cognitive factors. Consequently, the answer to Box B is "yes."

The next issue is whether Carlos suffers from legitimate academic, motor, or linguistic deficits (Box D). Just as was the case with Box A, the data are equivocal. His history suggests that he has developed skills, but his grades imply that he is failing to perform adequately with the skills he possesses. Paradoxically, his current teacher, as well as those who taught him before and his parents, describes a student with excellent study habits. Carlos's achievement test scores prove extremely informative. Carlos's scores represent a coherent pattern: better on rote and speeded tasks, worse on conceptually demanding tasks and those that require higher-order thinking. Specifically, Carlos read and computed well when working against a clock, but these tasks were fairly simple (and sentences and math problems were at an easy elementary level). He also identified words and spelled fairly well. Computational arithmetic skills were not very well developed, nor was his ability to extract meaning from sentences or answer reading comprehension questions. Likewise, despite spelling words correctly and displaying superior handwriting, the content of his writing was not especially well developed. It is noteworthy that scores on most intellectually demanding academic subtests matched Carlos's scores on WISC-IV indexes that measure general ability (i.e., VCI and PRI). Conversely, rote and speeded achievement subtest scores are higher, with values closer to Carlos's noncognitive index scores on the WISC-IV (i.e., WMI and PSI). Box D is tentatively answered "yes."

Box G questions if the academic problems are predominately in the language arts realm. Carlos's grades were excellent early and poorer later. He appears to do no better in math than in the language arts areas. The answer to Box G is "no." Nonetheless, he does not evidence academic problems that are predominantly in arithmetic, written expression, or handwriting. In fact, his problems, to the extent they are genuine, fail to fall along linguistic versus visual–spatial lines at all. The answer to Box I is thus also "no."

We turn finally to Box J. The question here concerns either the temporal or cross-subject matter nature of prospective problems. Correspondence with Carlos's situation should be clear immediately. The heart of his parents' concern is falling grades over time. If we consider the definition of a child with ISSS, we find a match with Carlos. He enjoys outstanding graphomotor and working memory development. These attributes probably aided his elevation to near the top of his primary-level classrooms. The kindergarten through third-grade curriculum values attention, efficiency, hand–eye coordination, and relatively low-level associative learning. Carlos, accordingly, thrived. In contrast, his splinter skill strengths represent a poor match for the increasingly high-level, analytical requirements of the middle school grades. He can identify words but may fail fully to comprehend their meanings; he can spell but not necessarily blend his well-spelled (and beautifully written) words into sophisticated passages. Because rote memorization and persistent work habits remain applicable to much elementary school math, Carlos continues to encounter some success here. Unlike many children with splinter skills, Carlos actually enjoys unexpectedly high skills in several domains, not just one. Consistent with most children with this amorphous condition, his outstanding strengths exclude executive functions and general ability (*g*).

Some children with ISSS also have Asperger's disorder or PDD, not otherwise specified. This was not the case with Carlos. Core characteristics of Asperger's were missing. He possessed reasonable social competency, although he was a bit aloof. He lacked the intensive, repetitive, overly focused verbal output of children with Asperger's disorder. He had none of the obsessive interests of children with PDD (or autism).

Intervention Plan

The following are suggested:

1. Carlos's parents initiated the evaluation, they expressed the most concern, and they required the most thorough explanation. In fact, most of the "intervention" consists of promoting understanding and, concomitantly, refuting underlying implicit misconceptions. Carlos has not "lost" skills. Almost certainly, he has continued to develop in all dimensions. The perception of a problem arose because Carlos's pattern of strengths meshed well with the early school curriculum but not with the later curriculum. Parents often believe that few intra-individual differences exist. If you're bright in school, you're bright in school. If you learn easily in third grade, you should learn just about as easily in sixth grade. Children with splinter skills demonstrate that this generalization is sometimes false. Carlos's parents needed to have these facts explained and their expectations for universal and easy success reviewed.

2. Carlos should be placed with teachers who emphasize associative learning, productivity, and convergent instruction approaches. Those that stress novel thinking, divergent problem solving, and insight probably represent a poor match for him.

3. Strategy training, such as learning planning and problem-solving steps via oral rehearsal, may work.

4. Carlos is encouraged to socialize with peers. Structured play activities may increase his social competence, refine his ability to acquire

friends when he chooses to do so, and provide cognitive and problem-solving models that may be currently lacking.

5. Carlos is not recommended for any special services.

Note of Explanation. Following the flowchart to reach conclusions about the presence of ISSS can be difficult. Diagnosticians are encouraged to keep the possibility of this pattern in mind even when the flowchart fails to lead them to this condition. The conundrum is that this pattern does not look either like a purely skill or a purely performance problem. Accordingly, deciding if Box D should be answered "yes" or "no" may be difficult. This was exactly the situation with Carlos. He had some academic deficits, especially compared to his outstanding development in several noncognitive spheres, but he also had problems using his skills fully—much like a student with a performance problem. The flowchart is a tool to help in problem solving, but it is not perfect.

CASE 10: TALIA

Background Information

Talia is a 15-year-old high school freshman. She has been a good student throughout her school career. She learned to read on time, consistently earned 100% on spelling tests during her elementary years, and mastered basic math facts and procedures. She has always enjoyed impeccable handwriting. Since beginning junior high, her semester grade point average has never dropped below 3.0, and she has never earned lower than a C on a report card. She has had regular school attendance. Although viewed as shy, she has always maintained friendships with one or two classmates.

Talia lives alone with her mother. Her parents were divorced 3 years ago, and she rarely sees her out-of-state father. About a year ago, her mother noticed increasing isolation, intensifying sleep problems, and weight loss associated with declining appetite. Equally troubling, Talia expresses pessimism about the future, little interest in going out with her friends, and intermittent bouts of irritability punctuated by periods of tearfulness. Her mother is concerned that her grades at school will suffer and consequently contacted the school psychologist for an evaluation.

Observation and Interview

At her mother's request, Talia met with the school psychologist. Talia appeared disheveled and lethargic, but she clearly wanted to cooperate. She downplayed her mother's concern, and, forcing a smile, indicated that her mother probably worries too much. With questioning, however, she confirmed the problems with sleeping, eating, energy, and pessimism previously reported by her mother. Although she denied suicidal ideation, she could think of few things in the future to look forward to and little of interest or enjoyment in her life now. She confirmed that she felt sad or ill-tempered most of the time. She wished that her mother would drop her concerns because she did not want to inconvenience her mother, who had many other "issues" to deal with, or school officials, who had other students more in need of assistance.

Analysis of Results

Talia does not need a comprehensive evaluation. The psychologist recognized that her problems concern probable depression, rather than a classroom problem. Although psychiatric problems sometimes mimic learning problems, and although it is important to remember that psychiatric problems can produce classroom failure, neither of these was the case with Talia. If the flowchart were followed beginning at Box A (Is this a classroom problem?), the answer would be "no." Accordingly, the rest of the flowchart is not appropriate. Instead, the DSM-IV-TR, among other sources, was consulted. Data supported a diagnosis of dysthymia (depression). Neither her mother's request for a psychoeducational evaluation nor Talia's wish to avoid imposing on others distracted the psychologist from her core problem. Talia was referred for mental health services for her personal benefit and to prevent her emotional problems from disrupting her long-standing success in the classroom. A diagnostic work-up was deferred to the receiving clinic. In light of sleep and appetite disruption, her mother was also encouraged to take her daughter to her pediatrician for a medical check up. If symptoms persist to marked degree, the team may eventually consider service eligibility under ED.

Talia's case illustrates that psychologists must be prepared to deal with all types of presenting problems, even if they envision their practice as restricted to academic ones. Before pursuing cognitive, information-processing, or work style issues, psychologists must implicitly rule out emotional and conspicuous medical problems by virtue of a "yes" answer to Box A. It is impossible to practice some aspects of psychology without minimal knowledge of competing childhood emotional and medical problems.

CASE 11: JEREMY

Background Information

Jeremy is a 9-year-old white male who was referred for evaluation by his parents and current third-grade teacher. The principal concern was "difficulty with handwriting and poor rate of work completion." In addition, Jeremy was reportedly averse to any type of handwriting task and had recently become resistant to attending school.

Jeremy was born at 40 weeks of gestational age via a spontaneous vaginal delivery, his Apgar scores were 9/10, and he left the nursery at 2 days without complications and came home, where he established a normal biological rhythm and an early attachment to parents. He walked, spoke his first words, and accomplished toilet training at normal ages. He has been viewed as slightly clumsy. He has consistently passed vision and hearing screenings. His mother volunteered that he has motor tics consisting of eye blinking and occasional shoulder shrugs. These reportedly wax and wane in intensity and seem to be more evident when Jeremy is "under stress."

Jeremy has attended his current suburban, fairly affluent school since kindergarten with near-perfect attendance until this academic year. He has missed 7 days through the first semester, typically because of complaints of nausea. His mother believes that he was afraid to go to school some days because of the prospect of failure and losing face. He seems to be frustrated by his inability to complete assignments. From kindergarten onward, handwriting has been the chief concern. The written work that he turns in is difficult to read; pencil pressure is too hard; much written work is left incomplete. His teacher now rates him as much below grade level in writing, somewhat below grade level in math, average in reading, and above grade level in science. According to her, Jeremy "takes extremely long to write his answers down or to share his ideas, even though he has excellent concepts." She has noted that he has become increasingly upset in math and frustrated when asked to write. On a standardized checklist, she indicated that Jeremy "completes most work, needs more assistance than classmates."

Jeremy lives with his biological mother and stepfather, who adopted him at age 18 months. There is an older full-brother who is 12 and reportedly does well in almost all school subjects. At home, Jeremy's parents have observed frequent complaints of aches and pains, fear of novel events, temper outbursts when frustrated, and moderate tendencies toward perfectionism. He has relatively few friends, seems to act younger than his age, and is a poor loser if things do not go his way. He is highly interested in science and loves to watch nature and wildlife-related programs on television. Family history is negative on mother's side for learning, developmental, or psychiatric disorders. His biological father, with whom he has regular contact, has been diagnosed with OCD and is treated with medication.

Observations

Jeremy was an age-appropriate-appearing 9-year-old who seemed apprehensive at the outset of the evaluation. He remained reticent during warm-up discussion that often elicits more interaction and some sense of comfort for many children. After approximately 10 minutes of the evaluation, he relaxed but remained quiet. He appeared well focused, and his effort was excellent. No signs of impulsivity, restlessness, social intrusion, or limit testing were seen. He was occasionally slow and deliberate in formulating both verbal responses and when constructing, drawing, or writing. No tics were noted.

Assessment Procedures

Wechsler Intelligence Scale for Children–IV; Wechsler Individual Achievement Test–II; NEPSY (Design Copying, Visuomotor Precision, Memory for Faces, Memory for Names, Narrative Memory, Phonological Processing); Grooved Pegboard Test; Behavior Assessment System for Children–2 (Parent Report Form, Teacher Report Form); informal assessment of curriculum material, parent interview, child interview. Scores on standardized instruments for Jeremy are listed in Table 5.10.

Analysis of Results

Regarding Box A, it is clear that Jeremy was referred for classroom learning issues. Both his teacher's and parents' questions were "Why isn't he learning better?" and "What can we do about it?" After answering the question about the prospect of an academic problem "yes," the rest of the flowchart can be used with Jeremy.

The next step was to establish if Jeremy's overall ability level was adequate to support the learning challenges of his current third-grade classroom. That is, we need to rule out general ability issues as the explanation for the referral. In Jeremy's case, WISC-IV scores proved instructive, although other sources of information could have helped support the same conclusion. Jeremy's FSIQ of 92 is average. This score, however, should not be taken at face value as an estimate of his cognitive ability. He scored substantially better on verbal reasoning, conceptual, and problem-solving tasks than he did on equivalent nonverbal and visual–spatial tasks (VCI = 128, 97th percentile; PRI = 88, 21st percentile). From these scores, we might estimate that Jeremy would be among the most cognitively able students in his class when activities involve language or discussion or depend heavily on linguistic processing. In contrast, activities that require visual–spatial and nonverbal competence may be hard for him. Based on his WISC-IV scores, an "average" expectation is not appropriate. Jeremy might be expected to do well on some things and to struggle on others. Indeed, his history agrees with test-based predictions; he has done excellently in science but poorly in writing. At any rate, our information is clearly sufficient to conclude that the answer to Box B's question is "yes."

TABLE 5.10. Summary of Assessment Scores for Jeremy

Name	Age	Sex	Dominant hand	Grade
Jeremy	9 years	Male	Right	3

Wechsler Intelligence Scale for Children–IV

Verbal Comprehension		*Perceptual Reasoning*		*Working Memory*		*Processing Speed*	
Similarities	16	Block Design	10	Digit Span	7	Coding	4
Vocabulary	17	Picture Concepts	7	Letter–Number Sequence	8	Symbol Search	4
Comprehension	11	Matrix Reasoning	7				

Scale	*Composite score*		*Percentile rank*
Verbal Comprehension	128 (120–133)	VCI	97th
Perceptual Reasoning	88 (81–97)	PRI	21st
Working Memory	86 (79–95)	WMI	18th
Processing Speed	68 (63–81)	PSI	2nd
Full Scale	92 (87–97)	FSIQ	30th
General Ability Index	108 (102–113)	GAI	70th

Wechsler Individual Achievement Test–II

WIAT-II subtests	*Scaled score*
Reading	
Word Reading	100
Reading Comprehension	102
Pseudoword Decoding	106
Mathematics	
Numerical Operations	96
Math Reasoning	110
Written Language	
Spelling	73
Written Expression	87

A Developmental Neuropsychological Assessment (NEPSY)

Phonological Processing	9
Visuomotor Precision	4
Design Copying	11
Memory for Faces	10
Memory for Names	9
Narrative Memory	9

Motor Exam

Pegboard

Dominant hand (right): 87 sec
Nondominant hand (left): 99 sec

(continued)

TABLE 5.10. *(continued)*

Behavior Assessment System for Children–2 (Parent Report)

Scale	Level
F	Acceptable
Response Pattern	Acceptable
Consistency	Acceptable
Hyperactivity	36
Aggression	37
Conduct Problems	40
Anxiety	67
Depression	53
Somatization	53
Atypicality	41
Withdrawal	56
Attention Problems	48
Adaptability	39
Social Skills	37
Leadership	34
Activities of Daily Living	42
Functional Communication	49

Behavior Assessment System for Children–2 (Teacher Report)

Scale	Level
F	Acceptable
Response Pattern	Acceptable
Consistency	Acceptable
Hyperactivity	41
Aggression	43
Conduct Problems	42
Anxiety	62
Depression	55
Somatization	58
Attention Problems	38
Learning Problems	56
Atypicality	43
Withdrawal	52
Adaptability	39
Social Skills	39
Leadership	40
Study Skills	45
Functional Communication	46

Turning to Box D, it is now necessary to determine if Jeremy has a legitimate academic skill deficiency in any of the crucial reading, computing, or writing skill strands or in any supportive skill, such as language or fine-motor performance. Background information certainly suggests that this might be the case. His teacher rated him as "far below grade level" in writing. Furthermore, his mother indicated that written work has been of poor quality since he was in kindergarten. Several work samples provided by his teacher also suggest a writing problem. For example, a recently completed worksheet requiring open-ended reactions to a story was quite hard to read, poorly organized, and without much punctuation. Interestingly, Jeremy's mother also submitted a work sample from arithmetic that contained poorly formed numerals and numerous erasures and was only partially complete. Although suggestive of a written expression problem, this information alone is inconclusive. It may be that Jeremy is merely inattentive or poorly motivated, and his written work suffers accordingly. It might also be the case that writing demands are excessive or that standards are set too high. To help address these issues and to confirm that a bona fide skill problem exists, Jeremy was administered standardized achievement tests that included writing. Working with him in a one-on-one situation permits assurance of full effort and cooperation and allows him to be compared precisely with age-mates.

Jeremy's writing scores (both his total Written Expression and Spelling) from the WIAT-II were below average. His Written Expression score, which reflects ideas and organization and depends on him writing with a pencil, was in the low-average range (standard score = 87). His Spelling score, which requires mastery of sound–symbol relationships or recall of entire word patterns while writing, was in the borderline range (standard score = 73). Both scores were significantly low compared to Jeremy's cognitive ability as reflected by verbal conceptual development. Both of these achievement subtests also align with his reported history and work samples. The answer to Box D is "yes." Looking at Jeremy's writing, it is obvious that it is nearly illegible, and when generating or rearranging sentences he lacked adequate punctuation, capitalization, and organization. The answer to Box G is "no." Jeremy's problems are not principally in the language arts subjects. It is then immediately possible to go to Box I and confirm that handwriting is significantly impaired. The answer to Box I is "yes." The flowchart suggests that Jeremy's problem may include elements of GU or NLD.

If one reviews the definitions of these two conditions, some degree of correspondence with both can be detected. Regarding the prospect of NLD, Jeremy does express significantly greater problems with visual–spatial and nonverbal material than linguistic and auditory material. His PRI is lower than his VCI, suggesting that he does better on cognitively related tasks that are verbal in nature. Similarly, his PSI is lower than his WMI, suggesting that he does better on attention, speed, and noncognitive tasks of auditory rather than visual or visual–motor nature. However, he did not demonstrate severe visual–spatial deficits on some subtests that typically prove hard for children with NLD. Specifically, he earned an average score on the Block Design subtest (scaled score = 10), and none of the designs he constructed evidenced severe problems recognizing patterns, discerning directions, or fitting parts into recognizable wholes. Likewise, his NEPSY Design Copying subtest score, derived from untimed reproduction of shapes, was average (scaled score = 11). Again, evidence of severe spatial confusion was missing when his shapes were checked. However, his pencil control appeared poor even here; his lines were heavily drawn and appeared to have been produced with an unsteady hand. Although Jeremy's social skills were not rated as very well developed by either his parents or teacher (see BASC-2 scores), he did not evidence (during the evaluation) the social clumsiness often characteristic of children with NLD, nor was his history descriptive of such severe problems. Finally, regarding the prospect of NLD, noteworthy computational arithmetic problems were absent from his history and were likewise not apparent in his current WIAT-II scores (Numerical Operations standard score = 96).

In contrast, Jeremy's history and current scores match most of the cardinal characteristics of GU. He has historically had trouble getting work done when it required writing or pencil use. He has had poor penmanship, as rated by his teachers. These problems are apparent in the current work sample supplied by his parents. His WISC-IV index scores agree with the emerging hypothesis of GU; his PSI standard score of 68 is especially concerning. When subtests that more precisely isolate graphomotor dexterity and speed are employed (NEPSY Visuomotor Precision), Jeremy's scores are noted to be quite low (scaled score = 4). Supplemental testing of manual dexterity without a pencil also showed problems. When Jeremy was required to pick up and place pegs individually into slotted openings (the Grooved Pegboard Test), he was quite slow with each hand (right and left hand scores approximately 2.5 and 2.0 standard deviations below average, respectively). Moreover, fine-motor skills, including those involving pencil use, appeared, subjectively, to be poorly executed. Jeremy seemed to grip his pencil tightly, to use odd angles to produce letters, and frequently to drop pegs. More directly related to classroom work, he appeared to lack comfort and automaticity when writing (letters were drawn rather than fluidly written). It is likely excessive effort would be needed to complete pencil-and-paper tasks at school. Furthermore, those tasks that include a graphomotor element are likely to be completed relatively slowly and to require that disproportionate attention be devoted to the motor portion of the task. When attention is inordinately devoted to motor output, relatively little focus may be available for attending to spelling, punctuation, or organization in written tasks. Graphomotor inefficiency might even cause problems in arithmetic if excessive attention is directed to numeral production and alignment rather than to executing the procedures and attending to the logic of ultimate answers.

Although many of Jeremy's classroom problems derive from graphomotor weaknesses, we have turned up additional information that should be considered when devising a plan to help him. He appears to be a temperamentally sensitive and anxious child. This was revealed in his parents' description of his behavior and his social interaction style over many years. It may also relate to a biological substrate shared with his biological father, who is being treated for OCD. Jeremy revealed during an interview that he is prone to worry. He articulated a variety of concerns seldom heard from children his age and whose presence often denotes a reflective, anxious approach to life. For example, he stated that he wished adults would stop pollution because it might "kill off all the animals," often worried before going to sleep if the sun would burn out, and was anxious that he would be in trouble at school for making too many mistakes. He identified being called on in class as among his greatest fears. Both parents and teacher confirmed the presence of anxiety; he was rated in the at-risk range on this dimension by both raters (BASC-2 Anxiety T scores: Parent = 67, Teacher = 62). It is plausible that Jeremy's heightened anxiety reflects both an inherent predisposition and the effects of chronic classroom problems. Struggling to get his written work done and concern (legitimately felt) that he may be scrutinized for poor work quality probably contribute to his feelings of stress and accompanying anxiety. These issues should be considered during planning. These same factors may contribute to limited social skills and relatively few friendships. Lack of self-confidence and subjective feelings of anxiety can preclude taking the initiative in social situations and lead to isolation. Isolation, in turn, can diminish one's sense of personal confidence and further contribute to anxious feelings. Intervening socially would also seem to be important. Finally, we note that Jeremy possesses numerous strengths; he is bright and has good verbal ability, a good memory, and well-developed reading skills. His family is ardently committed to help him progress.

Intervention Plan

Several straightforward recommendations can be made for Jeremy based on what we have learned.

1. First, he has obvious strengths that might be used to minimize problems with pencil-and-paper work and with writing and spelling. Since he reads and thinks very well, it would be helpful to have requirements for copying and writing drastically diminished and allow his capability to become evident. Among ways to do this would be for assignments and material from the blackboard to be given to him as printed material, thus eliminating his need to transcribe. Similarly, for written assignments in social studies or science, he may need permission to provide answers in a compressed (bullet point) format rather than in long narratives. At times, allowing him to provide responses verbally, such as to another knowledge-

able classmate, aide or teacher, may be called for. Sometimes children with such problems benefit from preparing longer assignments in an outline form and then producing a finished product as an oral, tape-recorded report. Seeking and reducing writing demands that constrain success in academic subjects, without specifying a priori all of the ways in which this would be done, would be strongly suggested.

2. Jeremy might be helped by teaching him to produce legible letters more quickly and efficiently. Thus, a remedial writing program such as outlined by Berninger and colleagues (see Chapter 3) would be suggested.

3. Even though such a program may make handwriting easier to produce, in the long run Jeremy may still struggle. Accordingly, teaching him an alternative means of writing by learning to keyboard was suggested. Unlike suggestions #1 and #2, however, teaching touch typing is a skill developed over time and would not be expected to provide immediate relief. Such a program is often best undertaken as a summer project. After extended practice, Jeremy may be able to use a word processing program with a spelling and grammar check to help him with written tasks. By middle school many children with Jeremy's type of writing problem use laptop computers.

4. He needs direct assistance in writing. In his case, this would need to begin with a task analysis to identify missing skills, followed by direct instruction and tutoring. In Jeremy's case, spelling needs to be incorporated into remedial activities.

5. Like many children who have encountered frustration at school, he needs sustained periods of success and copious positive feedback. This seems to be especially true given his at-risk status regarding anxiety. Capitalizing on his excellent reading skills, vast general knowledge, and interest in science would appear to be ways to find performance worthy of praise. Because Jeremy is concerned about being singled out for attention, it is probably best to commend him individually and/or praise his work by marking his papers.

6. A social skills training program may help. So would finding times for regular interactions with children his own age, even if parents initially had to arrange play dates.

7. To assure that these recommendations are implemented, Jeremy probably requires designation as a student with SLD. Specifically, he appears to meet criteria in the area of written expression.

CASE 12: MONA

Background Information

Mona is a 12-year-old white female whose only language is English. She was referred by her classroom teacher because of concern about low grades, especially in arithmetic. Several of her teachers also describe her as disorganized on complex tasks and as having marginal handwriting.

Mona's mother indicated that her daughter's health is perfect. She had recently been seen for a check-up by her pediatrician. She has always passed hearing and vision screenings provided at her school and, before that, during routine evaluations at her pediatrician's office. Mona's mother stated that she was born about 4 weeks early, but weighed 6 lbs, 1 oz., and was released home within 2 days of birth. She sat up, crawled, walked, and was toilet trained at normal times. Always viewed as talkative, Mona was described by her mother as having more well-developed language skills than her two older sisters, ages 13 and 15. As a preschooler, her parents remember that she loved to listen to them read stories but seldom engaged in coloring, puzzles, or other hands-on tasks. She was slow to learn to tie her shoes and did not ride a bicycle without training wheels until age 8 years.

Mona lives with her biological mother and stepfather, whom she has considered to be her father since age 3. Her biological father lives in another state, is remarried, and sees Mona and her sisters for about 1 month each summer. Her mother could not identify stress in the household or in the relationship between herself and Mona's stepfather that may contribute to school problems. Mona reportedly gets along well with both sisters, especially the eldest girl, who has consistently helped with math homework. Family history is reportedly negative for SLD and psychiatric disorders. There is a first cousin on her biological father's side with Down syndrome.

Mona attended public school from kindergarten through third grade, then transferred to a parochial school. This move was prompted by her parents' desire to see her receive a more structured classroom experience and to expose her to higher academic expectations. She was reportedly a good reader by the middle of first grade, but her handwriting was described as poor. Arithmetic was a problem early and continues to be so now. She reportedly has been slow to memorize math facts, confused about the order of operations, and inattentive to placement of numerals. For example, her third-grade teacher complained that Mona never paid attention to number columns; she required her to use a vertically placed marker made of construction paper to keep them straight. Now, as a sixth grader, she reportedly remains inconsistent in completing multiplace multiplication and long division problems. She has complained that fractions simply don't make sense to her. Her math grades were C's during fifth grade, but have been D's each grading period this year. Her mother is worried that she will fail this quarter. Her teacher has allowed her to work with a "math buddy" or increase the number of drills. Her mother has taken her to a tutor for the past few months. Although she scored well on spelling tests from first through fifth grade, Mona's teachers never viewed her as a good writer. According to her current teacher, "She produces a lot of written material, but her themes lack coherence." Mona has always disliked art and physical education but loves and excels at chorus.

Mona is described by both her mother and current teacher as immature. At home, she rarely seeks out her sisters' friends, instead preferring to talk and watch television with a third-grade neighbor. She is reluctant to try new activities. Unlike her sisters, she has never enjoyed sports. Attempts to introduce her to soccer, softball, bowling, and dance all failed. Parents believe that she was either confused by these activities or felt uncomfortable without them present to guide her. She has been viewed as slow to warm up socially and, perhaps, anxious.

Observations

Mona was a tall, well-groomed, 12-year-old who actually appeared older than her stated age. She had no stigmata or unusual physical characteristics. She was tentative at the outset of the evaluation and appeared anxious about what was expected of her. Even simple directions seemed to confuse her; she frequently looked for confirmation that she was performing tasks correctly. About 30 minutes into the evaluation, she appeared to relax noticeably. She demonstrated routine social amenities, such as proper greetings, but volunteered little personal information. Her attention span and cooperation were good. However, she used a chaotic, disorganized approach on several nonverbal tasks.

Assessment Procedures

Wechsler Intelligence Scale for Children–IV; Wechsler Individual Achievement Test–II; NEPSY (Design Copying, Visuomotor Precision, Memory for Faces, Memory for Names, Narrative Memory, Phonological Processing); Behavior Assessment System for Children–2 (Parent Report Form, Teacher Report Form); informal assessment of curriculum material, parent interview, child interview. Scores on standardized instruments for Mona are listed in Table 5.11.

Analysis of Results

It is easy to answer the first required question in our system by confirming that Mona was referred for academic concerns. Both her teacher and parents were concerned about her math performance. Box A was answered "yes." The rest of the flowchart is appropriate to use.

Turning to Box B, the inquiry about general cognitive competence,

TABLE 5.11. Summary of Assessment Scores for Mona

Name	Age	Sex	Grade
Mona	12 years	Female	6

Wechsler Intelligence Scale for Children–IV

Verbal Comprehension		*Perceptual Reasoning*		*Working Memory*		*Processing Speed*	
Similarities	12	Block Design	8	Digit Span	9	Coding	7
Vocabulary	12	Picture Concepts	7	Letter–Number Sequence	9	Symbol Search	8
Comprehension	11	Matrix Reasoning	8				

Scale	*Composite score*		*Percentile rank*
Verbal Comprehension	108 (101–114)	VCI	70th
Perceptual Reasoning	86 (79–95)	PRI	18th
Working Memory	94 (87–102)	WMI	34th
Processing Speed	85 (78–106)	PSI	16th
Full Scale	92 (87–97)	FSIQ	30th
General Ability Index	98 (92–104)	GAI	45th

Wechsler Individual Achievement Test–II

WIAT-II subtests	*Scaled score*
Word Reading	102
Reading Comprehension	91
Pseudoword Decoding	98
Numerical Operations	76
Math Reasoning	92
Spelling	85
Written Expression	78

A Developmental Neuropsychological Assessment (NEPSY)

Phonological Processing	12
Visuomotor Precision	9
Design Copying	6
Memory for Faces	9
Memory for Names	13
Narrative Memory	13

Behavior Assessment System for Children–2 (Parent Report)

Scale	*Level*
F	Acceptable
Response Pattern	Acceptable
Consistency	Acceptable
Hyperactivity	36

(continued)

TABLE 5.11. *(continued)*

Scale	Level
Aggression	38
Conduct Problems	39
Anxiety	57
Depression	43
Somatization	38
Atypicality	41
Withdrawal	38
Attention Problems	43
Adaptability	37
Social Skills	37
Leadership	32
Activities of Daily Living	36
Functional Communication	35

Behavior Assessment System for Children–2 (Teacher Report)

Scale	Level
F	Acceptable
Response Pattern	Acceptable
Consistency	Acceptable
Hyperactivity	44
Aggression	48
Conduct Problems	47
Anxiety	49
Depression	48
Somatization	51
Attention Problems	45
Learning Problems	66
Atypicality	47
Withdrawal	44
Adaptability	37
Social Skills	34
Leadership	36
Study Skills	44
Functional Communication	44

abundant background information and current ability scores help answer this question. Mona's developmental milestones, especially linguistic ones, were mastered on time, she has acquired competence in several academic subjects (e.g., basic reading), and she has successfully passed through many years of formal schooling, up to the sixth grade. Furthermore, her parents have never been concerned that she is cognitively delayed (notwithstanding her tendency to socialize with children younger than herself). Definitive information, however, comes from ability testing. Her WISC-IV FSIQ score of 92 is in the average range. Although based on this composite score she may be less cognitively developed than some of her classmates, her overall ability should be sufficient to allow her to succeed. Closer analysis suggests that Mona's composite (FSIQ) score may underestimate her ability. She expresses a significant discrepancy between VCI and PRI, the two cognitively related WISC-IV indices. Her VCI of 108 substantiates even more strongly than her FSIQ the conclusion that she is indeed cognitively able and that her classroom problems arise from something other than lack of overall ability. Thus, the answer to Box B is "yes."

Box D, regarding the prospect of a skill deficit, is addressed next. Several sources of information are pertinent. Each of Mona's teachers has identified her as struggling in math, and her current grades are D's. Mona's teacher brought work samples showing that she successfully completed only 55–65% of a recent assignment that was to be done independently (a set of worksheets). Group achievement test math scores, although unconvincing alone, further point to limited math skills (the last two group achievement test math clusters were at the 7th and 5th percentiles). Finally, Mona's Numerical Operations score on the WIAT-II of 76 strongly suggests poor skill development. This score was earned in a quiet setting, where problems with effort, attention, or understanding of directions were controlled. Interestingly, Mona did much better on Math Reasoning, suggesting that her math problems probably do not derive from lack of conceptual understanding as much as from executing procedures on paper. Besides computational arithmetic, Mona may suffer another genuine academic skill problem. She spelled adequately but produced a writing sample that was relatively poor. Her responses here were devoid of organization and were inconsistently punctuated. Her Written Expression scaled score of 78, like her Numerical Operations score, is low relative to her VCI on the WISC-IV. These discrepancies are both statistically significant and occur relatively rarely. Although not definitive of an SLD (i.e., our principal purpose is not to establish an ability–achievement discrepancy or address special education eligibility), her very low achievement scores compared to intact verbal skills suggest the atypical nature of her problem. The answer to Box D is, consequently, "yes." Box G, regarding the type of academic skill deficit, then proves immediately answerable. Her problems are not in language arts subjects. The answer to Box G is "no." Likewise, Box I is now readily addressed. It appears that Mona's problems concern computational arithmetic and complex writing. The "yes" answer to Box I then points to the prospect of NLD or GU.

Careful review of all of Mona's information suggests that her problem appears to match more accurately NLD than GU. Unlike most students with GU, at times her pencil-and-paper work is legible and she, herself, fails to complain about the effort necessary to complete written assignments. Furthermore, review of her work samples and her scores on graphomotor measures (e.g., NEPSY Visuomotor Precision) cannot localize her problem to the realm of pencil control and fine-motor output. In contrast, she has many characteristics of NLD. These include a VCI–PRI difference of 22 points, deficits in computational arithmetic, failure to organize complex tasks (such as writing a theme), mild problems with motor clumsiness, trouble with transitions, and some degree of social immaturity. Favorably, Mona possesses many strengths, including well-developed language skills and outstanding memory. Not surprisingly, she has always been able to acquire rote skills fairly well.

Intervention Plan

Several things may help Mona:

1. To the extent possible, using Mona's verbal abilities and diminishing visual–spatial requirements may help her. For example, tables and diagrams may prove harder to understand than clear, sequentially presented verbal explanations in subjects such as science and social studies. Placing her with teachers whose instructional styles include these characteristics may be wise as she enters junior high. Encouraging her current teacher to avoid assigning copying from the board, completing hands-on projects, or producing copious written work would be worth trying. She may benefit from taking oral, rather than written, tests.

2. In math, helping her rely on her cognitive/linguistic ability as a check for computational accuracy would seem wise. Thus, the steps to solve each mechanical arithmetic problem might be verbally expressed, memorized at a rote level, and subsequently applied in calculations. Similarly, turning a mechanical math task into a story-type problem of her own devising may improve her accuracy. This would allow her to determine if her written answers make real-world sense. Visual aids, such as the previously used marker to keep columns straight or graph paper, would also be worth trying. Because she is dramatically underachieving in computational arithmetic, because her deficits appear to be attributable to underlying processing problems (i.e., "a disorder in one or more of the basic psychological processes"), and because tutoring has failed to alleviate her deficits, she may qualify for special education services in the category of SLD. Her service needs seem best matched by resource placement, which would permit individual or small group instruction in math, coupled with classroom accommodations in written work.

3. Regarding writing, she probably needs a rubric that can help her approach each open-ended writing assignment. Once a set of procedures for organizing writing becomes overlearned and routine, her written performance may improve. Mona may also need a proviso to check her

work (e.g., always proofread), as she may miss visual detail and lack awareness of her own errors.

4. Many children with NLD find it hard to move from one task to another. Novelty may feel aversive and prove confusing. Thus, establishing a routine and predictable school day for Mona may be helpful. Likewise, employing instructional techniques that carefully build from one well-acquired skill to the next would seem to be a good match for her. Discovery approaches, or those that employ unclear expectations and no algorithm for problem solving, may be a poor match for Mona. By the same token, she has superior memory skills. As a way to promote success and as an antidote to frustration, placing her in some activities that require memorization of facts might be wise.

5. She may benefit from social skills training. Refining her pragmatic language skills also appears necessary. Self-monitoring in interpersonal situations may need to be explicitly taught. She should also be encouraged to mix with same-age children as a way of promoting long-term social competence. Given the risk for internalizing psychopathology, her emotional status should be closely monitored.

♦ ♦ ♦

Suggestions for Implementing the Classification and Intervention Planning System

♦

This chapter provides additional information to help you implement our system. It also outlines assessment and intervention planning practices developed over several years that may help school psychologists work more efficiently. Furthermore, we have found that these practices sometimes improve the quality of services for children (as well as parents and teachers) while simultaneously boosting school psychologists' job satisfaction. Some of the suggestions in this chapter concern just our system; others are general and applicable to any system that includes detailed data collection and psychometric testing. Obviously, local policies and practices can affect their viability and determine their ultimate implementation.

THE SCHOOL PSYCHOLOGIST'S ROLE

School psychologists, as holders of advanced degrees, almost always find themselves the most highly educated of those involved in formal evaluations. Their credentials are documented by educational and psychological certification and licensing processes (Pryzwansky, 1999). Moreover, they are likely to evaluate crucial domains that simply do not fall into other professionals' purview (see APA, Division 16, 1998; NASP, 2000). For example, use of tests of intelligence is generally restricted to psychologists. Likewise, memory, executive function, and personality are domains generally reserved for evaluation by psychologists. Besides these areas, many psychologists add linguistic, visual–spatial, motor, and academic tasks to their batteries. Use of extended batteries is especially common for psychologists whose training program included the neuropsychological bases of learning problems and for those who received supplemental formal or informal training in neuropsychological techniques (e.g., Hale & Fiorello, 2004). Although regulations vary by state, licensed psychologists (i.e., those authorized for independent practice by the local jurisdiction) and certified school psychologists often possess authority to document elements of an evaluation and establish eligibility unavailable to other team members. Accordingly, by historical precedence and credentialing, many psychologists assume lead roles. Unfortunately, little empirical research has addressed the leadership topic, and what is available suggests that school psychologists may actually lack specific training to support leadership role fulfillment (Huebner & Gould, 1991).

Among the various configurations of evaluation teams, those that have a designated leader seem to work most efficiently, regardless of whether the designee is a psychologist or not. A leader assures that the evaluation is conducted in a coherent manner, that all necessary assessment components are completed, and that data sufficient to support or rebut emergent hypotheses are collected. Rather than using identical evaluation teams in every instance, such as a psychologist, speech pathologist, occupational therapist, and special educator (so-called fixed team), a flexible team is often more efficient (Wodrich, 1986). Many times, psychologists possess special skills that make them the logical people to lead team efforts (Power, Atkins, Osborne, & Blum, 1994). That is, a psychologist may receive a referral from the pre-evaluation team and collect initial information. If his or her evaluation establishes that others need to be involved, such as a speech pathologist to address an articulation problem, then he or she contacts that professional, indicates the referral question to be answered by the supplemental evaluation, and ensures that data are collated and applied to the emerging hypotheses. Depending on the referral question, presenting problem, and child's age, any of several team members could be designated leader, although in many schools a psychologist or special educator is likely to assume this mantle.

Whether selected as leader or not, a school psychologist's prime task is to assure that the student is fully understood and that recommendations for treatment are produced. If possible, the plan is one supported by empirical evidence (see Stoiber & Kratochwill, 2000). As a school psychologist, you also have the responsibility to share test findings with parents and to adhere to various other obligations of the ethical codes of the NASP (2000) or the

APA (2002). Because you will not be working alone, it is generally wise to make clear to team members your perceptions of the evaluation task and to spell out the scope of your anticipated involvement. Disclosing your perceived responsibilities and stating your scope of practice, which can be done in a low-key but clear manner, cues other team members to share their positions on the same topics. If points of disagreement emerge, these can be discussed until resolved (alternatively, at least you will know about points of professional disagreement). Included may be issues of team leadership, information sharing with parents, and procedures for resolving conflicting opinions (e.g., about the nature and severity of an individual student's problems). If you decide to use the concepts outlined in this book and adopt the supporting rationale for assessment and planning, you may want to have your colleagues familiarize themselves with those concepts. Developing a common approach on key assessment and planning issues appears more easily accomplished early in the process of team formation; furthermore, shared norms may facilitate team effectiveness (Gutkin & Nemeth, 1997).

Regarding interdisciplinary work, speech pathologists, physical therapists, and occupational therapists are likely to use differing terminology to refer to various subtypes of learning or developmental problems. Unfortunately, outside of DSM-IV-TR (which minimally concerns academic disorders), no uniform nosological system exists for children with learning and developmental problems. Lack of a system that describes the common patterns of school failure is one reason for preparing this book and compiling descriptions of various patterns in a single place. Seeking to understand other professions' terminology can be quite instructive for school psychologists. For example, other professionals sometimes seek relatively fine-grained diagnoses, such as speech pathologists' references to word-finding problems or deficits in language pragmatics (Owens, 2004). A psychologist using this book's system might simply conclude that same child suffered from an SLI. The attributes of open-mindedness and commitment to learning from others are important for all diagnosticians working with children. Practicing school psychologists indicate that tolerance, empathy, self-knowledge, and self-confidence often develop only over the course of a career (Guest, 2000), but all psychologists, including those with little experience, can strive for these qualities in order to work well with their counterparts from other professions.

SOURCES OF INFORMATION

Face-to-Face Data Collection

Evaluations that include psychometric testing risk overemphasizing test scores. This is unfortunate because effective evaluations always depend upon a balance of information from both psychometric and nonpsychometric sources. Because test scores are important, it does not follow logically that other sources of information are unimportant, or vice versa. Regarding nonpsychometric information, three groups of individuals can provide valuable information: parents, teachers, and students. One of the best ways to acquire this information is from face-to-face interviews.

Parents

Parents enjoy a historical perspective unavailable to anyone else. Many parents, with proper questioning, describe the subtle character of problems and recall when they arose, as well as what seemed to ameliorate and exaggerate them. Similarly, parents often describe assets (some imagined, most real) unrecognized by others. Of course, parents sometimes have motives to minimize or maximize potential impairments. Parents may not be consciously aware of these tendencies. Parental reports may be slanted either to deny obvious problems or to describe substantial problems where none exist. But in the majority of cases, when parents are candid and their comments free of distortions, they reveal facts previously unknown to school personnel—family stresses (e.g., parents in the midst of separations or abusive home relations), cultural and linguistic background factors, and contributory health conditions (e.g., asthma, epilepsy, type-1 diabetes mellitus). Assuring that adequate instructional opportunities have been provided (regular attendance, a history of adequate academic engagement) is also essential. Parents can sometimes describe intervention efforts and their successes, obviously an important element in RTI consideration, although they should not be counted on to provide such information. Parents can also report the history of other family members with similar developmental, academic, or emotional problems, which might suggest the presence of a heritable disorder. Recognizing recurrent, biologically based patterns in families is likely to be increasingly important as the genetic contribution to many disorders becomes better understood (Plomin, Defries, Craig, & McGuffin, 2003). Accordingly, interviewing parents, typically after a structured social and developmental questionnaire is completed, is conventional practice. Many standard developmental questionnaires (e.g., Mercugliano, Power, & Blum, 1999; Sattler, 2001; Reynolds & Kamphaus, 2004) are available, and most school districts have standard forms routinely completed by parents. In addition, we have found access to a parent-completed BASC-2 to be quite helpful (see Chapter 1). Of course, useful information may not be forthcoming even after the most expertly conducted interviews, but interviews are the best hope of eliciting such information.

Favorably, school psychologists now appear to endorse the value of parental information, at least for some issues. For example, 82.3% of school psychologists recently indicated that they always involve parents when assessing for ADHD (Kilpatrick-Demaray et al., 2003). Importantly, collecting information during assessment may set the stage for information sharing later. Because parents will hear results at the process's conclusion, it is good to meet them near its start. Parental contact can be harder for school psychologists than for psychologists working in clinic settings, and this fact may sometimes prevent close psychologist–parent alliances from developing (Wodrich, 2004). Notwithstanding inconvenience and logistical barriers, parent contact is extremely valuable.

Teachers

Classroom teachers routinely provide invaluable information that complements, and sometimes contrasts with, parental information. What teachers typically lack in longitudinal perspective they more than make up for in two ways. First, they can recognize where students stand compared to their classmates. Unlike parents, they can indicate when a student's oral reading is truly deficient and can index (compared to current and past students) the problem's severity. The ability to detect outliers is especially crucial in a process that must determine if special services are needed and how much individual attention a student warrants (whether or not special services are used; Gresham, Reschly, & Carey, 1987; Weissberg et al., 1987). Second, teachers' professional understanding of the developmental/learning process permits fine-grained observation of existing deficits and delineation of situational factors that influence how these deficits are expressed in the classroom. For example, understanding of a third-grade student is greatly enhanced by teacher reports that he reads too fast, shuns word attack strategies, and guesses impulsively unless he is prompted to slow down. Accordingly, teacher interviews, often supplemented by checklists (e.g., Academic Performance Rating Scale [APRS], DuPaul et al., 1991; also see Shapiro, 2004), are helpful. Similarly, we find use of the teacher BASC-2 or Teacher Report Form (Achenbach & Rescorla, 2001) to be valuable (see Chapter 1).

Student

Child interviews should be conducted routinely, although their depth, focus, and complexity vary. Some students, especially those in junior high and above, recognize why school is hard and can describe the distinctive challenges they face. Self-disclosing older students typically provide concrete information, such as descriptions of their poor performance in math or English or their inability to write easily and clearly. Even young students can sometimes identify ways to make their learning easier (Blazer, 1999). Nonetheless, it is the rare student who is able to isolate and describe faithfully an underlying cognitive problem. In fact, perhaps even more than parents, students seem to misidentify information-processing problems. For instance, students sometimes complain about their poor memory (such as failure to recall facts in social studies), whereas test scores reveal that they actually lack background ideas (e.g., they possess a pattern of an SL or SLI). Such students' scores on measures of rote memory (e.g., memorization of word lists) may be perfectly average. Similarly, some students contend that school is hard for them because they read too slowly, although in reality they experience deficient word identification and word attack skills (e.g., may have a pattern consistent with PRD). Others say that their teachers talk so fast that they are unable to understand (suggesting the prospect of an SLI), whereas analysis of all information suggests that the real problem is an inability to transition from one activity to the next (e.g., deficit in processing novelty, indicating the possibility of NLD). In other words, patterns of success and failure contained in work samples, parent and teacher comments, and psychometric scores are generally more important in understanding learning problems than students' self-descriptions. Thus, child interviews only occasionally provide valuable information about the nature of underlying processing or cognitive deficits.

Identifying internalizing psychopathology is a different matter. Many children know what they feel and believe, but they may forgo sharing personal information (e.g., anxious or sad feelings, obsessive urges) with even their close confidants and parents. Consequently, this important information may be unrecognized by others. Accordingly, a skillful interview is generally the best method of eliciting these kinds of covert facts and personal feelings (Hope et al., 1999). In our system, CU is closely related to internalizing psychopathology. As a result, an interview is generally needed to confirm the presence of CU, which is involved in slow work completion, checking behavior, rituals, and worry (see Chapter 4). Standard interview forms are widely available (e.g., Sattler, 2001). Self-report rating scales (e.g., BASC-2; Personality Inventory for Youth, Lachar & Gruber, 1994) can also be used, although we have not found the information yielded by these techniques sufficient to justify their routine use.

In summary regarding interviews, hypotheses typically emerge from parental, teacher, and student interviews. Ideally, school psychologists consider the conditions listed in this book and their cardinal characteristics and follow the flowchart outlined in Figure 1.1/5.1. For example, suspicion of a reading problem triggers data collection from several sources. These data permit the psychologist to address general cognitive development, the legitimacy of the reading skill deficit, the presence of coexisting academic problems (i.e., the prospect of other language arts deficits), and whether emergent information is more indicative of phonological (PRD) or general language problems (SLI). Data collection might be driven, in part, by suspicion that PRD is present. As hypotheses arise, data collection follows a path that guarantees ample information to address each decision point (i.e., Boxes A–J) in Figure 1.1/5.1. Interview data are just one, but an important, potential information source.

Records

School psychologists are routinely taught to find valuable information in records, such as the contents of cumulative folders (see Nagle, 2002). As suggested earlier, all information should point toward the same diagnostic conclusion if a condition has been properly identified, and this applies to records as well. Various components of records provide potentially useful facts.

Report Card Grades

Report card grades are sometimes helpful, although this is more often true for students in junior high school and above. Grades are generally available in cumulative folders. If a student has a genuine academic deficit, then grades should reflect it. In other words, hypothesized literacy failures (which may suggest an underlying SLI or PRD) typically should be reflected in low marks in reading and writing but not in math. Unfortunately for our purposes, grades in the elementary years may be indicated to be satisfactory or better for all students. Without a meaningful distribution of grades, evidence of a struggling student is often impossible to glean from records. Furthermore, systems for indicating report card grades in the elementary years can seem inscrutable (especially for psychologists working with students from many different school districts); standard like grades are rarely used for the youngest students. Beginning in about the fifth or sixth grade in most settings, grades start to reflect more faithfully students' classroom status. Thus, early academic grades from report cards may not help much; later ones may be helpful.

Supplemental Report Card Information

Teachers' supplemental marks on report cards seem to have the opposite pattern, more value when assessing younger than older students. For example, students with ADHD almost always have indications of "fails to complete work," "lacks attention to detail," or "does not use time wisely" if these options are available for teachers to endorse. Once instruction becomes departmentalized (e.g., separate teachers for science, English, and social studies), such comments, which presuppose close observation of individual students, often disappear or lose their diagnostic value. Thus, attention or performance problems are often apparent in report cards in the early school years, but not later. The same may be true of emotional or interpersonal problems for the same reasons (i.e., they depend on close observation). High school teachers may be unaware that one of their many students is unhappy or lacks friends. On the other hand, junior high and high school teachers typically possess spreadsheets that indicate test scores and homework points. These data sources can pinpoint each student's current academic status. Thus, it may be quite easy to figure out if a low grade in math, for example, stems from missed assignments (perhaps attributable to ADHD) or poor test performance and inadequate mastery of math subject matter (perhaps due to NLD or a general cognitive problem).

Group Achievement Test Scores

Group achievement test scores offer another potential source of verification for emergent hypotheses, and these are generally kept in cumulative folders as well. High scores on group tests are routinely more instructive than low ones. Because students' success on mass-administered tests can be influenced by attention, linguistic, hand–eye coordination, and motivation problems, their results cannot be blindly accepted. Recall that group tests are sometimes administered in extremely large rooms where monitoring is limited and where students must listen carefully to directions and work without guidance or prompting. As a result, elementary students with SLI may fail to understand where to begin responding, how much time is available, or what to do in the face of uncertainty. Likewise, older students with ADHD may understand directions but stop working before time has elapsed or avoid carefully checking their optically scanned answer sheets to assure accuracy. Under these circumstances, a test intended to measure social studies knowledge, for example, can become a test of attention and perseverance. Such sources of error represent construct-irrelevant variance on content area tests (e.g., math, social studies, science; Messick, 1995). Accordingly, low scores on group achievement tests should be interpreted cautiously. Low scores in the presence of other evidence of poor academic skill development (e.g., work samples, teacher reports, individually administered tests) is expected, but low scores without such evidence do not automatically indicate the presence of true academic skill deficits.

High scores generally are more trustworthy. Students are unlikely to guess well enough to earn high scores without actually possessing skills. Moreover, few students copy their more academically able neighbors' answers and therefore score better than they should. Thus, students with adequate test scores are unlikely to be viewed by school psychologists as good candidates for detailed psychometric evaluations (Huebner, 1989).

Curriculum-Based Measurement Data

CBM is an excellent data source to help determine how well a student is functioning compared to grade-mates. Unfortunately, CBM may be available to the intervention team only if a school has chosen this method of assessment to screen for those students at-risk for learning problems. In the favorable scenario where school-wide CBM information is available, for example, a third grader referred to an intervention team due to poor reading can be evaluated on difficulty controlled, third-grade oral fluency probes, and objective information about his or her status compared to local norms can be established. Additionally, CBM data may benefit the intervention team and evaluating psychologist by serving as one basis of judging if a student is responding to intervention. This can be especially helpful if it is determined that a favorable RTI depends on special education services. For example, it may be possible in some cases to see acceptable RTI for a student outside the parameters of special education, whereas in other cases such a favorable response is attainable only if special services are accessed.

Health Records

Health records are also important to check. Some health information (such as hearing and vision screenings) may be evident in students' cumulative folders. A health condition able to affect classroom learning (such as asthma, type-1 diabetes mellitus, epilepsy) may be indicated there as well. In addition, a commonly used health, developmental, and social history form can bring out parents' indication of health problems (see Sattler, 2001). Checking the school nurse's record is wise. All of this is important because health problems have become increasingly recognized as able to mimic learning disabilities. When a chronic health problem is present, it is essential either to consult the child's physician regarding classroom implications or access educator-friendly information about the disorder (e.g., see Brown, 2004). The syndromes described in this book are not appropriate to use for children with chronic illness without considering the impact of a disease, its treatment (e.g., effects of medication), and children's adjustment to their illness.

Observation

Classroom Observations

Observing a student in class is often extremely helpful, even though several observations may be required to yield reliable conclusions (Doll & Elliott, 1994). Many formal, structured observation techniques exist, but their review is beyond the scope of this book (see Platzman et al., 1992). However, informal techniques are adequate for many students. Watching a student's work habits, reaction to academic challenges, and social interaction can be instructive, especially if the observer remembers to consider the possibility of the patterns listed in this book. In other words, classroom observations generally are made to look for specific patterns, not to collect undigested information about a student. Consistent with this point, two common weaknesses appear in reports of classroom observation, and these sometimes limit the ultimate usefulness of the direct observational data.

First, observations are often recorded as facts about overt behavior devoid of inferences. An example might be "Marcus listened to his teacher's directions, looked around the room for 15 seconds, then approached a classmate for clarification. He then returned to his seat and started working again, but after another 40 seconds looked around again briefly." Without comparisons to classmates or inferences about the effectiveness or appropriateness of a student's performance, the value of sterile information like this may be limited. Alternatively, properly analyzed observations of the same situation might speak directly to the prospect of a disorder, such as SLI or ADHD. Consider this observation: "Unlike any of his classmates, Marcus seemed to have trouble when his teacher gave verbal directions, resulting in hesitancy and repeated seeking of clarification from a fellow student." This single comment, when combined with others, may help to suggest SLI (Marcus struggles when he must listen to verbal directions) or NLD (Marcus becomes confused when he must make transitions). School psychologists are encouraged to trust their professional training and knowledge and to avoid acting as perfunctory recorders of decontextualized, uninterpreted student behavior.

Second, situational and task factors are often underemphasized in reports of observations. To support a system of identifying and planning based on syndromes, observations need to indicate under what conditions success and failure occur. For example, some students are described as inattentive, restless, or disruptive, suggesting the possibility of ADHD-C. Structured observations (such as outlined by Shapiro, 2004), however, can establish whether inattention intensifies during written assignments but abates when listening (but not writing) predominates. Such observations suggest the possibility of NLD or GU rather than ADHD-C. Other patterns of success and failure might imply the presence of alternative conditions. The point is that observations can occur in the context of emerging hypotheses and that the inferences drawn from observations can help support or refute these hypotheses. By using the comprehensive approach suggested in this book and attending to the conditions we describe, in-class observation can be consolidated with other information to support conclusions. Favorably, school psychologists appear routinely to use direct observation of students in natural settings, at least when behavioral or emotional problems are at issue (Shapiro & Heick, 2004). Unfavorably, simplistic or uninsightful observations sometimes provide little help in the quest to understand why an individual student is failing to learn. Of course, structured observations of antecedents, behaviors, and consequences are suggested during the pre-referral problem-solving process that generally precedes the search for special conditions.

Observations during Testing

As with in-class observations, testing-based observations support the broader task of diagnostic hypothesis testing. Unlike classroom observations, however, inferences based on test behavior suffer from limited ecological validity. That is, the child's requirements to understand directions, answer questions, inhibit impulses, sustain attention, and cooperate while working one-on-one with an adult are unlike most classroom demands. The good news is that these requirements are often sufficiently uniform to permit individual differences to become apparent. Indeed, there is some evidence to support the validity of factors such as motivation and persistence that arise during standardized test administrations (Glutting, Oakland, & McDermott, 1989). Using their individual universes of previously evaluated children as informal databases, school psychologists might recognize problems like limited ability to formulate answers or inhibit impulses, as well as greater-than-typical need for supplemental explanations. Using patterns described in this book as a guide, school psychologists can transfer their observations into secondary evidence for or against the chances of various conditions. Checklists (or open-ended questions organized into categories) to record observations are provided in most test record forms. For example, the WJ III Tests of Cognitive Abilities record form prompts examiners to rate students' test behavior on several dimensions (see Figure 6.1). Although these dimensions do not correspond to the conditions in our system, examiners' ratings nonetheless can be used to speak to the chances of one or more of the disorders in our system (see samples of open-ended observations from case examples in Chapter 5).

Outside Evaluations

Sometimes students are evaluated before school psychologists become involved. In fact, many psychologists, learning disability specialists, and educator-advocates focus their private practices on determining the educational needs of struggling students. Educational information may also arise from the diagnostic work of pediatricians, especially developmental pediatricians, many of whom view school learning as central to their practice, as well as primary care physicians (Shapiro & Gallico, 1993; American Academy of Pediatrics, 1999). Likewise, some neurologists concentrate on school problems or describe syndromes or diseases with school implica-

RICHARD W. WOODCOCK ♦ KEVIN S. MCGREW ♦ NANCY MATHER

Tests of Cognitive Abilities

STANDARD AND EXTENDED BATTERIES

W|J
|||

TEST RECORD

IDENTIFYING INFORMATION

Last Name __Heringa__ First Name __Mieke__

Sex: ☐ M ☒ F   ID __06114__

Date of Birth: __06__ / __21__ / __1996__
MM   DD   YYYY

School/Organization __Abbott Elementary School__

Teacher/Department __B. Martenson__

Adult Subjects: { Education (Years Completed) _____
Occupation _____

Date of Testing: __05__ / __02__ / __2005__
MM   DD   YYYY

Grade __3__ ___(Years Retained)___ Years Skipped _____ Years of Schooling _____)

Examiner's Name __M. Slack__

Normative Basis (Check one) ☒ Age ☐ Grade (K–12.9) ☐ 2-Year College (13–14.9) ☐ 4-Year College/University (13–18)

Additional Information

Does the subject have glasses?
☐ Yes ☒ No
Were they used during testing?
☐ Yes ☒ No

Does the subject have a hearing aid?
☐ Yes ☒ No
Was it used during testing?
☐ Yes ☒ No

Other Information _____

Year-Round School Only:
_____ Number of Days of Instruction in Year
_____ Number of Days Completed So Far

TEST SESSION OBSERVATIONS CHECKLIST

Check only one category for each item.

Level of conversational proficiency
- ☐ 1. Very advanced
- ☐ 2. Advanced
- ☐ 3. Typical for age/grade
- ☒ 4. Limited
- ☐ 5. Very limited

Level of cooperation
- ☐ 1. Exceptionally cooperative throughout the examination
- ☒ 2. Cooperative (typical for age/grade)
- ☐ 3. Uncooperative at times
- ☐ 4. Uncooperative throughout the examination

Level of activity
- ☐ 1. Seemed lethargic
- ☐ 2. Typical for age/grade
- ☒ 3. Appeared fidgety or restless at times
- ☐ 4. Overly active for age/grade; resulted in difficulty attending to tasks

Attention and concentration
- ☐ 1. Unusually absorbed by the tasks
- ☐ 2. Attentive to the tasks (typical for age/grade)
- ☒ 3. Distracted often
- ☐ 4. Consistently inattentive and distracted

Self-confidence
- ☐ 1. Appeared confident and self-assured
- ☒ 2. Appeared at ease and comfortable (typical for age/grade)
- ☐ 3. Appeared tense or worried at times
- ☐ 4. Appeared overtly anxious

Care in responding
- ☐ 1. Very slow and hesitant in responding
- ☐ 2. Slow and careful in responding
- ☐ 3. Prompt but careful in responding (typical for age/grade)
- ☒ 4. At times responded too quickly
- ☐ 5. Impulsive and careless in responding

Response to difficult tasks
- ☐ 1. Noticeably increased level of effort for difficult tasks
- ☐ 2. Generally persisted with difficult tasks (typical for age/grade)
- ☒ 3. Attempted but gave up easily
- ☐ 4. Would not try difficult tasks at all

Do you have any reason to believe this testing session may not represent a fair sample of the subject's abilities? ☒ No
☐ Yes. These results may not be a fair estimate because ... _____

Were any modifications made to the standardized test procedures during this administration? ☒ No
☐ Yes. The following modifications were made: _____

FIGURE 6.1. Facesheet to Woodcock–Johnson III Tests of Cognitive Ability. From Woodcock, McGrew, and Mather (2001). Copyright © 2001 by The Riverside Publishing Company. First page of test record form from the Woodcock-Johnson® III (WJ III®) reproduced with permission of the publisher. All rights reserved.

tions (Erenberg, 1991). In considering information from all of these sources, open-mindedness coupled with circumspection is key.

Specifically, school-based practitioners are counseled against out-of-hand negative reactions. Rejecting others' work because of its unfamiliar language and format or its reliance on unrecognized diagnostic tools can be reflexive. Many outside evaluations contain wonderful insights, and much helpful information sometimes can be found; unbiased reading and careful consideration of the content of these evaluations is advised. Even the best outside evaluations, however, accomplish only part of the task. School teams are still required to figure out how to integrate findings into the context of a specific school. Furthermore, some outside evaluations fail to adopt a broad mind-set, and many represent less than the full evaluation advocated here. For example, some evaluations lack recommendations and instead focus on a student's eligibility for special education services. In these instances, school psychologists (and the local school team) are still obliged to collect sufficient information so that they can understand the child fully. When outside evaluations appear, it is important for school psychologists to recognize what they offer and avoid being distracted by special education eligibility statements. Even when outside evaluations reach unacceptable conclusions about service eligibility, the same evaluation might successfully illuminate the cause of school problems. School-based professionals, therefore, should strive to back away from initial overfocus on legal issues that often leave parents and school officials at loggerheads.

These points aside, some outside evaluations are not at all helpful, and their conclusions should be largely discounted. Evaluations that are especially inadequate are those that merely make a case for special education services (some of these are clearly slanted to make parents happy) but fail to address the nature of the child's underlying problems and strengths. In these cases, students probably require a full evaluation of the type described in this book. Likewise, evaluations that document one of the conditions in this book but are plainly incomplete or poorly executed need to be questioned. For example, an evaluation using only a WISC-IV and an achievement battery might inappropriately conclude that a student suffers from an NLD. Without background information, observation or interview to address social skills, and a more complete psychometric base, this conclusion is likely to be premature. Accordingly, beginning an intervention plan for such a student with the supposition that his or her problems derive from NLD would be misguided. This child would need supplemental assessment and use of a decision-making process to confirm the nature of his or her problem. Be careful about outside evaluations.

This warning is especially pertinent for ADHD and all of the other performance-related conditions outlined in Chapter 4. If an outside evaluation leaves unaddressed certain questions, findings from it may be erroneous (or at least incomplete). As shown in Figure 1.1/5.1 (Box B and D), general cognitive deficits and lack of academic skills should be ruled out before ADHD (or OCD, depression, etc.) is ruled in (for example, see Hoff, Doepke, & Landau, 2002; Kutcher et al., 2004). Yet school-based professionals may encounter children with such a diagnosis already affixed by a nonschool professional before IQ, information-processing, or academic components are considered. When an incomplete evaluation is received from outside the school, the school team is left with unresolved questions: Might this student's failure spring from weak academic skills rather than attention problems? Might he or she struggle because of an undetected cognitive or information-processing problem? Although not all students with an ADHD (or other psychiatric) diagnosis require full psychometric evaluations, consideration must be given routinely to academic skills and to confirming that there is no obvious cognitive delay. That is, background information should be reviewed and parents carefully questioned about academic skills and cognitive development in all cases. Because most ADHD diagnoses are established by primary care physicians, who almost never assess cognitive or academic skills directly (AAP, 2000; Williams, Klinepeter, Palmes, Pulley, & Foy, 2004), school psychologists should expect to encounter this situation. Besides wariness for ADHD, a disorder whose rate has grown dramatically in recent years, school-based professionals should be vigilant of other mushrooming diagnoses (e.g., bipolar disorder, Asperger's disorder). School psychologists might be dubious in instances where the condition's presence is not well documented, a limited evaluation was conducted, unconventional procedures were used, or a practitioner possesses only unconventional credentials.

WHEN AND WHERE TO TEST

Schools are wonderful places to observe students, consult with teachers, oversee intervention plans, and provide in-service training. But many of them are poor places in which to conduct valid and time-efficient psychometric testing. Three reasons seem to underlie this unfortunate fact. First, children come to school with a specific mind-set unless they are advised beforehand to the contrary. That is, most children arrive at school expecting to follow their regular schedule of attendance taking, lunch money collecting, calendar drills, and the like. They know which lessons occur when, and they may be looking forward to ones they especially like. In other words, they recognize when recess happens and when a special event, such a birthday party, is on the schedule. Consequently, unplanned, and especially impromptu, removal by a stranger for testing can be anxiety producing, bewildering, and disappointing. Likewise, campus-based evaluations often leave the student distracted as he or she continues to think about the prospect of missing events; he or she may repeatedly try to convince the examiner to finish the evaluation so as to be able to return to class. Such factors can compromise test validity.

Second, psychologists sometimes must perform standardized evaluations in substandard settings and without access to a full array of testing equipment. We have both been forced to work at tables that prohibit proper arrangement of test materials, in rooms that are too hot or too cold, and in settings where interruptions (such as by teachers looking for supplies or overhead announcements) are impossible to prevent. Itinerant school psychologists know that it is impossible to carry with them all of the material that might be needed for an evaluation. A special ability test needed to round out an evaluation too often seems to be left at another location. For comprehensive evaluations, where hypotheses emerge and require confirmation with specialized instruments, this limitation can be painfully restrictive. Incomplete or nonstandard evaluations, both threats to validity, may ensue.

Third, campus-based evaluations sometimes suffer by leaving parents out of the process for too long. Although special education rules appear to mandate direct pre-evaluation contact between some members of the evaluation team and parents (U.S. Department of Education, 1997), early contact between parent and school psychologist per se is not universal. Psychoeducational evaluations are risky if they begin by a psychologist simply going to a classroom, being introduced, and then bringing a student to a testing location. Besides inducing anxiety and puzzlement, this manner of evaluation sometimes fails to convey that parents and school are working together to accomplish something important to both. If parental contact is not made at the time of testing, important situational information may also be missed. For example, parents can indicate if a student is not feeling well, is especially anxious, missed a medication dosage, or is not wearing his or her prescription lenses. Parental contact at the commencement of testing can protect evaluation validity.

The antidote to all of these problems is increased advance planning before evaluations and intensified organization during them. In the extreme (or ideal), a designated centralized student study center provides the venue for psychometric testing. Psychometric labs with custom tables, adjustable chairs, adequate lighting, and soundproofing would be provided at such a site. Such a configuration also allows all test material and test record forms to be shelved within reach. Having used this setting in a clinic, we both can attest to the startling gain in efficiency it provides. A valid assessment is also much easier to accomplish in a specifically configured evaluation setting. A setup like this may require so much scheduling and transportation as to make it impossible to adopt for most public schools. Few schools do this now or are likely to in the future. We would be remiss, however, in failing to point out that the ease and speed of psychometric testing is so great under ideal circumstances that benefit is likely, even if overhead and transportation costs were fully accounted for. In other words, the extra cost of these line items may be compensated for by greatly increased numbers of evaluations and concomitantly reduced school psychologists' cost. There is now a nationwide shortage of school psychologists (Curtis, Grier, & Hunley, 2004) that approaches crisis severity in some locations. Optimum efficiency (and economy) provided by creating specialized assessment settings may be worth investigating in some of these locations. As presently conducted, school-based evaluations are extremely time consuming (see Lichtenstein & Fischetti, 1998, for a breakdown of time and activities).

Because acquiring an idealized setup is unlikely, approximations of the ideal might be considered. The advantages of advance scheduling and direct parental contact alone can be substantial. For example, we have found great benefit from scheduling evaluations that start at 8:00 A.M. and asking parents to bring their child to school for the appointment. For many parents, this would mean an early drop-off time for their son or daughter. Of course, many parents are unable to do this; however, many others not only agree, but also appreciate a chance to meet the psychologist, share information (briefly), and learn directly what can be accomplished by such an assessment. Equally important, face-to-face contact between psychologist and parent clearly conveys the evaluation's collaborative nature. This fact often allays students' anxiety. We typically suggest that students are scheduled for evaluations that run from 8:00 A.M. until noon. Special arrangements will be made for a later lunch (if needed). Many parents choose to send a snack. Similarly, the student is informed that he or she will not be attending school that morning because of a special appointment, much like an appointment with a dentist or eye doctor. Reassurances that no shots will be given and that he or she has done nothing wrong are provided routinely. Most children 8 years or older can be evaluated in a single setting if all material is available, if they understand from the outset that they are expected to work throughout the morning, and if distractions are eliminated and 5-minute breaks are provided every hour. To make this timeline work, the evaluator needs to be fully proficient in administering the relevant tests. Equally important, the school psychologist must express an enthusiastic and engaging style. All of these things are necessary. For example, if examiners are slow and unsure about administration, the process slows enormously, the child becomes bored, and the assessment will have to stop earlier or risk being invalid. Under these circumstances, multiple testing sessions will probably be needed. Likewise, a stiff examiner who fails to build rapport and does not engage the student in between-task conversation has little chance of finding a student eager to work all morning. Mentoring by a psychologist with an effective interpersonal style and proficient test-administration skills can be remarkably helpful, especially for beginning school psychologists.

Besides benefiting the student, this approach often enhances psychologists' sense of professionalism. In other words, legitimate sense of one's importance is promoted by use of executive-type scheduling, early contact in a professional-to-parent format, and structured (rather than haphazard) access to a student. Resistance from teachers, who wish to preserve sacred instruction time, can usually be circumvented. Key to such an approach is to adopt scheduled evaluations as routine practice, emphasize that one morning of instruction only will be missed for the psychological portion of the evaluation, indicate that other professionals also schedule their time, and, perhaps most important, demonstrate that working this way produces quick evaluation turn-around.

SHARING FINDINGS WITH PARENTS

For many school psychologists, psychoeducational evaluations have been historically synonymous with establishing special education eligibility. Students have been tested to see if they qualify for special education. Accordingly, parental meetings, including those during which one might share evaluation results, often follow basic administrative guidelines. For example, it is common for school psychologists to have two contacts with parents. The first is a pre-evaluation meeting (perhaps by phone, but sometimes not at all if other team members execute this meeting) to outline evaluation procedures and to explain that special education services may be in the offing. The second is a multidisciplinary conference to discuss evaluation findings and address eligibility. In many parts of the country, these meetings are legalistic in tone and comprise many team members. Not infrequently, candid and open discussion is difficult.

School psychologists, of course, cannot abandon their administrative obligations, nor can they fail to honor administrative guidelines that were promulgated to protect students' and parents' rights. Nonetheless, ethical and practice imperatives may be impossible to satisfy by merely following the administrative steps required by local schools. School psychologists are encouraged to adopt the task of "assessment to understand students" and uncouple it from their parallel administrative (special education-related) duties (see Chapter 1). Psychologists are obliged to share evaluation findings with parents in a manner that guarantees their understanding and enables results to benefit the child. As a result, many parents require a pre-multidisciplinary, post-testing evaluation conference. We encourage such a meeting. This meeting permits candid sharing of results, some of which are so sensitive and emotionally laden as to warrant a conference free from administrative formality. This would be the case, for example, if test findings suggest mental retardation in a previously undiagnosed child. In addition, by meeting alone (or with one or two directly related team members), results can be explained in a way that helps parents understand without consuming the time of other team members. Complicated or complex evaluation findings may also trigger a separate meeting. Such meetings can be time-efficient because the need to hear detailed evaluation findings and to delve into details and simplified explanations are different for parents and members of the professional evaluation team. With a pre-multidisciplinary conference, psychologists can adjust their explanation of findings to parents' level of understanding without other team members present. Although pre-multidisciplinary conferences can be logistical headaches, they are generally worth the inconvenience.

The *Standards for Educational and Psychological Testing*, written in part by the American Psychological Association, call for results to be shared with the client or a responsible party (American Educational Research Association, 2002). The task is to promote understanding, but the means vary. A college student seeking vocational guidance who completed an interest inventory often needs to learn his or her results with a literal description. In contrast, parents of an elementary student who was administered six tests (each with many subtests) require something different. It is impossible and counterproductive to explain every score on every subtest. We have tried it ourselves, and we have witnessed unsuccessful attempts by others many times. Providing parents with this much information, which is invariably couched in psychological jargon, is apt to leave them confused. Most of the lay public, presumably including parents, conceptualizes cognitive ability fairly globally (Furnham, 2004), and much of what is attempted by detailed explanation runs contrary to this conceptualization. An alternative to extremely detailed score reporting is proposed, and it follows the logic of this book's overall organization. Specifically, parents seem to understand evaluation findings, including those from psychometric tests, when they address four major questions:

1. Is the problem due to general cognitive ability?
2. Is the problem due to lack of productivity in a student who actually possesses academic skills?
3. Is the problem one of failure to acquire academic (or related language or fine-motor) skills, and what weaknesses in development underlie this failure?
4. Is there really a problem at all (of the type included in our system)?

That is, parent conferences can follow the decision-making process that you have already used.

If psychologists indicate that the evaluation was conducted to answer these questions, focused information can be shared to address each question. Often, this can be done in a top-down approach. For example:

> We evaluated Adam so that we could understand why school has been so hard for him. Results of our evaluation, including tests, told us the following. First, Adam is bright enough to read and write better than he currently does. There is no problem with his overall thinking ability. Second, just as you and his teacher suspected, his reading and spelling skills are much poorer than those of other students his age. Third, there are underlying problems in how Adam understands and uses language that make school hard for him. Lack of general language development seems to be at the heart of his inability to learn some school subjects. Now, let us show you some of the information that led us to this conclusion.

Beginning with an overview (top-down approach), school psychologists then can convey findings with just enough detail to allow parents to understand, but not feel overwhelmed. As an example, the following might be said:

> We first wanted to make sure that Adam's current level of overall ability was okay. When you told us about his development and his school records were checked, we doubted if this was the problem. He has shown a lot of mechanical ability historically and is very good in math. He was administered an individual test, an IQ test, that measured his current ability in four areas. He did at least average in three of them. He showed above-average development in recognizing patterns and solving problems that did not involve words. He also scored in the average range on short-term memory, such as remembering number sequences, and in an area that required him to work quickly with a pencil. He did have trouble on the part of the IQ test that required him to use language to solve problems or to describe relationships. Also, his vocabulary was not very large or sophisticated. Even though the verbal portions of IQ testing were low, we know that lack of overall ability is not his problem.

The questions about academic skill development and narrow cognitive deficits can be handled in the same manner, with the amount of detail and number of examples modified as necessary. Explanations that repeatedly return to the key decision points seem to help parents see the big picture. Parents can be reminded that evaluations are designed to answer questions and that this is how the team proceeded to answer the important questions about their child.

A top-down approach, however, is not advised in at least two situations. The first of these is any of the IQ-related conditions outlined in

Chapter 2. Because parents often harbor misconceptions about IQ, are so quick to doubt the validity of ability scores, and are apt to mistrust an examiner who is ascribing low IQ to their child, a bottom-up approach may be needed. The bottom-up approach involves review of each IQ subtest. Parents are told the test's content, may be given samples (hypothetical, not real items), and are given their child's precise score (as it appears on the face of the test record form, a computer printout, or a specially prepared graph). For each subtest, such as on the WISC-IV, parents are told that scores reflect current functioning and depend on cognitive maturity, inherent ability as it becomes manifest, environmental influences, and individual factors, such as motivation and curiosity. Parents are provided an on-the-spot mini-course in the measurement of mental ability. This degree of detail is also provided for scores on achievement tests and, for children with mental retardation, adaptive behavior scales. Using a bottom-up approach, psychologists must decide how much information to provide about special ability tests (e.g., measures of phonological processing, fine-motor speed). Typically, we simply state that many other tests, such as those involving memory, hand–eye coordination, or attention, fell in the same range and are compatible with our general conclusions (if this is indeed the pattern found). Outlier scores, especially high ones, generally are shared as well. A candid explanation is provided about why outlier scores fail to alter the overall conclusion of general ability (e.g., "Your daughter did better on measures of rote memory, as you can see from these scores, but every task that required judgment, analysis, or problem solving produced scores at the same level"). Background and nonpsychometric information are typically covered in this process as well. The bottom-up approach helps parents appreciate the depth and complexity of the evaluation. Equally important, it can defuse the negative reactions of some parents by clarifying the meaning of test scores. Specifically, parents see what is meant by general cognitive ability, why this ability is so important for school success, where their child currently scores, and that present scores measure neither innate intelligence nor guarantee future scores. If mental retardation is concluded to be present, a host of related misconceptions about that diagnosis can be addressed at this time.

A second indication for the bottom-up approach is the dubious and/or openly hostile parent (regardless of the presence of an IQ-related condition). Such a parent may be angry because he or she believes that the school is identifying a problem that does not exist. Strong parental denial may be present. Alternatively, another parent may be angry because his or her child is not deemed eligible for special education services. An ardent desire to secure services is sought because it is believed that creating eligibility and awarding more intensive instruction are the only hope for success. As might be suspected from the discussion above, the detailed nature of the bottom-up approach often conveys respect for parents (e.g., the parent may think, "Thank you for taking so much time and concern to see that I understand"). It can also communicate that a psychologist is available to help the child be better understood and treated at school, not just to address special education placement. Furthermore, many parents' negative attitudes arise because of genuine confusion about the nature of their child's problem. A comprehensive review of what has been found can contribute to understanding that may have long been elusive.

Because it is generally helpful to conclude by reviewing the same four questions mentioned above, psychologists may need to highlight salient findings as they are presented during use of a bottom-up approach (e.g., "Try to remember what that pattern of low scores on language-related subtests looked like because we will come back to their importance later." Subsequent discussion of SLI can be supported). That is, after scores are reviewed, parents may be directed to consider whether the data support an IQ-related, performance-related, or narrow-information processing problem. This would be done with the previously reviewed WISC-IV pattern visible to help answer the question "Is the problem one of failure to acquire academic (or related language or fine-motor) skills, and what weaknesses in development underlie this failure?" In other words, at the conclusion of score review, parents still need to be directed back to conclusions, and findings still need to be summarized in a clear manner by the psychologist. Having parents consider the four questions above is often a necessary vehicle for understanding how the diagnostic conclusion was reached.

School psychologists are advised to remember, again, that students should be evaluated so that they can be understood and helped. Patterns are recognized and labels used to facilitate this process. Psychologists need to decide when to share names of conditions (such as those included here) with parents. Sometimes describing the overt manifestations of NLD *and* the NLD term helps parents. With complete information such as this, parents may better conceptualize their child's assets and liabilities and better remember these elements over time. On the other hand, some parents misunderstand or obsess about terms, and for them providing labels may be counterproductive. Many of the terms used here are heuristic and provide convenient ways for diagnosticians to organize their thinking and planning, but they may not be widely used (or recognized by others, especially GU and CU). Accordingly, it may be unwise to share specific terms. Professional judgment obviously is necessary in each instance.

Two exceptions to professionals' latitude in reporting labels exist. The first is ADHD (both ADHD-C and ADHD-I). Because a host of interventions exist for this condition, parents are entitled to know that it is present. Similarly, if MiMR (or any level of mental retardation) is documented, then parents must be told this fact unequivocally. Beyond service entitlement, a mental retardation designation may compel supplemental evaluations, such as genetic studies (see Wodrich & Kaplan, 2005). For each of these conditions (ADHD and MiMR), which must be definitely confirmed, we list specific criteria to be satisfied, whereas for all other conditions in this book we merely list characteristics (see discussion in Chapter 1). Some psychologists struggle to overcome squeamishness in sharing findings. To practice fully and effectively, bad news at times has to be conveyed. Concerning developmental evaluations, British psychiatrist Jeremy Turk (2004) offered the following compassionate but cogent statement: "Nobody wants to learn bad news, but it is a lot better than no news at all. At least you know where you stand" (p. 16). This statement seems apropos to many sensitive school psychologist–parent encounters.

The line between assessment and intervention is sometimes drawn too starkly. In reality, therapeutic outcome may arise from well-conducted parent conferences, in part because previous misunderstanding can be removed and a student's behavior may be reframed in a more positive light (Bowman & Goldberg, 1983). Thus, some barriers to effective treatment may be removed by the assessment process itself. In other instances, follow-up treatment depends on school psychologists' using their behavioral intervention skills. When school–home collaboration is required to deal with conduct or academic problems, conjoint behavioral therapy may be indicated. Relationships established during a parent conference might provide a springboard to begin such therapy that was impossible previously (see Freer & Watson, 1999; Sheridan et al., 2001). Other shorter-duration collaboration between home and school that has been endorsed by parents, such as school psychologists providing "how to" suggestions (Christensen, Hurley, Sheridan, & Fenstermacher, 1997), may also be enabled by conferences that leave parents receptive to suggestions.

SHARING INFORMATION WITH OTHER TEAM MEMBERS

Premultidisciplinary, posttesting evaluation conferences with parents often speed up and focus any subsequent formal meetings about special education eligibility and programming. Typically, psychologists share condensed evaluation findings, as do other team members during multidisciplinary conferences concerning special services eligibility, and then decisions are made. It is not usually necessary or advisable to share detailed psychometric scores during such meetings. Whether key decision points from our flowchart (Figure 1.1/5.1) are reviewed, together with the information that supports conclusions, depends on how findings are shared with other team members, as discussed below.

Practitioners appear to be split on whether assessment information should be pooled and decisions made before the multidisciplinary team meeting if special education eligibility is at issue. Moreover, special education rules invest authority in the team problem-solving process, which includes parents. Accordingly, in order to satisfy both the spirit and letter of administrative guidelines, summary decisions about the nature of students' problems and what to do about them should be withheld until an intact multidisciplinary meeting (with parents present) is held.

Nonetheless, summative conclusions are one thing, and formative hypothesis generation and testing are quite another. In reality, most team members will discuss findings as they arise (indeed, this step helps determine the direction of data collection), and accordingly there will be few surprises at the time of a formal multidisciplinary meeting. Shared professional responsibility in planning is also important in promoting teachers' ongoing implementation of treatment recommendations. Keeping a student's homeroom teacher involved in all aspects of the evaluation and planning process is essential because most children will remain in their homeroom after being evaluated, even if they are found eligible for special services. Too often, children who receive special services, including those afforded resource instruction, are provided no classroom accommodations by their regular teacher (Wilson, Gutkin, Hagen, & Oats, 1998).

A related matter concerns documentation of evaluation findings and whether just one document (including psychological findings) or several documents, including a separate psychoeducational report, are prepared. Local and administrative factors are determinative here. One caveat, however, is that a single multidisciplinary document may lack coherence so that readers can follow the flow of what was done, from the reason for assessment through evaluation procedures to findings, summary, and recommendations. On the other hand, we have found that concentrating on a search for the problems underlying school failure, as advocated throughout this book, helps keep documentation concise. Furthermore, documents that answer the big questions succinctly can be read and understood by team members (or by those outside the team) more readily than reports that are excessively descriptive. Reports that emphasize test scores, rather than interpreted data as they speak to key decision points, are often hard to understand (see Wodrich, 1997, for examples). As the importance of documenting previous attempts to remedy the problem becomes imperative (e.g., the RTI model), generation of coherent records may become even more problematic.

FINAL REMINDER: NO SYSTEM IS COMPLETE, AND CHILDREN ARE INDIVISIBLE

In this book, we describe common patterns associated with classroom failure in a way that is designed to help school-based professionals. Clearly, other patterns exist that might have been included, and there are other classification/organizational systems that might be used. Practicing school psychologists (and graduate students) are encouraged to read about these alternatives and to keep an open mind. For example, learning problems and their neuropsychological bases are presented by Hale and Fiorello (2004); the relationship of brain function (and dysfunction) and academic performance is covered by Berninger and Richards (2002); systemic and theory-related approaches are presented by Flanagan and Ortiz (2001) as well as Naglieri (1997) and colleagues (Das, Naglieri, & Kirby, 1994). Professionals' understanding can only be enriched by additional information about individual differences and how differences on these dimensions influence academic success.

Contemporary practitioners are also encouraged to familiarize themselves with DSM-IV-TR, the recognized guide for emotional and psychiatric disorders. Even if averse to establishing mental health diagnoses themselves, school psychologists will encounter many children who already bear such diagnoses. Of course, we argue that children with emotional problems should be recognized by school psychologists just as much as those with pure learning problems. In fact, as seen with NLD, CU, and ADHD, the distinction between problems designated learning and those designated emotional is somewhat artificial.

Equally important, children typically experience diffuse rather than circumscribed, clear-cut problems. Accordingly, school psychologists cannot conduct evaluations that concern only learning problems because children with primary psychiatric problems also will be encountered. Thus, it is interesting to read psychoeducational evaluations that restrict the reason for evaluation to "evaluate to determine the possible presence of a specific learning disability." This referral question's narrow focus makes it illogical. An emotional problem must be ruled out (in essence, Box A in our flowchart, Figure 1.1/5.1) before a learning problem is ruled in. Just as many children with emotional problems as learning problems should be identified, at least according to some psychiatric prevalence figures (e.g., Friedman, Kutash, & Newman, 2001). In reality, however, one-sixth as many students are identified for ED as for SLD services (U.S. Department of Education, 2002). Furthermore, even when a legitimate SLD is detected, emotional problems may also exist. As practitioners, psychologists should be cognizant that stress, frustration, loss of face, and demoralization often accompany academic failure. As scientists, psychologists should recognize the high comorbidity rates of emotional and learning problems. This information begs for school psychologists to embrace diverse sources of information, avoid narrow conceptualizations, and strive to understand all aspects of the children that we are committed to help.

References

♦

Abikoff, H., Hechtman, L., Klein, R. G., Gallagher, R., Fleiss, K., Etcovitch, J., et al. (2004). Social functioning in children with ADHD treated with long-term methylphenidate and multimodal psychosocial treatment. *Journal of the American Academy of Child and Adolescent Psychiatry, 43*, 820–829.

Abikoff, H., Hechtman, L., Klein, R. G., Weiss, G., Fleiss, K., Etcovitch, J., et al. (2004). Symptomatic improvement in children with ADHD treated with long-term methylphenidate and multimodal psychosocial treatment. *Journal of the American Academy of Child and Adolescent Psychiatry, 43*, 802–811.

Abrantes, A. M., Brown, S. A., & Tomlinson, K. L. (2003). Psychiatric comorbidity among outpatient substance abusing adolescents. *Journal of Child and Adolescent Substance Abuse, 13*, 83–101.

Achenbach, T. M., & Rescorla, L. A. (2001). *Manual for the ASEBA School-Age Forms and Profiles.* Burlington, VT: University of Vermont, Research Center for Children, Youth, & Families.

Adams, G. B., & Burke, R. W. (1999). Children and adolescents with obsessive–compulsive disorder: A primer for teachers. *Childhood Education* (Fall), 2–7.

Adams, G. B., Waas, G., March, J. S., & Smith, M. C. (1994). Obsessive–compulsive disorder in children and adolescents: The role of the school psychologist in identification, assessment, and treatment. *School Psychology Quarterly, 9*, 274–294.

Adams, W., & Sheslow, D. (1995). *Wide Range Assessment of Visual Motor Abilities.* Wilmington, DE: Wide Range.

Adams, W., & Sheslow, D. (2003). *The Wide Range Assessment of Memory and Learning–2nd Edition.* Wilmington, DE: Wide Range.

Allport, G. W. (1940). The psychologist's frame of reference. *Psychological Bulletin, 37*, 1–28.

American Academy of Child and Adolescent Psychiatry. (1998a). Practice parameters for the assessment and treatment of children and adolescents with language and learning disorders. *Journal of the American Academy of Child and Adolescent Psychiatry, 37*, 46S–62S.

American Academy of Child and Adolescent Psychiatry. (1998b). Practice parameters for the assessment and treatment of children and adolescents with obsessive–compulsive disorder. *Journal of the American Academy of Child and Adolescent Psychiatry, 37,* 27S–45S.

American Academy of Pediatrics. (1999). The pediatrician's role in development and implementation of an individual education plan (IEP) and/or an individual family service plan (IFSP). *Pediatrics, 104,* 124–127.

American Academy of Pediatrics. (2000). Clinical practices guidelines: Diagnosis and evaluation of the child with attention-deficit/hyperactivity disorder. *Pediatrics, 105,* 1158–1170.

American Academy of Pediatrics. (2001). Clinical practice guidelines: Treatment of the school-age child with attention-deficit/hyperactivity disorder. *Pediatrics, 108,* 1033–1044.

American Academy of School Psychology. (2004). Statement on comprehensive evaluation for learning disabilities. *Trainer's Forum, 23*(4), 13–15.

American Association on Mental Retardation. (2002). *Mental retardation: Definition, classification, and system of supports* (10th ed.). Washington, DC: Author.

American Association on Mental Retardation. (2004a). *AAMR/ARC position statements: Early intervention.* Retrieved from www.aamr.org/Policies/pos_early_intervention.shtml

American Association on Mental Retardation. (2004b). *AAMR/ARC position statements: Family support.* Retrieved from www.aamr.org/Policies/pos_fam_support.shtml

American Educational Research Association. (2002). *Standards for educational and psychological testing.* Washington, DC: Author.

American Psychiatric Association. (2000). *Diagnostic and statistical manual of mental disorders* (4th ed.). Washington, DC: Author.

American Psychological Association [APA]. (2002). Ethical principles of psychologists and code of conduct. *American Psychologist, 57,* 1060–1073.

American Psychological Association [APA], Division 16. (1998). Specialty of school psychology recognized. *The School Psychologist, 52,* 108–109.

Anastopoulos, A. D. (2000). The MTA study and parent training in managing ADHD. *ADHD Report, 8,* 7–9.

Anastopoulos, A. D., Shelton, T. L., DuPaul, G. J., Guevremont, D. C. (1993). Parent training for attention-deficit/hyperactivity disorder: Its impact on parent functioning. *Journal of Abnormal Child Psychology, 21,* 581–596.

Anderson, P. (2002). Assessment and development of executive function (EF) during childhood. *Child Neuropsychology, 8,* 71–82.

Andrews, T. J., & Naglieri, J. A. (1994). Aptitude-treatment interactions reconsidered. *Comminique, 22*(6), 8–9.

Antshel, K. M., & Remer, R. (2003). Social skills training in children with attention-deficit/hyperactivity disorder: A randomized-controlled clinical trial. *Journal of Clinical Child and Adolescent Psychology, 32,* 153–165.

Arter, J. A., & Jenkins, J. R. (1979). Differential diagnosis-prescriptive teaching: A critical appraisal. *Review of Educational Research, 49,* 517–555.

Assesmany, A., McIntosh, D. E., Phelps, L., & Rizza, M. G. (2001). Discriminant validity of the WISC-III with children classified as ADHD. *Journal of Psychoeducational Assessment, 19,* 137–147.

Baker, S., Gersten, R., & Lee, D. S. (2002). A synthesis of empirical research on teaching mathematics on low-achieving students. *The Elementary School Journal, 103,* 51–73.

Barkley, R. A. (1997a). *ADHD and the nature of self-control.* New York: Guilford Press.

Barkley, R. A. (1997b). *Defiant children: A clinician's manual for assessment and parent training* (2nd ed.). New York: Guilford Press.

Barkley, R. A. (2000). *Taking charge of ADHD: The complete, authoritative guide for parents* (rev. ed.). New York: Guilford Press.

Barkley, R. A. (2001). The inattentive type of ADHD as a distinct disorder: What remains to be done. *Clinical Psychology: Science and Practice, 8,* 489–493.

Barkley, R. A. (2002). Psychosocial treatments for attention-deficit/hyperactivity disorder in children. *Journal of Clinical Psychiatry, 63*(Suppl. 12), 36–43.

Barkley, R. A. (2004). Adolescents with attention-deficit/hyperactivity disorder: An overview of empirically based treatments. *Journal of Psychiatric Practice, 10,* 39–56.

Barkley, R. A. (2006). *Attention-deficit hyperactivity disorder: A handbook for diagnosis and treatment* (3rd ed.). New York: Guilford Press.

Barkley, R. A., DuPaul, G. J., & McMurray, M. B. (1991). Attention deficit disorder with and without hyperactivity: Clinical response to three dose levels of methylphenidate. *Pediatrics, 87,* 519–531.

Barkley, R. A., & Grodzinsky, G. M. (1994). Are tests of frontal lobe functions useful in the diagnosis of attention-deficit disorder? *Clinical Neuropsychologist, 8,* 121–139.

Barkley, R. A., Murphy, K. R., DuPaul, G. J., & Bush, T. (2002). Driving in young adults with attention-deficit/hyperactivity disorder: Knowledge, performance, adverse outcomes, and the role of executive function. *Journal of the International Neuropsychological Society, 8,* 655–672.

Baron, I. S. (2000). Clinical implications and practical applications of child neuropsychological evaluations. In K. O. Yeates, M. D. Ris, & H. G. Taylor (Eds.), *Pediatric neuropsychology: Research, theory, and practice* (pp. 439–456). New York: Guilford Press.

Barrett, P., Healy-Farrell, L., & March, J. S. (2004). Cognitive-behavioral family treatment of childhood obsessive–compulsive disorder: A controlled trial. *Journal of the American Academy of Child and Adolescent Psychiatry, 43,* 46–62.

Batshaw, M. L. (Ed.). (2002). *Children with disabilities* (5th ed.). Baltimore: Brookes.

Beery, K. E., Buktenica, N. A., & Beery, N. A. (2004). *The Beery–Buktenica Developmental Test of Visual–Motor Integration* (5th ed.). Minneapolis: Pearson Assessments.

Beitchman, J. H., Wilson, B., Johnson, C., Atkinson, L., Young, A., Adlaf, E., et al. (2001). Fourteen-year follow-up of speech/language-impaired and control children: Psychiatric outcome. *Journal of the American Academy of Child and Adolescent Psychiatry, 40,* 75–82.

Benazon, N. R., Ager, J., & Rosenberg, D. R. (2002). Cognitive-behavioral therapy in treatment-naïve children and adolescents with obsessive–compulsive disorder: An open trial. *Behaviour Research and Therapy, 40,* 529–539.

Benner, G. J., Nelson, J. R., & Epstein, M. H. (2002). Language skills and children with EBD: A literature review. *Journal of Emotional and Behavior Disorders, 10,* 43–59.

Berninger, V. W. (1994). *Reading and writing acquisition: A development neuropsychological perspective.* Madison, WI: Brown.

Berninger, V. W. (2000). Development of language by hand and its connections to language by ear, mouth, and eye. *Topics of Language Disorders, 20,* 65–84.

Berninger, V. W. (2004). Understanding the "graphia" in developmental dysgraphia: A developmental neuropsychological perspective for disorders in producing written language. In D. Dewey & D. E. Tupper (Eds.), *Developmental motor disorders: A neuropsychological perspective* (pp. 328–350). New York: Guilford Press.

Berninger, V. W., & Richards, T. L. (2002). *Brain literacy for educators and psychologists.* Boston: Academic Press.

Berninger, V. W., Vaughn, K. B., Abbott, R. D., Abbott, S. P., Woodruff-Rogan, L., Brooks, A. et al. (1997). Treatment of handwriting problems in beginning writers: Transfer from handwriting to composition. *Journal of Educational Psychology, 89*, 652–666.

Biederman, J. (1998). Resolved: Mania is mistaken for ADHD in prepubertal children. *Journal of the American Academy of Child and Adolescent Psychiatry, 37*, 1091–1093.

Biederman, J. (2003). Pharmacotherapy for attention-deficit/hyperactivity disorder (ADHD) decreases the risk for substance abuse: Findings from a longitudinal follow-up of youths with and without ADHD. *Journal of Clinical Psychiatry, 64*(Suppl. 11), 3–8.

Biederman, J., Faraone, S., Mick, E., Wozniak, J., Chen, L., Ouellette, C., et al. (1996). Attention-deficit hyperactivity disorder and juvenile mania: An overlooked comorbidity? *American Academy of Child and Adolescent Psychiatry, 35*, 997–1008.

Biederman, J., Faraone, S. V., Weber, W., Russell, R., Rater, M., & Park, K. (1997). Correspondence between DSM-III-R and DSM-IV attention-deficit hyperactivity disorder. *Journal of the American Academy of Child and Adolescent Psychiatry, 36*, 1682–1687.

Bigler, E. D. (1989). On the neuropsychology of suicide. *Journal of Learning Disabilities, 22*, 180–185.

Bigler, E. D., Clark, E., & Farmer, J. E. (1997). *Childhood traumatic brain injury: Diagnosis, assessment, and intervention*. Austin, TX: PRO-ED.

Bishop, D. V. M. (2000). Pragmatic language impairment: A correlate of SLI, a distinct subgroup, or part of the autistic continuum? In D. V. M. Bishop & L. B. Leonard (Eds.), *Speech and language impairments in children: Causes, characteristics, intervention and outcome* (pp. 99–112). Philadelphia: Psychology Press Limited.

Bishop, D. V. M., & Snowling, M. J. (2004). Developmental dyslexia and specific language impairment: Same or different? *Psychological Bulletin, 130*(6), 858–886.

Blachowicz, C., & Ogle, D. (2001). *Reading comprehension: Strategies for independent learners*. New York: Guilford Press.

Blazer, B. (1999). Developing 504 classroom accommodation plans: A collaborative systemic parent–student–teacher approach. *Teaching Exceptional Children, 32*, 28–33.

Boder, E., & Jarrico, S. (1982). *The Boder Test of Reading–Spelling Patterns*. San Antonio, TX: The Psychological Corporation.

Boll, T. (1993). *Children's Category Test manual*. San Antonio, TX: The Psychological Corporation.

Botting, N., & Conti-Ramsden, G. (2004). Characteristics of children with specific language impairment. In L. Verhoeven & H. van Balkom (Eds.), *Classification of developmental language disorders: Theoretical issues and clinical implications* (pp. 23–38). Mahwah, NJ: Erlbaum.

Bowman, P., & Goldberg, M. (1983). "Reframing": A tool for the school psychologist. *Psychology in the Schools, 20*, 210–214.

Bramlett, R. K., Murphy, J. J., Johnson, J., Wallingsford, L., & Hall, J. D. (2002). Contemporary practices in school psychology: A national survey of roles and referral problems. *Psychology in the Schools, 39*, 327–335.

Brody, N. (1997). Intelligence, schooling, and society. *American Psychologist, 52*, 1046–1050.

Brody, N. (1999). What is intelligence? *International Review of Psychiatry, 11*, 19–25.

Brooks, A., Todd, A. W., Tofflemoyer, S., & Horner, R. H. (2003). Use of functional assessment and a self-management system to increase academic engagement and work completion. *Journal of Positive Behavior Interventions, 5,* 144–152.

Brown, D., Pryzwansky, W. B., & Schulte, A. C. (2001). *Psychological consultation: Introduction to theory and practice* (5th ed.). Boston: Allyn & Bacon.

Brown, R. T. (Ed.). (2004). *Handbook of pediatric psychology in school settings.* Mahwah, NJ: Erlbaum.

Bruininks, R. H., Woodcock, R. W., Weatherman, R. E., & Hill, B. K. (1996). *Scales of Independent Behavior—Revised.* Itasca, IL: Riverside.

Bullock, J., Pierce, S., & McClellan, L. (1989). *TOUCH MATH.* Colorado Springs, CO: Innovative Learning Concepts.

Burns, M. K., & Symington, T. (2002). A meta-analysis of prereferral intervention teams: Student and systemic outcomes. *Journal of School Psychology, 40,* 437–447.

Burt, C. (1937). *The backward child.* London: University of London Press.

Butler, F. M., Miller, S. P., Lee, K., & Pierce, T. (2001). Teaching mathematics to students with mild-to-moderate mental retardation: A review of the literature. *Mental Retardation, 39,* 20–31.

Byrne, B., & Fielding-Barnsley, R. (1991). Evaluation of a program to teach phonemic awareness to young children. *Journal of Educational Psychology, 83,* 451–455.

Camarata, S., & Yoder P. (2002). Language transitions during development and intervention: Theoretical implications for developmental neuroscience. *International Journal of Developmental Neuroscience, 20,* 459–465.

Carlson, C. L., & Mann, M. (2000). Attention-deficit/hyperactivity disorder, predominantly inattentive subtype. *Child and Adolescent Psychiatric Clinics of North America, 9,* 499–510.

Carlson, C. L., & Mann, M. (2002). Sluggish cognitive tempo predicts a different pattern of impairment in the attention-deficit/hyperactivity disorder, predominantly inattentive type. *Journal of Child and Clinical Child and Adolescent Psychology, 31,* 123–129.

Carlson, C. L., Mann, M., & Alexander, D. K. (2000). Effects of reward and response cost on the performance and motivation of children with ADHD. *Cognitive Therapy and Research, 24,* 87–98.

Carroll, J. B. (2000). Commentary on profile analysis. *School Psychology Quarterly, 15,* 449–456.

Catts, H. W., Fey, M. E., & Tomblin, J. B. (2002). A longitudinal investigation of reading outcomes in children with language impairments. *Journal of Speech, Language, and Hearing Research, 45*(6), 1142–1157.

Catts, H. W., Gillispie, M., Leonard, L. B., Kail, R. V., & Miller, C. A. (2002). The role of speed of processing, rapid naming, and phonological awareness in reading achievement. *Journal of Learning Disabilities, 35,* 510–525.

Chhabildas, N., Pennington, B. F., & Willcutt, E. G. (2001). A comparison of the neuropsychological profiles of the DSM-IV subtypes of ADHD. *Journal of Abnormal Child Psychology, 29,* 529–540.

Christensen, S. L., Hurley, C. M., Sheridan, S. M., & Fenstermacher, K. (1997). Parents' and school psychologists' perspectives on parent involvement activities. *School Psychology Review, 26,* 111–130.

Conners, C. K. (1997). *Conners' Rating Scales—Revised Technical Manual.* North Tonawanda, NY: Multi-Health Systems.

Conners, C. K., Epstein, J., & March, J. (2001). Multi-modal treatment of ADHD (MTA): An alternative outcome analysis. *Journal of the American Academy of Child and Adolescent Psychiatry, 40,* 159–167.

Conners, C. K., March, J. S., Frances, A., Wells, K. C., & Ross, R. (2001). Treatment of attention-deficit/hyperactivity disorder: Expert consensus guidelines. *Journal of Attention Disorders, 4,* S1–S128.

Conners, F. A. (1992). Reading instruction for students with moderate mental retardation: Review and analysis of research. *American Journal on Mental Retardation, 96,* 577–597.

Conners, K. (2000). *Conner's Continuous Performance Test II—Manual.* North Tonawanda, NY: Multi-Health Systems.

Cornoldi, C., Rigoni, F., Tressoldi, P. E., & Vio, C. (1999). Imagery deficits in nonverbal learning disabilities. *Journal of Learning Disabilities, 32,* 48–57.

Cox, D. J., Merkel, R. L., Penberthy, J. K., Kovatchev, B., & Hankin, C. S. (2004). Impact of methlyphenidate delivery profiles on driving performance of adolescents with attention-deficit/hyperactivity disorder: A pilot study. *Journal of the American Academy of Child and Adolescent Psychiatry, 43,* 269–275.

Curtis, M. J., Grier, J. E. C., & Hunley, S. A. (2004). The changing face of school psychology: Trends in data and projections for the future. *School Psychology Review, 33,* 49–66.

D'Amato, R. C. (2003). School psychology is not what it used be: Thoughts from the new editor concerning our "futures" and *School Psychology Quarterly. School Psychology Quarterly, 18*(1), iii–xii.

Das, J. P., Naglieri, J. A., & Kirby, J. R. (1994). *Assessment of cognitive processes: The PASS theory of intelligence.* Boston: Allyn & Bacon.

Davila, R. (1994). ADHD and eligibility for special services. In D. L. Wodrich, *Attention-deficit/hyperactivity disorder: What every parent wants to know* (pp. 175–191). Baltimore: Brookes.

Dekker, M. C., & Koot, H. M. (2003a). DSM-IV disorders in children with borderline to moderate intellectual disability I: Prevalence and impact. *Journal of the American Academy of Child and Adolescent Psychiatry, 42,* 915–922.

Dekker, M. C., & Koot, H. M. (2003b). DSM-IV disorders in children with borderline to moderate intellectual disability I: Child and family predictors. *Journal of the American Academy of Child and Adolescent Psychiatry, 42,* 923–931.

De la Paz, S., & Graham, S. (1997). The effects of dictation and advanced planning instruction on the composing of students with writing and learning problems. *Journal of Educational Psychology, 89,* 203–222.

Delis, D. C., Kaplan, E., & Kramer, J. H. (2001). *Delis Kaplan Executive Function System: Examiner's manual.* San Antonio, TX: Psychological Corporation.

Delis, D. C., Kramer, J. H., Kaplan, E., & Ober, B. A. (1994). *California Verbal Learning Test Manual: Children's Version.* San Antonio, TX: The Psychological Corporation.

Demaray, M. K., Elting, J., & Schaefer, K. (2003). Assessment of attention-deficit/hyperactivity disorder (ADHD): A comparative evaluation of five commonly used, published rating scales. *Psychology in the Schools, 40,* 341–361.

Denckla, M. B. (1994). Measurement of executive function. In G. R. Lyon (Ed.), *Frames of reference for the assessment of learning disabilities: New views on measurement issues* (pp. 117–142). Baltimore: Brookes.

DeShazo-Barry, T., Lyman, R. D., & Grofer-Klinger, L. (2002). Academic underachievement and attention-deficit/hyperactivity disorder: The negative impact of symptom severity on school performance. *Journal of School Psychology, 40,* 259–283.

Doll, B., & Elliott, S. N. (1994). Representativeness of observed preschool social behaviors: How many data are enough? *Journal of Early Education, 18,* 227–238.

Dombrowski, S. C., Kamphaus, R. W., & Reynolds, C. R. (2004). After the demise of the discrepancy: Proposed learning disabilities diagnostic criteria. *Professional Psychology: Research and Practice, 35*, 364–372.

Dunn, L. M., & Dunn, L. M. (1997). *Norms booklet for the Peabody Picture Vocabulary Test—Third Edition.* Circle Pines, MN: American Guidance Service.

DuPaul, G. J., & Eckert, T. L. (1997). The effects of school-based interventions for attention-deficit/hyperactivity disorder: A meta-analysis. *School Psychology Review, 26*, 5–27.

DuPaul, G. J., Power, T. J., Anastopoulos, A. D., & Reid, R. (1998). *ADHD Rating Scale–IV: Checklists, norms, and clinical interpretation.* New York: Guilford Press.

DuPaul, G. J., Rapport, M. D., & Perriello, L. M. (1991). Teacher ratings of academic skills: The development of the academic performance rating scale. *School Psychology Review, 20*, 284–300.

DuPaul, G. J., Volpe, R. J., Jitendra, A. K., Lutz, J. G., Lorah, K. S., & Gruber, R. (2004). Elementary school students with ADHD: Predictors of academic achievement. *Journal of School Psychology, 42*, 285–301.

Dykens, E. M. (2002). Are jigsaw puzzle skills "spared" in persons with Prader-Willi syndrome? *Journal of Child Psychology and Psychiatry, 43*, 343–352.

Dykens, E. M., Hodapp, R. M., & Finucane, B. M. (2000). *Genetics and mental retardation syndromes: A new look at behavior and interventions.* Baltimore: Brookes.

Ehri, L. C., Nunes, S., Willows, D., Schuster, B., Yaghoub-Zadeh, Z., & Shanahan, T. (2001). Phonemic awareness instruction helps children learn to read: Evidence from the National Reading Panel's meta-analysis. *Reading Research Quarterly, 36*, 250–287.

Elliott, S. N., Busse, R. T., & Shapiro, E. S. (1999). Intervention techniques for academic performance problems. In T. Gutkin & C. R. Reynolds (Eds.), *The handbook of school psychology* (3rd ed., pp. 664–685). New York: Wiley.

Elwood, R. W. (1993). Clinical discrimination and the use of neuropsychological tests: An appeal to Bayes' theorem. *The Clinical Neuropsychologist, 7*, 224–233.

Erenberg, G. (1991). Learning disabilities: An overview. *Seminars in Neurology, 11*(1), 1–6.

Evans, J. J., Floyd, R. G., McGrew, K. S., & LeForgee, M. H. (2002). The relations between measures of Cattell–Horn–Carroll (CHC) cognitive abilities and reading achievement during childhood and adolescence. *School Psychology Review, 31*, 246–262.

Federal Register. (1999). [34 *Code of Federal Regulations* X300.7(c)(6)].

Feldman, G. M., Kelly, R. M., & Diehl, V. A. (2004). An interpretative analysis of five commonly used processing speed measures. *Journal of Psychoeducational Assessment, 22*, 151–163.

Firman, K. B., Beare, P., & Loyd, R. (2002). Enhancing self-management in students with mental retardation: Extrinsic versus intrinsic procedures. *Education and Training in Mental Retardation and Developmental Disabilities, 37*, 163–171.

Fisher, N. J., DeLuca, J. W., & Rourke, B. P. (1997). Wisconsin Card Sorting Test and Halstead Category Test performances of children and adolescents who exhibit the syndrome of nonverbal learning disabilities. *Child Neuropsychology, 3*, 61–70.

Fitzgerald, J. (2001). Can minimally trained college volunteers help young at-risk children to read better? *Reading Research Quarterly, 36*, 28–46.

Flanagan, D. P. (2000). Wechsler-based CHC cross-battery assessment and reading achievement: Strengthening the validity of interpretations drawn from Wechsler test scores. *School Psychology Quarterly, 15*, 295–329.

Flanagan, D. P., McGrew, K. S, & Ortiz, S. O. (2000). *The Wechsler intelligence scales and Gf-Gc theory: A contemporary approach to interpretation.* Needham Heights, MA: Allyn & Bacon.

Flanagan, D. P., & Ortiz, S. (2001). *Essentials of cross-battery assessment.* New York: Wiley.

Fletcher, J. M. (1989). Nonverbal learning disabilities and suicide: Classification leads to prevention. *Journal of Learning Disabilities, 22,* 176–179.

Fletcher, J. M., & Reschly, D. J. (2004). Changing procedures for identifying learning disabilities: The danger of perpetuating old ideas. *The School Psychologist, 59,* 10–15.

Floyd, R. G., Shaver, R. B., & McGrew, K. S. (2003). Interpretation of the Woodcock–Johnson III Tests of Cognitive Abilities: Acting on evidence. In F. A. Schrank & D. P. Flanagan (Eds.), *WJ III clinical use and interpretation: Scientist–practitioner perspectives* (pp. 1–46). London: Academic Press.

Forness, S. R. (2001). Special education and related services: What have we learned from meta-analysis? *Exceptionality, 9,* 185–197.

Forum for Child and Family Statistics. (2004). *America's Children 2004.* Retrieved February 24, 2005, from www.childstats.gov/ac2004/edu.asp

Frankenberger, C. (2005). Nonverbal learning disabilities: An emerging profile. Retrieved July 1, 2005, from www.nldonline.com

Franklin, M. E., Kozak, M. J., Cashman, L. A., Coles, M. E., Rheingold, A. A., & Foa, E. B. (1998). Cognitive-behavioral treatment of pediatric obsessive–compulsive disorder: An open clinical trial. *Journal of the American Academy of Child and Adolescent Psychiatry, 37,* 412–419.

Franklin, M. E., Rynn, M., Foa, E. B., & March, J. S. (2003). Treatment of obsessive–compulsive disorder. In M. A. Reinecke, F. M. Dattilio, & A. Freeman (Eds.), *Cognitive therapy with children and adolescents: A casebook for clinical practice* (2nd ed., pp. 162–184). New York: Guilford Press.

Freeman, S. F. N. (2000). Academic and social attainments of children with mental retardation in general education and special education settings. *Remedial and Special Education, 21,* 3–19.

Freer, P., & Watson, T. S. (1999). A comparison of parent and teacher acceptability ratings of behavioral and conjoint behavioral consultation. *School Psychology Review, 28,* 672–684.

Friedman, R. M., Kutash, K., & Newman, C. C. (2001). *Data trends: Summaries of current research findings in the children's mental health field.* Retrieved October 19, 2004, from datatrends.fmhi.usf.edu/2001Datatrends.pdf

Fuchs, D., Fuchs, L. S., Mathes, P. G., & Simmons, D. C. (1997). Peer-assisted learning strategies: Making classrooms more responsive to diversity. *American Educational Research Journal, 34,* 174–204.

Fuchs, D., Fuchs, L., Thompson, A., Svenson, E., Yen, L., Al Otaiba, S., et al. (2001). Peer-assisted learning strategies in reading: Extensions for kindergarten, first grade, and high school. *Remedial and Special Education, 22,* 15–21.

Fuchs, D., Mock, D., Morgan, P. L., & Young, C. L. (2003). Responsiveness-to-intervention: Definitions, evidence, and implications for the learning disabilities construct. *Learning Disabilities Research and Practice, 18,* 157–171.

Fuchs, L. S., Fuchs, D., & Kazdan, S. (1999). Effects of peer-assisted learning strategies on high school students with serious reading problems. *Remedial and Special Education, 20,* 309–318.

Fuchs, L. S., Fuchs, D., Yazdian, L., & Powell, S. R. (2002). Enhancing first-grade children's mathematical development with peer-assisted learning strategies. *School Psychology Review, 31,* 569–583.

Furnham, A. (2004). Are lay people lumpers or splitters? The factor structure of, and sex differences related to, self-rated and other-related abilities. *Learning and Individual Differences, 14*, 153–168.

Geary, D. C. (2003). Learning disabilities in arithmetic: Problem-solving differences and cognitive deficits. In H. L. Swanson, K. R. Harris, & S. Graham (Eds.), *Handbook of learning disabilities* (pp. 199–212). New York: Guilford Press.

Geller, D. A., Biederman, J., Reed, E. D., Spencer, T., & Wilens, T. E. (1995). Similarities in response to fluoxetine in the treatment of children and adolescents with obsessive–compulsive disorder. *Journal of the American Academy of Child and Adolescent Psychiatry, 34*, 36–44.

Geller, D. A., Biederman, J., Stewart, S. E., Mullin, M., Martin, A., Spencer, T. et al. (2003). Which SSRI? A meta-analysis of pharmacotherapy trials in pediatric obsessive–compulsive disorder. *American Journal of Psychiatry, 160*, 1919–1928.

Geller, D. A., Hoog, S. L., Heiligenstein, J. H., Ricardi, R. K., Tamura, R., Kluszynski, S., et al. (2001). Fluoxetine treatment for obsessive–compulsive disorder in children and adolescents: A placebo-controlled clinical trial. *Journal of the American Academy of Child and Adolescent Psychiatry, 40*, 773–779.

Gill, C. B., Klecan-Aker, J., Roberts, T., & Fredenburg, K. A. (2003). Following directions: Rehearsal and visualization strategies for children with specific language impairment. *Child Language Teaching and Therapy, 19*, 85–101.

Gillon, G., & Dodd, B. (1995). The effects of training phonological, semantic, and syntactic processing skills in spoken language on reading ability. *Language, Speech, and Hearing in Schools, 26*, 58–68.

Gillon, G., & Dodd, B. (1997). Enhancing the phonological processing skills of children with specific reading disability. *European Journal of Disorders of Communication, 32*, 67–90.

Gillon, G. T. (2004). *Phonological awareness: From research to practice.* New York: Guilford Press.

Glascoe, F. P. (1997). Parents' concern about children's development: Prescreening technique or screening test? *Pediatrics, 99*, 522–528.

Glutting, J. J., Oakland, T., & McDermott, P. A. (1989). Observing child behavior during testing: Constructs, validity, and situational generality. *Journal of School Psychology, 27*, 155–164.

Goldstein, S., & Reynolds, C. R. (Eds.). (1999). *Handbook of neurodevelopmental and genetic disorders in children.* New York: Guilford Press.

Good, R. H., & Kaminski, R. A. E. (2002). *Dynamic indicators of basic early literacy skills* (6th ed.). Eugene, OR: Institute for the Development of Educational Achievement.

Gordon, M. (1991). *The Gordon Diagnostic System.* Boulder, CO: Clinical Diagnostic Systems.

Gottfredson, L. S. (1997). Why g matters: The complexity of everyday life. *Intelligence, 24*, 79–132.

Grados, M. A., & Riddle, M. A. (1999). Obsessive–compulsive disorder in children and adolescents: Treatment guidelines. *CNS Drugs, 12*, 257–277.

Grados, M. A., & Riddle, M. A. (2001). Pharmacological treatment of childhood obsessive–compulsive disorder: From theory to practice. *Journal of Clinical Child Psychology, 30*, 67–79.

Graham, S., Berninger, V., Abbott, R., Abbott, S., & Whitaker, D. (1997). The role of mechanics in composing of elementary school students: A new methodological approach. *Journal of Educational Psychology, 89*, 170–182.

Graham, S., Harris, K. R., & Fink, B. (2000). Is handwriting causally related to learning to write? Treatment of handwriting problems in beginning writers. *Journal of Educational Psychology, 92,* 620–633.

Graham, S., & Weintraub, N. (1996). A review of handwriting research: Progress and prospects from 1980 to 1994. *Educational Psychology Review, 8,* 7–87.

Greenberg, L. M., Corman, C. L., & Kindschi, C. L. (1997). *Test of Variables of Attention—Manual.* Los Alamitos, CA: Universal Attention Disorders.

Greene, R., Biederman, J., Faraone, S., Monuteaux, M., Mick, E., DuPre, E., et al. (2001). Social impairment in girls with ADHD: Patterns, gender comparisons, and correlates. *Journal of the American Academy of Child and Adolescent Psychiatry, 40,* 704–710.

Greenwood, C. R., Horton, B. T., & Utley, C. A. (2002). Academic engagement: Current perspectives on research and practice. *School Psychology Review, 31,* 328–349.

Greenwood, C. R., Terry, B., Marquis, J., & Walker, D. (1994). Confirming a performance-based instructional model. *School Psychology Review, 23,* 652–668.

Gresham, F. M., MacMillan, D. L., & Bocian, K. M. (1996). Learning disabilities, low achievement, and mild mental retardation: More alike than different? *Journal of Learning Disabilities, 29,* 570–581.

Gresham, F. M., MacMillan, D. L., & Siperstein, G. N. (1995). Critical analysis of 1992 AAMR definition: Issues for school psychologists. *School Psychology Quarterly, 10,* 1–19.

Gresham, F. M., Reschly, D. J., & Carey, M. P. (1987). Teachers as "tests": Classification accuracy and concurrent validation in the identification of learning disabled students. *School Psychology Review, 16,* 543–553.

Grigorenko, E. L., Klin, A., Pauls, D. L., Senft, R., Hooper, C., & Volkmar, F. (2002). A descriptive study of hyperlexia in a clinically referred sample of children with developmental delays. *Journal of Autism and Developmental Disorders, 32,* 3–12.

Guadalupe v. Tempe Elementary School District, 587 F.2d 1022 (9th Cir. 1978).

Guastello, E. F., Beasley, T. M., & Sinatra, R. C. (2000). Concept mapping effects on science content comprehension of low-achieving inner-city seventh graders. *Remedial and Special Education, 21,* 356–365.

Guest, K. E. (2000). Career development of school psychologist. *Journal of School Psychology, 38,* 237–257.

Guralnick, M. J. (2000). Early childhood intervention: Evolution of a system. *Focus on Autism and Other Developmental Disabilities, 15,* 68–79.

Gutkin, T. B., & Nemeth, C. (1997). Selected factors impacting decision making in prereferral intervention and other school-based teams: Exploring the intersection between school and social psychology. *Journal of School Psychology, 35,* 195–216.

Gyns, J. A., Willis, W. G., & Faust, D. (1995). School psychologists' diagnoses of learning disabilities: A study of illusory correlation. *Journal of School Psychology, 33,* 59–73.

Haddad, F. A., Garcia, Y. E., Naglieri, J. A., Grimditch, M., McAndrews, A., & Eubanks, J. (2003). Planning facilitation and reading comprehension: Instructional relevance of the PASS theory. *Journal of Psychoeducational Assessment, 21,* 282–289.

HaileMariam, A., Bradley-Johnson, S., & Johnson, C. M. (2002). Pediatrician's preferences of ADHD information from schools. *School Psychology Review, 31,* 94–105.

Hale, J. B., & Fiorello, C. A. (2004). *School neuropsychology: A practitioner's guidebook.* New York: Guilford Press.

Hallowell, E. M., & Ratney, J. J. (1994). *Driven to distraction: Recognizing and coping with attention-deficit disorder from childhood through adulthood.* New York: Touchstone.

Hammill, D., & Larson, S. (1996). *Test of Written Language* (3rd ed.). Austin, TX: PRO-ED.

Hanushek, E. A., Kain, J. F., & Rivkin, S. G. (1998). *Does special education raise academic achievement for students with disabilities?* National Bureau of Economic Research, Working Paper No. 6690, Cambridge, MA.

Harpaz-Rotem, I., & Rosenheck, R. A. (2004). Changes in outpatient psychiatric diagnoses in privately insured children and adolescents from 1995 to 2000. *Child Psychiatry and Human Development, 34,* 329–340.

Heaton, R. K., Chelune, G. J., Talley, J. L., Kay, G. G., & Curtiss, G. (1993). *Wisconsin Card Sorting Test Manual: Revised and Expanded.* Lutz, FL: Psychological Assessment Resources.

Hechtman, L., Abikoff, H., Klein, R. G., Greenfield, B., Etcovitch, J., Cousins, L., et al. (2004). Children with ADHD treated with long-term methylphenidate and multimodal psychosocial treatment: Impact on parental practices. *Journal of the American Academy of Child and Adolescent Psychiatry, 43,* 830–838.

Hechtman, L., Abikoff, H., Klein, R. G., Weiss, G., Respitz, C., Kouri, J., et al. (2004). Academic achievement and emotional status of children with ADHD treated with long-term methylphenidate and multimodal psychosocial treatment. *Journal of the American Academy of Child and Adolescent Psychiatry, 43,* 812–819.

Hetzroni, O. E., & Shavit, P. (2002). Comparison of two instructional strategies for acquiring form and sound of Hebrew letters by students with mild mental retardation. *Education and Training in Mental Retardation and Developmental Disabilities, 37,* 273–282.

Hinshaw, S. (2001). Is the inattentive type of ADHD a separate disorder? *Clinical Psychology: Science and Practice, 8,* 498–501.

Hodapp, R. M., Evans, D., & Gray, F. L. (1999). Intellectual development in children with Down syndrome. In J. A. Rondal, J. Perera, & L. Nadel (Eds.), *Down syndrome: A review of current knowledge* (pp. 124–132). London: Whurr.

Hodgens, J. B., Cole, J., & Boldizar, J. (2000). Peer-based differences among boys with ADHD. *Journal of Clinical Child Psychology, 29,* 443–452.

Hoff, K. E., Doepke, K, & Landau, S. (2002). Best practices in the assessment of children with attention-deficit/hyperactivity disorder: Linking assessment to intervention. In A. Thomas & J. Grimes (Eds.), *Best practices in school psychology IV* (Vol. 2, pp. 1129–1150). Bethesda, MD: National Association of School Psychologists.

Hoff, K. E., Ervin, R. A., & Friman, P. C. (2005). Refining functional behavioral assessment: Analyzing the separate and combined effects of hypothesized controlling variables during ongoing classroom routines. *School Psychology Review, 34,* 45–57.

Hoffman, J. B., & DuPaul, G. J. (2000). Psychoeducational interventions for children and adolescents with attention-deficit/hyperactivity disorder. *Child and Adolescent Psychiatric Clinics of North America, 9,* 647–661.

Hope, T. L., Adams, C., Reynolds, L., Powers, D., Perez, R. A., & Kelley, M. L. (1999). Parent vs. self-report: Contributions toward diagnosis of adolescent psychopathology. *Journal of Psychopathology and Behavioral Assessment, 21,* 349–363.

Horner, R. H. (2000). Positive behavior supports. *Focus on Autism and Other Developmental Disabilities, 15,* 97–105.

Hoskyn, M., & Swanson, H. L. (2000). Cognitive processing of low achievers and children with reading disabilities: A selective meta-analytic review of the published literature. *School Psychology Review, 29,* 102–119.

House, A. E. (2002). *DSM-IV diagnosis in the schools* (rev. ed.). New York: Guilford Press.

Howe, N. L., Bigler, E. D., Lawson, J. S., & Burlingame, G. M. (1999). Reading disability subtypes and the Test of Memory and Learning. *Archives of Clinical Neuropsychology, 14,* 317–339.

Hoza, B. (2001). Psychosocial treatment issues in the MTA: A reply to Greene and Ablon. *Journal of Clinical Child Psychology, 30,* 126–130.

Huebner, E. S. (1989). Factors influencing the decision to administer psychoeducational tests. *Psychology in the Schools, 26,* 365–370.

Huebner, E. S., & Gould, K. (1991). Multidisciplinary teams revisited: Current perceptions of school psychologists regarding team functioning. *School Psychology Review, 20,* 428–434.

Individuals with Disabilities Education Act of 1997, 20 U.S.C. §§ 1400-1491 (1997).

Jitendra, A. K., Edwards, L. L., Sacks, G., & Jacobson, L. A. (2004). What research says about vocabulary instruction for students with learning disabilities. *Exceptional Children, 70,* 299–322.

Jones, D., & Christensen, C. A. (1999). Relationship between automaticity in handwriting and students' ability to generate written text. *Journal of Educational Psychology, 91,* 44–49.

Jones, K. L. (1997). *Smith's recognizable patterns of human malformation* (4th ed.). Philadelphia: W. B. Saunders.

Jones, S. (1999). LD in-depth: Dysgraphia accommodations and modifications. *Learning Disabilities OnLine.* Retrieved July 1, 2005, from www.Indonline.org/Id_indepth/writing/dysgraphia.html

Juel, C., Griffith, P. L., & Gough, P. B. (1986). Acquisition of literacy: A longitudinal study of children in first and second grade. *Journal of Educational Psychology, 78,* 243–255.

Kail, R. (2000). Speed of information processing: Developmental changes and links to intelligence. *Journal of School Psychology, 38,* 51–61.

Kamphaus, R. W. (1993). *Clinical assessment of children's intelligence.* Boston: Allyn & Bacon.

Kamphaus, R. W., Reynolds, C. R., & Imperato-McCammon, C. (1999). Role of diagnosis and classification in school psychology. In C. R. Reynolds & T. B. Gutkin (Eds.), *The handbook of school psychology* (3rd ed., pp. 292–306). New York: Wiley.

Kaufman, A. S., & Kaufman, N. L. (1993). *Kaufman Adolescent and Adult Intelligence Test: Manual.* Circle Pines: MN: American Guidance Service.

Kavale, K. A., Kaufman, A. S., Naglieri, J. A., & Hale, J. B. (2005, Winter). Changing procedures for identifying learning disabilities: The danger of poorly supported ideas. *The School Psychologist,* 16–25.

Kazdin, A. E. (2001). *Behavior modification in applied settings* (6th ed.). Belmont, CA: Wadsworth/Thomson Learning.

Kazdin, A. E., & Weisz, J. R. (Eds.). (2003). *Evidence-based psychotherapies for children and adolescents.* New York: Guilford Press.

Kiernan, W. (2000). Where we are now: Perspectives on employment of persons with mental retardation. *Focus on Autism and Other Developmental Disabilities, 15,* 90–96, 115.

Kilpatrick-Demaray, M., Schaefer, K., & Delong, L. (2003). Attention-deficit/hyperactivity disorder (ADHD): A national survey of training and current assessment practices in the schools. *Psychology in the Schools, 40,* 583–597.

Korkman, M., Kirk, U., & Kemp, S. (1998). *A Developmental Neuropsychological Assessment (NEPSY) manual.* San Antonio, TX: The Psychological Corporation.

Kranzler, J. H. (1997). Educational and policy issues related to the use and interpretation of intelligence tests in the schools. *School Psychology Review, 26,* 150–162.

Kratochwill, T. R., & Bergan, J. R. (1990). *Behavioral consultation and therapy.* New York: Plenum.

Kratochwill, T. R., & McGivern, J. E. (1996). Clinical diagnosis, behavioral assessment, and functional analysis: Examining the connection between assessment and intervention. *School Psychology Review, 25,* 342–355.

Kratochwill, T. R., & Stoiber, K. C. (2002). Evidence-based interventions in school psychology: Conceptual foundations of the procedural and coding manual of Division 16 and the Society for the Study of School Psychology Task Force. *School Psychology Quarterly, 17,* 341–389.

Kupersmidt, J. B., Coie, J. D., & Dodge, K. A. (1990). The role of peer relationships in the development of disorder. In S. R. Asher & J. D. Coie (Eds.), *Peer rejection in childhood* (pp. 274–305). New York: Cambridge University Press.

Kutcher, S., Aman, M., Brooks, S. J., Buitelaar, J., van Dallen, E., Fegert, J., et al. (2004). International consensus statement on attention-deficit/hyperactivity disorder practice suggestions. *European Neuropsychopharmacology, 14,* 11–28.

Lachar, D., & Gruber, C. P. (1994). *Manual for the Personality Inventory for Youth (PIY): A self-report manual to the Personality Inventory for Children (PIC).* Los Angeles: Western Psychological Services.

Lafayette Instrument Company. (n.d.). *Grooved pegboard.* Lafayette, IN: Author.

Leonard, L. B. (1998). *Children with specific language impairment.* Cambridge, MA: MIT Press.

Lewis, B., Freebairn, L., & Taylor, H. G. (2000). Follow-up of children with early expressive phonology disorders. *Journal of Learning Disabilities, 25,* 586–597.

Lewis, B., Freebairn, L., & Taylor, H. G. (2002). Correlates of spelling abilities in children with early speech sound disorders. *Reading and Writing: An Interdisciplinary Journal, 15,* 389–407.

Lewis, R. B., Graves, A. W., Ashton, T. M., & Kieley, C. L. (1998). Word processing tools for students with learning disabilities: A comparison of strategies to increase text entry speed. *Learning Disabilities Research and Practice, 13,* 95–108.

Lichtenstein, R., & Fischetti, B. A. (1998). How long does a psychoeducational evaluation take? An urban Connecticut study. *Professional Psychology: Research and Practice, 29,* 144–148.

Liebowitz, M. R., Turner, S. M., Piacentini, J., Biedel, D. C., Clarvit, S. R., Davies, S. O., et al. (2002). Fluoxetine in children and adolescents with OCD: A placebo-controlled trial. *Journal of the Amercian Academy of Child and Adolescent Psychiatry, 41,* 1431–1438.

Lin, S. J., Crawford, S. Y., & Lurvey, P. L. (2005). Trend and area variation in amphetamine prescription usage among children and adolescents treated in Michigan. *Social Science and Medicine, 60,* 617–626.

Lindamood, P., & Lindamood, P. (1998). *The Lindamood phoneme sequencing program for reading, spelling, and speech.* Austin, TX: PRO-ED.

Little, L. (2001). Peer victimization of children with Asperger spectrum disorders. *Journal of the American Academy of Child and Adolescent Psychiatry, 40,* 995–996.

Lyon, G. R., & Flynn, J. M. (1991). Educational validation studies with subtypes of learning-disabled readers. In B. P. Rourke (Ed.), *Neuropsychological validation of learning disability subtypes* (pp. 223–242). New York: Guilford Press.

Lyon, R., Stewart, N., & Freedman, D. (1982). Neuropsychological characteristics of empirically derived subgroups of learning disabled readers. *Journal of Clinical Neuropsychology, 4,* 343–365.

Lyon, R., Watson, B., Reitta, S., Porch, B., & Rhodes, J. (1981). Selected linguistic and perceptual deficits of empirically derived subgroups of learning disabled readers. *Journal of School Psychology, 19,* 152–166.

MacMillan, D. L., Gresham, F. M., Bocian, K. M., & Lambros, K. M. (1998). Current plight of borderline students: Where do they belong? *Education and Training in Mental Retardation and Developmental Disabilities, 33,* 83–94.

Maheady, L., Harper, G. F., & Mallette, B. (2001). Peer-mediated instruction and interventions and students with mild disabilities. *Remedial and Special Education, 22,* 4–14.

Mann, V. A. (2003). Language processes: Keys to reading disability. In H. L. Swanson, K. R. Harris, & S. Graham (Eds.), *Handbook of learning disabilities* (pp. 213–228). New York: Guilford Press.

Manning, S. C., & Miller, D. C. (2001). Identifying ADHD subtypes using the Parent and Teacher Rating Scales of the Behavior Assessment Scale for Children. *Journal of Attention Disorders, 5,* 41–51.

March, J. S. (1995). Cognitive-behavioral psychotherapy for children and adolescents with OCD: A review and recommendations for treatment. *Journal of the American Academy of Child and Adolescent Psychiatry, 34,* 7–18.

March, J. S., & Mulle, K. (1998). *OCD in children and adolescents: A cognitive-behavioral treatment manual.* New York: Guilford Press.

Margalit, M., & Roth, Y. B. (1989). Strategic keyboard training and spelling improvement among children with learning disabilities and mental retardation. *Educational Psychology, 9,* 321–329.

Masi, G., Marcheschi, M, & Pfanner, P. (1998). Adolescents with borderline intellectual functioning: Psychopathological risk. *Adolescence, 33,* 416–425.

Mathes, P. G., Fuchs, D., & Fuchs, L. S. (1997). Cooperative story mapping. *Remedial and Special Education, 18,* 20–27.

Mathes, P. G., Howard, J. K., Allen, S. H., & Fuchs, D. (1998). Peer-assisted learning strategies for first-grade readers: Responding to needs of diverse learners. *Reading Research Quarterly, 33,* 62–94.

Mazzocco, M. M. M. (2001). Math learning disability and math LD subtypes: Evidence from studies of Turner Syndrome, fragile X syndrome, and neurofibromatosis type 1. *Journal of Learning Disabilities, 34,* 520–533.

McBurnett, K., Pfiffner, L. J., & Frick, P. J. (2001). Symptom properties as a function of ADHD type: An argument for continued study of sluggish cognitive tempo. *Journal of Abnormal Child Psychology, 29,* 207–213.

McCabe, P. C. (2005). Social and behavioral correlates of preschoolers with specific language impairment. *Psychology in the Schools, 42,* 373–387.

McCarney, S. B. (1995). *Early Childhood Attention-Deficit Disorders Evaluation Scale.* Colombia, MO: Hawthorne Educational Services.

McCurdy, M., Skinner, C. H., Grantham, K., Watson, T. S., & Hindman, P. M. (2001). Increasing on-task behavior in an elementary student during mathematics seatwork by interspersing additional brief problems. *School Psychology Review, 30,* 23–32.

McKinney, J. D. (1990). Longitudinal research on the behavioral characteristics of children with learning disabilities. In J. Torgesen (Ed.), *Cognitive and behavioral characteristics of children with learning disabilities* (pp. 115–138). Austin, TX: PRO-ED.

Meichenbaum, D. (1985). Teaching thinking: A cognitive-behavioral perspective. In S. F. Chipman, J. W. Segal, & R. Glaser (Eds.), *Thinking and learning skills,* Vol. 2: *Research and open questions* (pp. 407–426). Hillsdale, NJ: Erlbaum.

Mercugliano, M., Power, T. J., & Blum, N. J. (1999). *The clinician's practical guide to attention-deficit/hyperactivity disorder.* Baltimore: Brookes.

Mervis, C. B. (2003). Williams syndrome: 15 years of psychological research. *Developmental Neuropsychology, 23,* 1–12.

Messick, S. (1995). Validity of psychological assessment: Validation of inferences from persons' responses and performances as scientific inquiry into score meaning. *American Psychologist, 50,* 741–749.

Meyer, G. J., Finn, S. E., Eyde, L. D., Kay, G. G., Moreland, K. L., Dies, R. R., et al. (2001). Psychological testing and psychological assessment: A review of evidence and issues. *American Psychologist, 56,* 128–156.

Milich, R., Balentine, A. C., & Lynam, D. R. (2001). ADHD, combined type and ADHD, predominantly inattentive type are distinct and unrelated disorders. *Clinical Psychology: Science and Practice, 8,* 463–488.

Molina, B. S. G., & Pelham, W. E. (2003). Childhood predictors of adolescent substance use in a longitudinal study of children with ADHD. *Journal of Abnormal Psychology, 112,* 497–507.

Morris, R. D., Steubling, K. K., Fletcher, J. M., Shaywitz, S. E., Lyon, G. R., Shankweiler, D. P., et al. (1998). Subtypes of reading disability: Variability around a phonological core. *Journal of Educational Psychology, 90,* 347–373.

MTA Cooperative Group. (1999a). A 14–month randomized clinical trial of treatment strategies for attention-deficit/hyperactivity disorder. *Archives of General Psychiatry, 56,* 1073–1086.

MTA Cooperative Group. (1999b). Moderators and mediators of treatment response for children with attention-deficit/hyperactivity disorder. *Archives of General Psychiatry, 56,* 1088–1096.

Nagle, R. J. (2002). Best practices in planning and conducting needs assessment. In A. Thomas & J. Grimes (Eds.), *Best practices in school psychology IV* (Vol. 1, pp. 265–279). Bethesda, MD: National Association of School Psychologists.

Naglieri, J. A. (1997). *Cognitive Assessment System: Administration and scoring manual.* Itasca, IL: Riverside.

Naglieri, J. A. (1999). *Essentials of CAS assessment.* New York: Wiley.

Naglieri, J. A. (2000). Can profile analysis of ability test scores work?: An illustration using the PASS theory and CAS with an unselected cohort. *School Psychology Quarterly, 15,* 419–433.

National Association of School Psychologists [NASP]. (2000). *Professional conduct manual: Principles for professional ethics guidelines for the provision of school psychological services.* Retrieved October, 5, 2004, from www.nasponline.org/pdf/PCM1100.pdf

National Association of School Psychologists [NASP]. (2003). *NASP recommendations for IDEA reauthorization: Identification and eligibility determination for students with specific learning disabilities.* Bethesda, MD: Author.

Nigg, J. T., Blaskey, L. G., Huang-Pollock, C., & Rappley, M. D. (2002). Neuropsychological executive functions and DSM-IV ADHD subtypes. *Journal of the American Academy of Child and Adolescent Psychiatry, 41,* 59–66.

Nowicki, E. A. (2003). A meta-analysis of the social competence of children with learning disabilities compared to classmates of low and average to high achievement. *Learning Disability Quarterly, 26,* 171–188.

Nunes, T., Bryant, P., & Olsson, J. (2003). Learning morphological and phonological spelling rules: An intervention study. *Scientific Studies in Reading, 7,* 289–307.

Nyborg, H. (Ed.). (2003). *The scientific study of general intelligence: Tribute to Arthur R. Jensen.* Amsterdam: Pergamon.

Olson, R., Forsberg, H., Wise, B., & Rack, J. (1994). Measurement of word recognition, orthographic, and phonological skills. In G. R. Lyon (Ed.), *Frames of reference for the assessment of learning disabilities: New views on measurement issues* (pp. 243–268). Baltimore: Brookes.

Ostrander, R., Weinfurt, K. P., Yarnold, P. R., & August, G. J. (1998). Diagnosing attention-deficit disorders with the Behavioral Assessment System for Children and the Child Behavior Checklist: Test and construct validity analyses using optimal discriminant classification trees. *Journal of Consulting and Clinical Psychology, 66,* 660–672.

Owens, R. E., Jr. (2004). *Language disorders: A functional approach to assessment and intervention* (4th ed.). Boston: Pearson Education.

Parker, Z., & Stewart, E. (1994). School consultation and the management of obsessive–compulsive personality in the classroom. *Adolescence, 29,* 563–574.

Patton, J. R., & Dunn, C. (1998). *Transition from school to young adulthood: Basic concepts and recommended practices.* Austin, TX: PRO-ED.

Patton, J. R., Polloway, E. A., & Smith, T. E. C. (2000). Educating students with mild mental retardation. *Focus on Autism and Other Developmental Disabilities, 15,* 80–89.

Pearson, D. A., Santos, C. W., Roache, J. D., Casat, C. D., Loveland, K. A., Lachar, D., et al. (2003). Treatment effects of methylphenidate on behavioral adjustment in children with mental retardation and ADHD. *Journal of the American Academy of Child and Adolescent Psychiatry, 42,* 209–216.

Pelham, W. E. (2001). Are ADHD/I and ADHD/C the same or different?: Does it matter? *Clinical Psychology: Science and Practice, 8,* 502–506.

Pelham, W. E., Wheeler, T., & Chronis, A. (1998). Empirically supported psychosocial treatments for attention-deficit/hyperactivity disorder. *Journal of Clinical Child Psychology, 27,* 190–205.

Pellegrino, L. (2002). Cerebral palsy. In M. L. Batshaw (Ed.), *Children with disabilities* (5th ed., pp. 443–466). Baltimore: Brookes.

Pennington, B. F. (2002). *The development of psychopathology: Nature and nurture.* New York: Guilford Press.

Petti, V. L., Voelker, S. L., Shore, D. L., & Hayman-Abello, S. E. (2003). Perception of nonverbal emotion cues by children with nonverbal learning disabilities. *Journal of Developmental and Physical Disabilities, 15,* 23–36.

Pfiffner, L. J., & Barkley, R. A. (1998). Treatment of ADHD in school settings. In R. A. Barkley, *Attention-deficit hyperactivity disorder: A handbook for diagnosis and treatment* (2nd ed., pp. 458–490). New York: Guilford Press.

Pfiffner, L. J., Calzada, E., & McBurnett, K. (2000). Interventions to enhance social competence. *Child and Adolescent Psychiatric Clinics of North America, 9,* 689–709.

Phelps, L. (Ed.). (1998). *Health-related disorders in children and adolescents: A guidebook for understanding and educating.* Washington, DC: American Psychological Association.

Phelps, L. (Ed.). (in press). *Chronic health-related disorders in children: Collaborative medical and psychoeducational interventions.* Washington, DC: American Psychological Association.

Piacentini, J., Bergman, R. L., Jacobs, C., McCracken, J. T., & Kretchman, J. (2002). Open trial of cognitive-behavioral therapy for childhood obsessive–compulsive disorder. *Journal of Anxiety Disorders, 16,* 207–219.

Piacentini, J., Bergman, R. L., Keller, M., & McCracken, J. (2003). Functional impairment in children and adolescents with obsessive–compulsive disorder. *Journal of Child and Adolescent Psychopharmacology, 13,* 61–70.

Piacentini, J., & Langley, A. K. (2004). Cognitive-behavioral therapy for children who have obsessive–compulsive disorder. *Journal of Clinical Psychology, 60,* 1181–1194.

Platzman, K. A., Stoy, M. R., Brown, R. T., Coles, C. D., Smith, I. E., & Falek, A. (1992). Review of observational methods in attention-deficit/hyperactivity disorder (ADHD): Implications for diagnosis. *School Psychology Quarterly, 7,* 155–177.

Plomin, R., Defries, J. C., Craig, I. W., & McGuffin, P. (Eds.). (2003). *Behavioral genetics in the postgenomics era.* Washington, DC: American Psychological Association.

Poe, M. D., Burchinal, M. R., & Roberts, J. E. (2004). Early language and the development of children's reading skills. *Journal of School Psychology, 42,* 315–332.

Power, T. J., Atkins, M. S., Osborne, M. L., & Blum, N. J. (1994). The school psychologist as manager of programming for ADHD. *School Psychology Review, 23,* 279–291.

Pritchard, D. A., Livingston, R. B., Reynolds, C. R., & Moses, J.A. (2000). Modal profiles for the WISC-III. *School Psychology Quarterly, 15,* 400–418.

Proctor, B. E., Floyd, R. G., & Shaver, R. B. (2005). Cattell–Horn–Carroll broad cognitive ability profiles of low math achievers. *Psychology in the Schools, 42,* 1–12.

Pryzwansky, W. B. (1999). Accreditation and credentialing systems of school psychologists. In C. R. Reynolds & T. B. Gutkin (Eds.), *The handbook of school psychology* (3rd ed., pp. 1145–1158). New York: Wiley.

Psychological Corporation. (2002). *Wechsler Individual Achievement Test* (2nd ed.). San Antonio, TX: Author.

Public Law 108-446. (2004). *The Individuals with Disabilities Education Act amendments of 2004.*

Rabiner, D. L., Malone, P. S., and the Conduct Problems Prevention Research Group. (2004). The impact of tutoring on early reading achievement for children with and without attention problems. *Journal of Abnormal Child Psychology, 32,* 273–284.

Raiford, S. E., Weiss, L. G., Rolfhus, E., & Coalson, D. (2005). *Wechsler Intelligence Scale–IV: Technical Report #4: General ability index.* San Antonio, TX: Harcourt Assessment.

Rapin, I. (1996). Practitioner review: Developmental language disorders: A clinical update. *Journal of Child Psychology and Psychiatry, 37,* 643–655.

Rapoport, J. L. (1989). The children speak. In J. L. Rapoport (Ed.), *Obsessive–compulsive disorder in children and adolescents* (pp. 151–165). Washington, DC: American Psychiatric Press.

Rapport, M. D., Denney, C., DuPaul, G. J., & Gardner, M. J. (1994). Attention-deficit disorder and methylphenidate: Normalization rates, clinical effectiveness, and response prediction in 76 children. *Journal of the American Academy of Child and Adolescent Psychiatry, 33,* 882–893.

Rashotte, C. A., MacPhee, K., & Torgesen, J. K. (2001). The effectiveness of a group reading instruction program with poor readers in multiple grades. *Learning Disability Quarterly, 24,* 119–134.

Rathvon, N. (1999). *Effective school interventions: Strategies for enhancing academic achievement and social competence.* New York: Guilford Press.

Reitan, R. M., & Wolfson, D. (1992). *Neuropsychological evaluation of older children.* Tucson, AZ: Neuropsychological Press.

Reschly, D. J. (1997). Diagnostic and treatment utility of intelligence tests. In D. P. Flanagan, J. L. Genshaft, & P. L. Harrison (Eds.), *Contemporary intellectual assessment: Theories, tests, and issues* (pp. 437–456). New York: Guilford Press.

Reynolds, C. R., & Kamphaus, R. W. (2003). *Reynolds Intellectual Assessment Scales and the Reynolds Intellectual Screening Test: Professional manual.* Lutz, FL: Psychological Assessment Resources.

Reynolds, C. R., & Kamphaus, R. W. (2004). *Behavior Assessment System for Children— Second Edition*. Circle Pines, MN: American Guidance Service.

Riccio, C. A., & French, C. L. (2004). The status of empirical support for treatments of attention deficits. *The Clinical Neuropsychologist, 18,* 528–558.

Riccio, C. A., & Hynd, G. W. (1993). Developmental language disorders in children: Relationship with learning disability and attention-deficit/hyperactivity disorder. *School Psychology Review, 22,* 696–709.

Riccio, C. A., Reynolds, C. R., Lowe, P., & Moore, J. J. (2002). The continuous performance test: A window on the neural substrates for attention? *Archives of Clinical Neuropsychology, 17,* 235–272.

Riddle, M. A., Scahill, L., King, R. A., Hardin, M. T., Anderson, G. M., Ort, S. I., et al. (1992). Double-blind, crossover trial of fluoxetine and placebo in children and adolescents with obsessive–compulsive disorder. *Journal of the American Academy of Child and Adolescent Psychiatry, 31,* 1062–1069.

Robertson, C., & Salter, W. (1997). *The phonological awareness test.* East Moline, IL: LinguiSystems.

Rohrbreck, C. A., Ginsburg-Block, M. D., Fantuzzo, J. W., & Miller, T. R. (2003). Peer-assisted learning interventions with elementary school students: A meta-analytic review. *Educational Psychology, 95,* 240–257.

Roman, M. A. (1998). The syndrome of nonverbal learning disabilities: Clinical description and applied aspects. *Current Issues in Education, 1.* Retrieved April 20, 2005, from cie.ed.asu.edu/volume1/number7

Root, R. W., & Resnick, R. J. (2003). An update on the diagnosis and treatment of attention-deficit/hyperactivity disorder in children. *Professional Psychology: Research and Practice, 34,* 34–41.

Rourke, B. P. (1989). *Nonverbal learning disabilities: The syndrome and the model.* New York: Guilford Press.

Rourke, B. P. (1994). Neuropsychological assessment of children with learning disabilities: Measurement issues. In G. R. Lyon (Ed.), *Frames of reference for the assessment of learning disabilities: New views on measurement issues* (pp. 475–514). Baltimore: Brookes.

Rourke, B. P. (1995). *Syndrome of nonverbal learning disabilities: Neurodevelopmental manifestations.* New York: Guilford Press.

Rourke, B. P., Ahmad, S. A., Collins, D. W., Hayman-Abello, B. A., Hayman-Abello, S. E., & Warriner, E. M. (2002). Child clinical/pediatric neuropsychology: Some recent advances. *Annual Review of Psychology, 53,* 309–339.

Rourke, B. P., & Conway, J. A. (1997). Disabilities of arithmetic and mathematical reasoning: Perspectives from neurology and neuropsychology. *Journal of Learning Disabilities, 30,* 34–46.

Rourke, B. P., & Findlayson, M. A. J. (1978). Neuropsychological significance of variations in patterns of academic performance: Verbal and visual–spatial abilities. *Journal of Abnormal Child Psychology, 6,* 121–133.

Rourke, B. P., & Strang, J. D. (1978). Neuropsychological signifiance of variations in patterns of academic performance: Motor, psychomotor, and tactile–perceptual abilities. *Journal of Pediatric Psychology, 3,* 62–66.

Rourke, B. P., Young, G. C., & Leenarrs, A. A. (1989). A childhood learning disability that predisposes those afflicted to adolescent and adult depression and suicide risk. *Journal of Learning Disabilities, 22,* 169–175.

Safran, S. P. (2001). Asperger syndrome: The emerging challenge to special education. *Exceptional Children, 67*(2), 151–160.

Safran, S. P., Safran, J. S., & Ellis, K. (2003). Intervention ABCs for children with Asperger syndrome. *Topics in Language Disorders, 23,* 154–165.

Salvia, J., & Ysseldyke, J. E. (1998). *Assessment* (7th ed.). Boston: Houghton Mifflin.

Sattler, J. (2001). *Assessment of children: Cognitive applications* (4th ed.). San Diego, CA: Sattler.

Sax, L., & Kautz, K. J. (2004). Who first suggests the diagnosis of attention-deficit/ hyperactivity disorder? *Annals of Family Medicine, 1,* 171–174.

Schmitt, A. J., & Wodrich, D. L. (2004). Validation of a Developmental Neuro- psychological Assessement (NEPSY) through comparison of neurological, scholas- tic concerns, and control groups. *Archives of Clinical Neuropsychology, 19,* 1077– 1093.

Schrank, F. A., Flanagan, D. P., Woodcock, R. W., & Mascolo, J. T. (2002). *Essentials of WJ III cognitive abilities assessment.* New York: Wiley.

Schreerenberger, R. C. (1983). *History of mental retardation.* Baltimore: Brookes.

Schuele, C. M. (2004). The impact of developmental speech and language impairments on the acquisition of literacy skills. *Mental Retardation and Developmental Dis- abilities Research Reviews, 10,* 176–183.

Schulte, A. C., Osborne, S. S., & Erchul, W. P. (1998). Effective special education: A United States dilemma. *School Psychology Review, 27,* 66–76.

Semel, E., Wiig, E. H., & Secord, W. A. (2003). *Clinical evaluation of language funda- mentals* (4th ed.). San Antonio, TX: Harcourt Assessment.

Semrud-Clikeman, M. (2001). *Traumatic brain injury in children and adolescents: Assessment and intervention.* New York: Guilford Press.

Shapiro, B. K., & Gallico, R. P. (1993). Learning disabilities. *Pediatric Clinics of North America, 40*(3), 491–505.

Shapiro, E. S. (2004). *Academic skills problems: Direct assessment and intervention* (3rd ed.). New York: Guilford Press.

Shapiro, E. S., Angello, L. M., & Eckert, T. L. (2004). Has curriculum-based assessment become a staple of school psychology practice? An update and extension of knowl- edge, use, and attitudes from 1990 to 2000. *School Psychology Review, 33,* 249– 257.

Shapiro, E. S., & Heick, P. F. (2004). School psychologist assessment practices in the evaluation of students referred for social/behavioral/emotional problems. *Psychol- ogy in the Schools, 41,* 551–561.

Shapiro, E. S., & Kratochwill, T. R. (Eds.). (1988). *Behavioral assessment in schools: Conceptual foundations and practical applications.* New York: Guilford Press.

Share, D. L., & Stanovich, K. E. (1995). Cognitive processes in early reading develop- ment: A model of acquisition and individual differences. *Issues in Education: Con- tributions from Educational Psychology, 1,* 1–57.

Shaw, S. R. (1999). Part 1: School psychology and slow learners. The devolution of inter- est in slow learners: Can we continue to ignore? [Electronic version]. *Communiqué, 28.* Retrieved December 15, 2004, from www.nasponline.org/publications/ cq283slowlearn.html

Shaw, S. R. (2000a). Part 3: School psychology and slow learners. Academic interven- tions for slow learners [Electronic version]. *Communique, 28.* Retrieved December 15, 2004, from www.nasponline.org/publications/cq285slowlearn.html

Shaw, S. R. (2000b). Part 4: School psychology and slow learners. Slow learners and mental health issues [Electronic version]. *Communique, 28.* Retrieved December 15, 2004, from www.nasponline.org/publications/cq286slowlearn.html

Shaw, S. R. (2001). IDEA '97 and "Slow Learners." *National Mental Health and Educa-*

tion Center. Retrieved December 15, 2004, from www.naspcenter.org/teachers/ IDEA_slow.html

Shaw, S. R., & Gouwens, D. A. (2002). Chasing and catching slow learners in changing times [Electronic version]. *Communique, 31.* Retrieved December 15, 2004, from www.nasponline.org/publications/cq314slowlearner.html

Shaywitz, S. (2003). *Overcoming dyslexia: A new and complete science-based program for reading problems at any level.* New York: Vintage Books.

Sheridan, S. M., Eagle, J. W., Cowan, R. J., & Mickelson, W. (2001). The effects of conjoint behavioral consultation: Results of a 4–year investigation. *Journal of School Psychology, 39,* 361–385.

Shinn, M. R. (Ed.). (1998). *Advanced applications of curriculum-based measurement.* New York: Guilford Press.

Siperstein, G. N., & Leffert, J. S. (1997). Comparison of socially accepted and rejected children with mental retardation. *American Journal on Mental Retardation, 101,* 339–351.

Skinner, C. H., Wallace, M. A., & Neddenriep, C. E. (2002). Academic remediation: Educational applications of research on assignment preference and choice. *Child and Family Behavior Therapy, 24,* 51–65.

Snow, C. E. (2002). *Reading for understanding. Toward an R&D program in reading comprehension.* Santa Monica, CA: Rand.

Sohlberg, M. M., Johnson, L., Paule, L., Raskin, S. A., & Mateer, C. A. (1993). *Attention process training–II: A program to address attentional deficits for persons with mild cognitive dysfunction.* Puyallup, WA: Association for Neuropsychological Research and Development.

Sparrow, S. S., Cicchetti, D. V., & Balla, D. A. (2005). *Vineland-II Adaptive Behavior Scales.* Circle Pines, MN: American Guidance Service.

Spearman, R. C. (1904). "General intelligence": Objectively determined and measured. *American Journal of Psychology, 15,* 201–292.

Spencer, T. J., Biederman, J., Wozniak, J., Faraone, S. V., Wilens, T. E., & Mick, E. (2001). Parsing pediatric bipolar disorder from its associated comorbidity with the disruptive disorders. *Biological Psychiatry, 49,* 1062–1070.

Sprague, R. L., & Sleator, E. K. (1977). Methylphenidate in hyperkinetic children: Differences in dose effects on learning and social behavior. *Science, 198,* 1274–1276.

Squire, L. R., & Schacter, D. L. (2003). *Neuropsychology of memory* (3rd ed.). New York: Guilford Press.

Stage, S. A., Abbott, R. D., Jenkins, J. R., & Berninger, V. W. (2003). Predicting response to early reading intervention from verbal IQ, reading-related language abilities, attention ratings, and verbal IQ–word reading discrepancy: Failure to validate discrepancy method. *Journal of Learning Disabilities, 36,* 24–33.

Stein, M. T., Klin, A., & Miller, K. (2004). When Asperger syndrome and a nonverbal learning disability look alike. *Journal of Developmental and Behavioral Pediatrics, 25,* S59–S64.

Sternberg, R. J., & Grigorenko, E. L. (2002). Difference scores in the identification of children with learning disabilities: It's time to use a different method. *Journal of School Psychology, 40,* 65–83.

Stoiber, K. C., & Kratochwill, T. R. (2000). Empirically supported interventions and school psychology: Rationale and methodological issues—Part I. *School Psychology Review, 15,* 75–105.

Stromme, P., & Diseth, T. H. (2000). Prevalence of psychiatric diagnoses in children with mental retardation: Data from a population-based study. *Developmental Medicine and Child Neurology, 42,* 266–270.

Swanson, H. L. (1999). Reading research for students with LD: A meta-analysis of intervention outcomes. *Journal of Learning Disabilities, 32,* 504–532.

Swanson, H. L., Hoskyn, M., & Lee, C. (1999). *Interventions for students with learning disabilities: A meta-analysis of treatment outcomes.* New York: Guilford Press.

Taub, G. E., & McGrew, K. S. (2004). Confirmatory factor analysis of Cattell–Horn–Carroll theory and cross-age invariance of the Woodcock–Johnson Tests of Cognitive abilities. *School Psychology Quarterly, 19,* 72–87.

Telzrow, C. F., & Bonar, A. M. (2002). Responding to students with nonverbal learning disabilities. *Teaching Exceptional Children, 34,* 8–13.

Torgesen, J. K., Alexander, A. W., Wagner, R. K., Rashotte, C. A. Voeller, K. K. S., & Conway, T. (2001). Intensive remedial instruction for children with severe reading disabilities: Immediate and long-term outcomes from two instructional approaches. *Journal of Learning Disabilities, 34,* 33–58, 78.

Torgesen, J. K., & Bryant, B. (1994). *Test of Phonological Awareness.* Austin, TX: PRO-ED.

Torgesen, J. K., & Mathes, P. G. (2000). *A basic guide to understanding, assessing, and teaching phonological awareness.* Austin, TX: PRO-ED.

Torgesen, J. K., Wagner, R. K., Rashotte, C. A., Rose, E., Lindamood, P., & Conway, T., et al. (1999). Preventing reading failure in young children with phonological processing disabilities: Group and individual responses to instruction. *Journal of Educational Psychology, 91*(4), 579–593.

Tsatsanis, K. D., Foley, C., & Donehower, C. (2004). Contemporary outcome research and programming guidelines for Asperger syndrome and high-functioning autism. *Topics in Language Disorders, 24,* 249–259.

Turk, J. (2004). The importance of diagnosis. In D. Dew-Hughes (Ed.), *Educating children with fragile X syndrome* (pp. 132–143). London: RoutledgeFalmer.

U.S. Department of Education. (1997). Individuals with Disabilities Education Act amendments of 1997. Retrieved October 17, 2004, from www.ed.gov/policy/speced/leg/idea/idea.pdf

U.S. Department of Education. (2002). *Twenty-fourth annual report to Congress on implementation of IDEA.* Retrieved October 19, 2004, from www.ed.gov/about/reports/annual/osep/2002/index.html

U.S. Department of Education. (2003). *Identifying and treating attention-deficit/hyperactivity disorder: A resource for school and home.* Jessup, MD: Author.

Upshur, R. E. G. (2000). Two techniques for teaching the estimation of prior probabilities. *Teaching and Learning in Medicine, 12,* 141–144.

Valas, H. (1999). Students with learning disabilities and low-achieving students: Peer acceptance, loneliness, self-esteem, and depression. *Social Psychology of Education, 3,* 173–192.

Van Balkom, H., & Verhoeven, L. (2004). Pragmatic disability in children with specific language impairments. In L. Verhoeven & H. van Balkom (Eds.), *Classification of developmental language disorders: Theoretical issues and clinical implications* (pp. 283–305). Mahwah, NJ: Erlbaum.

Vaughn, M. L., Riccio, C. A., Hynd, G. W., & Hall, J. (1997). Diagnosing ADHD (predominately inattentive type and combined subtypes): Discriminant validity of the Behavior Assessment System for Children and the Achenbach Parent and Teacher Rating Scales. *Journal of Clinical Child Psychology, 26,* 349–357.

Vaughn, S., & Fuchs, L. S. (2003). Redefining learning disabilities as inadequate response to instruction: The promise and potential problems. *Learning Disabilities Research and Practice, 18,* 137–146.

Wagner, R. K., Torgesen, J. K., & Rashotte, C. A. (1999). *Comprehensive Test of Phonological Processing.* Austin, TX: PRO-ED.

Waschbusch, D. A., Pelham, W. E., Jr., Jennings, R., Greiner, A. R., Tarter, R. E., & Moss, H. B. (2002). Reactive aggression in boys with disruptive behavior disorders: Behavior, physiology, and affect. *Journal of Abnormal Child Psychology, 30,* 641–656.

Watkins, M. W. (2000). Cognitive profile analysis: A shared professional myth. *School Psychology Quarterly, 15,* 465–479.

Watkins, M. W., & Glutting, J. J. (2000). Incremental validity of WISC-III profile elevation, scatter, and shape information for predicting reading and math achievement. *Psychoeducational Assessment, 12,* 402–408.

Wechsler, D. (1997). *Wechsler Memory Scale—Third Edition: Administration and Scoring Manual.* San Antonio, TX: The Psychological Corporation.

Wechsler, D. (2002). *Wechsler Individual Achievement Test—Second Edition.* San Antonio, TX: The Psychological Corporation.

Wechsler, D. (2003). *Wechsler Intelligence Scale for Children—Fourth Edition: Administration and Scoring Manual.* San Antonio, TX: The Psychological Corporation.

Wechsler, D., Kaplan, E., Fein, D., Kramer, J., Morris, R., Delis, D., et al. (2004). *Wechsler Intelligence Scale for Children Fourth Edition—Integrated: Administration and Scoring Manual.* San Antonio, TX: The Psychological Corporation.

Wehmeyer, M. L., Sands, D. J., Knowlton, H. E., & Kozleski, E. B. (2002). *Teaching students with mental retardation: Providing access to the general curriculum.* Baltimore, MD: Brookes.

Weiler, M. D., Holmes-Bernstein, J., Bellinger, D. C., & Waber, D. P. (2000). Processing speed in children with attention-deficit/hyperactivity disorder, inattentive type. *Child Neuropsychology, 6,* 218–234.

Weiler, M. D., Holmes-Bernstein, J., Bellinger, D. C., & Waber, D. P. (2002). Information-processing deficits in children with attention-deficit/hyperactivity disorder, inattentive type, and children with reading disability. *Journal of Learning Disorders, 35,* 448–461.

Weiner, B. (1985). An attributional theory of achievement motivation and emotion. *Psychological Review, 92,* 548–573.

Weintraub, N., & Graham, S. (2000). The contribution of gender, orthographic, finger function, and visual–motor process: Prediction of handwriting status. *Occupational Therapy Research Journal, 20,* 121–140.

Weismer, S. E. (1997). The role of stress in language processing and intervention. *Topics in Language Disorders, 17,* 41–52.

Weissberg, R. P., Cowen, E. L., Lotyczewksi, B. S., Boike, M. F., Orara, N., Stalonas, P., et al. (1987). Teacher ratings of children's problem and competence behaviors: Normative and parametric characteristics. *American Journal of Community Psychology, 15,* 387–401.

Wheeler-Maedgen, J., & Carlson, C. L. (2000). Social functioning and emotional regulation in the attention-deficit/hyperactivity subtypes. *Journal of Clinical Child Psychology, 29,* 30–42.

Wilens, T. E. (2004). Attention-deficit/hyperactivity disorder and the substance use disorders: The nature of the relationship, subtypes at risk, and treatment issues. *Psychiatric Clinics of North America, 27,* 283–301.

Williams, J., Klinepeter, K., Palmes, G., Pulley, A., & Foy, J. M. (2004). Diagnoses and treatment of behavioral health disorders in pediatric practice. *Pediatrics, 114,* 601–606.

Williams, J. K., Richman, L. C., & Yarbrough, D. B. (1992). Comparison of visual–

spatial performance strategy training in children with Turner syndrome and learning disabilities. *Journal of Learning Disabilities, 25,* 658–664.

Williams, K. T. (1997). *Expressive Vocabulary Test.* Circle Pines, MN: American Guidance Service.

Wilson, C. P., Gutkin, T. B., Hagen, K. M., & Oats, R. G. (1998). General education teacher's knowledge and self-reported use of classroom interventions for work with difficult-to-teach students. *School Psychology Quarterly, 13,* 45–62.

Wilson, M. S., & Reschly, D. J. (1996). Assessment in school psychology training and practice. *School Psychology Review, 25,* 9–23.

Wise, B. W., Ring, J., & Olson, R. K. (1999). Training phonological awareness with and without explicit attention to articulation. *Journal of Experimental Child Psychology, 72,* 271–304.

Wodrich, D. L. (1986). The terminology and purposes of assessment. In D. L. Wodrich & J. E. Joy (Eds.), *Multidisciplinary assessment of children with learning disabilities and mental retardation* (pp. 1–29). Baltimore: Brookes.

Wodrich, D. L. (1997). *Children's psychological testing: A guide for nonpsychologists* (3rd ed.). Baltimore: Brookes.

Wodrich, D. L. (2000). *Attention-deficit/hyperactivity disorder: What every parent wants to know* (2nd ed.). Baltimore: Brookes.

Wodrich, D. L. (2004). Professional beliefs related to the practice of pediatric medicine and school psychology. *Journal of School Psychology, 42,* 265–284.

Wodrich, D. L., & Barry, C. T. (1991). A survey of school psychologists' practices for identifying mentally retarded students. *Psychology in the Schools, 28,* 165–171.

Wodrich, D. L., & Kaplan, A. K. (2005). Indications for seeking a medical consultation. *Journal of Applied School Psychology, 22*(1), 1–28.

Wodrich, D. L., & Kush, J. C. (1998). The effect of methylphenidate on teachers' behavioral ratings in specific school situations. *Psychology in the Schools, 35,* 81–88.

Wodrich, D. L. (1999). School psychologists: Strategic allies in the contemporary practice of primary care pediatrics. *Clinical Pediatrics, 38,* 597–606.

Wodrich, D. L., Stobo, N., & Trca, M. (1998). Three ways to consider educational performance when determining serious emotional disturbance. *School Psychology Quarterly, 13,* 228–240.

Wolraich, M. L., Felice, M. E., & Drotar, D. (1996). *The classification of child and adolescent mental diagnoses in primary care. Diagnostic and statistical manual for primary care (DSM-PC), Child and adolescent version.* Elk Grove, IL: American Academy of Pediatrics.

Woodcock, R. W., McGrew, K. S., & Mather, N. (2001). *Woodcock–Johnson III Tests of Cognitive Abilities and Tests of Achievement.* Itasca, IL: Riverside.

World Health Organization. (1990). *International classification of diseases and related health problems* (10th rev.). Geneva: Author.

Worling, D. E., Humphries, T., & Tannock, R. (1999). Spatial and emotional aspects of language inferencing in nonverbal learning disabilities. *Brain and Language, 70,* 220–239.

Young, A. R., Beitchman, J. H., Johnson, C., Douglas, L., Atkinson, L., Escobar, M., et al. (2002). Young adult academic outcomes in a longitudinal sample of early identified language impaired and control children. *Journal of Child Psychology and Psychiatry and Allied Disciplines, 43,* 635–645.

Zigmond, N., Jenkins, J., Fuchs, L., Deno, S., Fuchs, D., Baker, J. N., et al. (1995). Special education in restructured schools: Findings from three multi-year studies. *Kappan, 76,* 531–535.

Index

♦